7

ADVANCES IN ORAL RADIOLOGY

Allan B. Reiskin

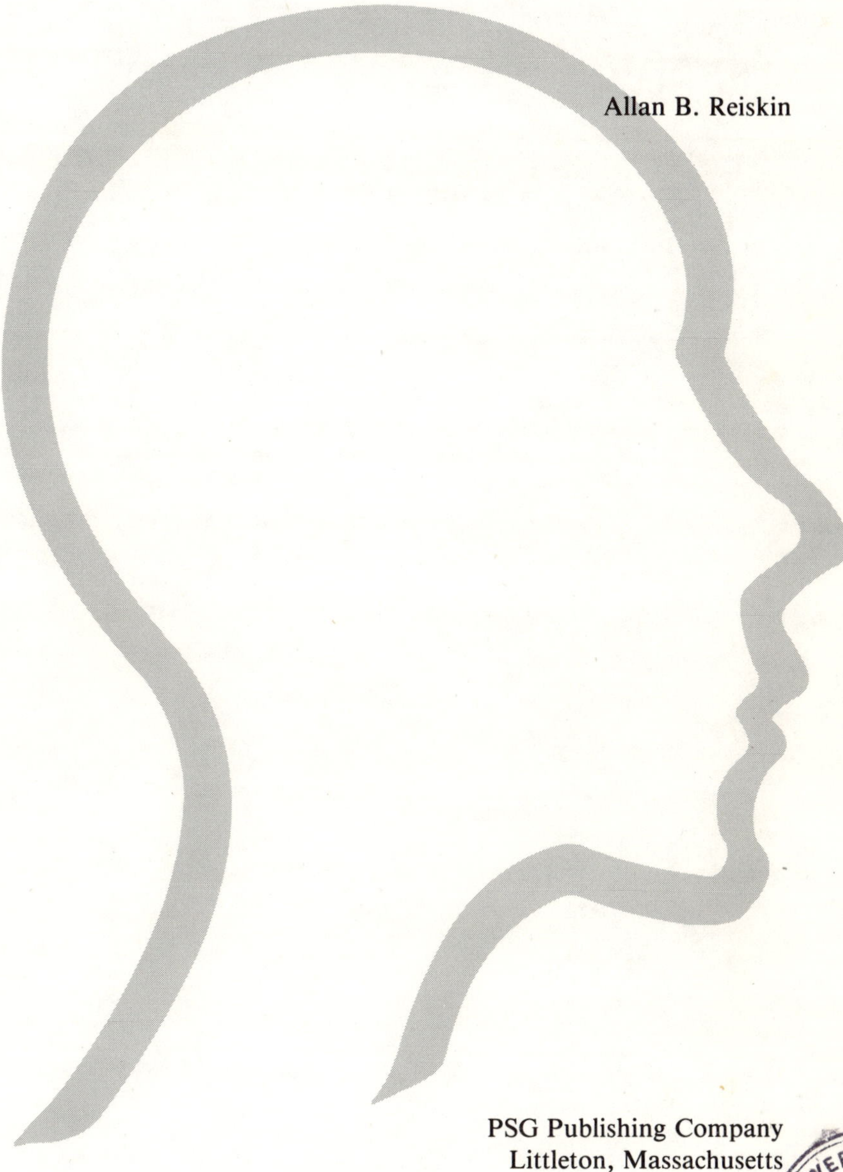

PSG Publishing Company
Littleton, Massachusetts

ADVANCES IN ORAL RADIOLOGY

Postgraduate Dental Handbook Series, Volume 12

Volume Editor

Allan B. Reiskin, BA, DDS, DPhil (Oxon)
Professor of Radiology
Department of Oral Diagnosis
University of Connecticut Health Center
School of Dental Medicine
Farmington

Series Editor

Alvin F. Gardner, DDS, MS, PhD, FICD
Washington, DC

Library of Congress Cataloging in Publication Data

Reiskin, Allan B
Advances in oral radiology.

(Postgraduate dental handbook series ; 12)
Includes bibliographical references and index.
1. Mouth--Radiography. 2. Teeth--Radiography. I. Freedman, Michael L. II. Lurie, Alan G. III. Title. IV. Series.
RK309.R44 616.3'1'0757 79-21095
ISBN 0-88416-165-X

Printed in the United States of America.

International Standard Book Number: 0-88416-165-X

Series International Standard Book Number: 0-88416-174-9

Library of Congress Catalog Card Number: 79-21095

CONTRIBUTORS

Michael L. Freedman, PhD
Associate Professor of Radiology
Department of Oral Diagnosis
University of Connecticut Health Center
School of Dental Medicine
Farmington

Alan G. Lurie, DDS, PhD
Associate Professor of Radiology
Department of Oral Diagnosis
University of Connecticut Health Center
School of Dental Medicine
Farmington

Allan B. Reiskin, BA, DDS, DPhil (Oxon)
Professor of Radiology
Department of Oral Diagnosis
University of Connecticut Health Center
School of Dental Medicine
Farmington

CONTENTS

FOREWORD

During the past decade there has been a gratifying increase in new knowledge in the art and science of dentistry from general practitioners of dentistry and dental specialists. The biological and dental sciences are in a period of explosive growth whose rate has been particularly increased in basic dental sciences with clinical applications and in clinical dentistry by the diversification of experimental methods in dental procedures.

Dental sciences are currently considered as multidimensional with great individual differences. Dental scientists and practitioners know that the adaptation of techniques from other fields of science is not simple, usually indirect, and inapplicable unless radically revised, extended, or reformulated for dentistry. The basic experimental methods originating in the clinical dental sciences may now be joined by the methods of the biological and physical sciences, and made technically feasible by the introduction of modern electronics and computers.

It is the goal of the Postgraduate Dental Handbook Series to present critical analyses, based on impressive clinical and research experience. This series provides basic dental sciences with clinical applications and clinical dental sciences in a correlated fashion. Similarly, it provides the most current concepts in clinical dentistry of direct value to practitioners, specialists, students, and hygienists throughout the world. By bringing together all of our knowledge, volumes in the Postgraduate Dental Handbook Series will fill a critical need felt by many clinicians and investigators.

Dr. Allan B. Reiskin, Professor of Radiology and Head of the Division of Oral Radiology in the Department of Oral Diagnosis of the School of Dental Medicine at the University of Connecticut Health Center, presents the methods and techniques for the most effective solutions to the clinical problems in oral radiology confronting the dental practitioner. He is a dental educator and researcher who has succeeded in producing an eminently readable, comprehensive work in the field of dental radiology.

The present work reveals fresh insights based upon knowledge of the latest research in the field of radiology. Dr. Reiskin has directed his insights in radiology to the general practitioner of dentistry, and has selected stimulating and informative topics in radiology for discussion which are both scientific and consistently practical. All of the topics receive highly critical attention with the most important areas clearly emphasized. The discussions of the mechanisms of radiologic diagnosis are highly critical, yet concise, with numerous important relationships based upon fundamental radiologic principles. In this monograph, the author has come to grips with the problems which have plagued the dental practitioner taking the radiographs of the dental patient, thereby providing the general practitioner of dentistry with a specialized assessment of the most important features and problems in modern dental radiology.

Sophisticated modern dental radiology techniques are presented not as isolated disciplines or free-standing entities but from the viewpoint of their usefulness and limitations in dental practice.

It is hoped that this up-to-date monograph on modern dental radiology, together with future radiologic research, will provide the bridge to a new era in the holistic treatment of the dental patient. The editor of the Postgraduate Dental Handbook Series expresses his gratitude and appreciation to the author and to the contributors who assumed this vital task for dentistry.

Alvin F. Gardner, Series Editor

ACKNOWLEDGMENT

The author acknowledges the support and encouragement of his family and colleagues in the Division of Oral Radiology.

INTRODUCTION

The interpretive and technical aspects of dental radiology have necessarily suffered on several accounts. First, radiology is not a recognized specialty within the dental profession. Compared to the recognized disciplines, it receives relatively little attention in the undergraduate curriculum. Second, every dentist provides his own x-ray services and will have a depth of experience which is directly related to the characteristics and size of his own patient population. Third, most disease found in the jaws is chronic and benign, rarely leading to procedures that require histologic examination. Confirmation of a radiographic diagnosis is, therefore, infrequent. Fourth, the dental marketplace is quite small and has not provided a significant economic stimulus to manufacturers to apply today's space age technology to designing equipment for dental radiographic procedures.

Expertise in dental radiology is, therefore, limited. A few individuals in large institutions have had an opportunity to analyze thousands of patient examinations each year. Unfortunately, even within institutions, the ability to record, confirm, catalog, and study the results of many patient examinations is severely restricted.

Although dental radiography has not changed dramatically in the last 70 years, we are on the threshold of major alterations in practice patterns. There is a growing consciousness about the potential hazards of exposure to ionizing radiation, and there is increasing recognition of the limitations of currently used technical procedures. This book will attempt to provide a limited insight into developing trends in dental radiology, from a technologic and interpretive point of view. It is our hope and expectation that the information contained within these pages will be of value to practitioners, who will find it necessary to modify their practice patterns in the future.

Allan B. Reiskin

INTRODUCTION

SECTION I

TECHNOLOGY

1 The X-Ray System

In selecting x-ray equipment for an office, several important factors should be taken into account. First, one can rarely afford the luxury of choosing individual pieces of equipment. Rather, the entire system, including the radiation source, the image receptor, the devices used for processing the image, and all of the accessories or devices used for controlling or interconnecting these major components, should be considered as a unit. Second, the specific diagnostic needs of the practice should be identified. Equipment required in an orthodontic practice may be unsuitable for a general dentist. The needs of one oral surgeon might vary dramatically from those of his colleagues, depending upon whether the practice is restricted to exodontia and minor surgical procedures or includes a broad range of problems such as orthognathic surgery, chronic progressive diseases, and trauma. The needs of the periodontist may vary to a small but significant degree from those of an endodontist. Third, there is a growing recognition by both professionals and health care consumers that the risks associated with exposure to ionizing radiation may be significantly greater than have been estimated in the past. Therefore, patient exposure or system speed, as well as other safety features, are considerations that cannot be overlooked.[1]

Proprietary recommendations would be inappropriate here. Furthermore, data needed for such recommendations do not exist. No data bank is available to consumers that specifies the frequency-of-repair record for any particular brand or model of any component of any x-ray system. It is necessary, therefore, to rely on a careful analysis of the specifications that manufacturers are legally obligated to provide and to weigh judiciously the experience of colleagues and dealers. In the latter case, however, a prospective purchaser should remember that colleagues may be reluctant to acknowledge publicly what they themselves regard as an error in judgement, and that dealers are motivated by the profitability of a sale, as well as by such considerations as the long-term prospects that accrue from the acquisition of a new and regular customer.

X-RAY SYSTEMS

The potential importance of x-ray diagnosis in the healing arts was recognized immediately by Roentgen and his contemporaries. Medical and dental applications were demonstrated within a period of two weeks following the reported discovery of x-rays.[2] Unfortunately, the power of this diagnostic modality was so overwhelming that many health professionals remained satisfied for decades with the performance of devices that did not differ significantly in concept from those described by Roentgen, Edison, and Coolidge. However, we are now in a period of transition. Dental radiology is beginning to incorporate many of the technologic advances that have been applied in medicine. This technology should be evaluated within the context of cost, safety, and effectiveness, as well as in terms of convenience.

The most common type of x-ray system in dental practice today employs a single phase generator using self-rectified tube and stationary anode. Such generators are used with a variety of films as image receptors. Essentially all films require postexposure manual processing in wet chemicals. In practices with larger numbers of patients or with special needs, the use of panoramic x-ray equipment is more common, although some evidence suggests that this modality may not be well understood by its users (Reiskin, In preparation). A growing trend exists toward the use of machine processing of films rather than wet tanks or manual development.

In dealing with this major factor, the x-ray system, characteristics known to be of significant technical importance in currently used systems will be described. Brief descriptions of devices used in other branches of the healing arts, and in nondestructive industrial testing, that may soon find its way into dentistry will follow.

X-RAY GENERATORS

The most common type of x-ray generator uses alternating current as its power source. Current is supplied to the filament in the x-ray tube. Electrons from the filament are drawn to a target by a high voltage placed between the filament and the target (Figure 1-1). Alternating current is produced by electromagnetic induction and, as the name implies, the polarity or direction of the current is constantly changing, or alternating. The flow of alternating current graphs as a sine wave with each pulse or cycle having a positive and a negative component (Figure 1-2). The flow of electrons from the filament to the target in an x-ray tube depends upon

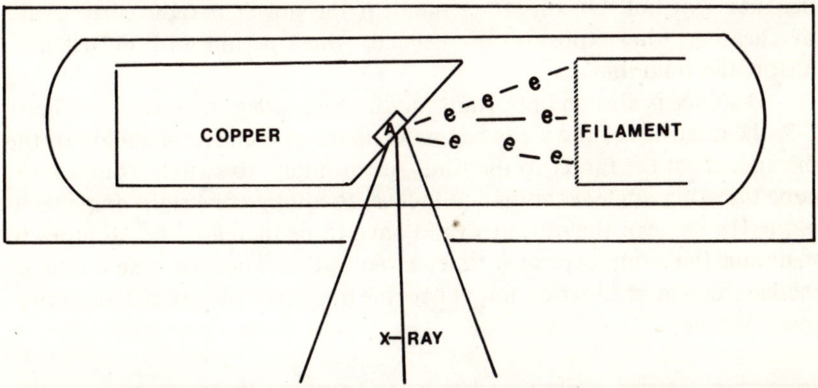

Figure 1-1 Schematic representation of a dental x-ray tube. Electrons from the heated filament are drawn to the target or anode (A) by a high potential difference. As electrons strike the anode, x-rays are produced.

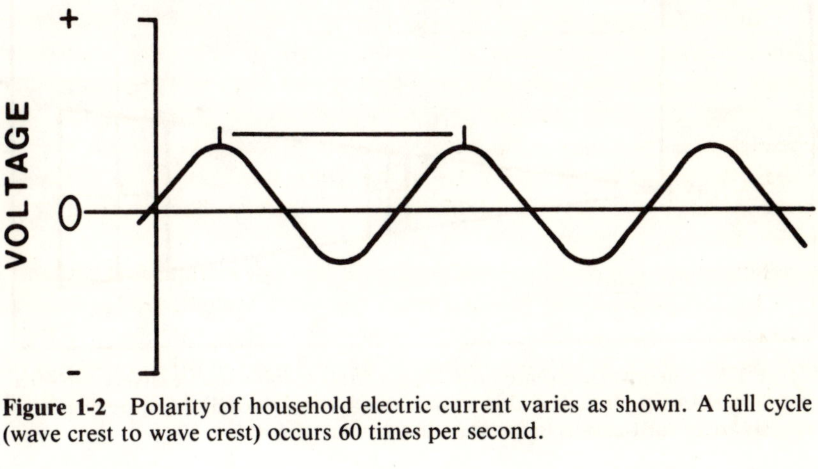

Figure 1-2 Polarity of household electric current varies as shown. A full cycle (wave crest to wave crest) occurs 60 times per second.

the polarity of both the target and filament. Like charges repel each other and unlike charges attract. Negatively-charged electrons are drawn from the filament to the target only when the target has a positive charge. Since the bombardment of the target by electrons generates x-rays, they are produced only when the target is positive, or for half of each cycle. Furthermore, the power fluctuates as the polarity changes, so that peak voltage exists for a limited period during each half cycle. This type of system is not efficient, since most of the energy from the bombardment of the target with electrons produces heat, with a relatively insignificant amount of energy being transformed into x-rays. In order to obtain a sufficient number of x-ray photons of adequate energy, the x-ray tube must be able to dissipate the heat. If the heat is not dissipated quickly enough, the tube will fail. On the other hand, if the power is reduced to avoid overheating, long exposures are needed, which permit motion that may distort the final image.

Distance is also an important factor to consider. As shown in Figure 1-3, the intensity of the x-ray beam decreases as the inverse square of the distance from the target to the film. Accordingly, to switch from a short cone bisecting angle technique (4 inches) to a long cone right angle technique (16 inches), the output would have to be increased by 16 times to maintain the same exposure time. Even if the exposure time could be increased, heat production might become one problem and patient movement another.

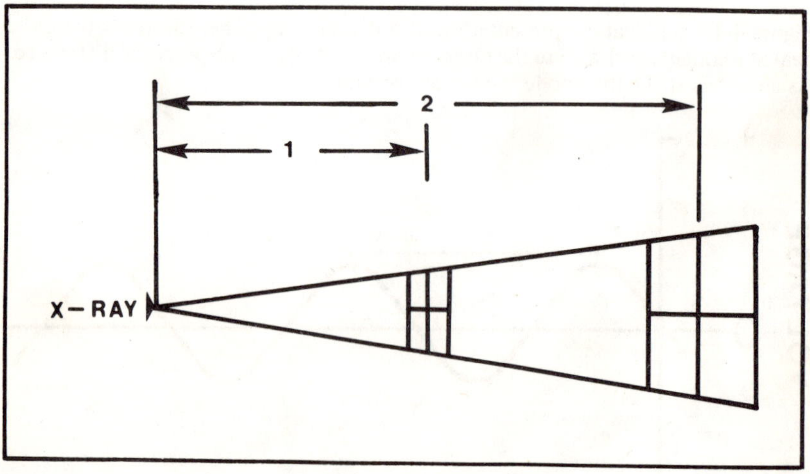

Figure 1-3 The inverse square law. X-rays from a point source diverge. Notice that the number of photons within a given area at one unit of distance are dispersed over an area four times as large when the distance doubles.

The number of x-ray photons produced depends primarily on the current applied to the filament (the milliamperage); the greater the milliampere rating of the x-ray generator, the more photons produced per unit time. The energy of each x-ray photon depends on the kilovoltage. As a general rule, a higher kilovoltage provides more useable photons. Ideally, x-ray machines should have high tube currents and high but variable kilovoltages. For reasons to be discussed elsewhere, a small target is also desirable.

The capacity of an x-ray generator can be evaluated in several ways. First, manufacturers include in the operator's manual a recommended duty cycle. This duty cycle is based on the combined effects of heat production, cooling capacity, and time. For example, a manufacturer may recommend that at a specific kilovoltage, milliampere, and time setting, an interval of 10 seconds or 10 minutes be allowed between exposures. Exposures made at shorter time intervals or at higher kilovoltage, milliampere, or time settings may cause overheating. If the overheating is minimal, the target may be softened and etched by the bombardment of electrons. Small quantities of the target can evaporate and be deposited on the glass envelope of the tube, thereby increasing its filtration and reducing overall output. Both the quality and the quantity of x-rays are diminished when the duty cycle is continuously or severely exceeded.

Table 1-1 describes the duty cycles of nine different x-ray machines. The duty cycle, in each case, is based on the manufacturer's recommended setting for an 8-inch target-to-film distance. At one extreme 310 exposures are allowed within a 10-minute interval; at the opposite extreme only 16 exposures are allowed within a 10-minute interval.

Table 1-1
Duty Cycles of Selected X-Ray Machines

Unit	kVp*	mamp†	Time (seconds)	Maximum no. exposures per 10 minutes
1	90	15	0.10	310
2	70	15	0.25	160
3	70	15	0.25	160
4	90	15	0.10	200
5	70	15	0.25	120
6	70	15	0.25	80
7	65	10	0.40	21
8	56	7	?	20
9	65	7½	?	16

*kVp–kilovolts (peak)
†mamp–milliampere

The meaning of the duty cycle is apparent if one looks at a few patterns of utilization. First, a well-trained, competent, x-ray technician can expose intraoral films at a rate of approximately two to three films per minute or 20 to 30 films per 10 minutes. This rate is well below the duty cycle of some machines but at the fringe or above the duty cycle of others. Tube life certainly depends on how frequently a duty cycle is approached or exceeded. Second, switching from a short to a long cone technique entails a substantial increase in exposure times. Consequently, the duty cycle could be exceeded in routine use in several machines unless time for cooling is allowed between exposures. Third, the adequacy of some machines for extraoral examinations is dubious. The production of a diagnostic cephalometric film at a 5-foot target-to-object distance requires from 7 to 35 milliampere/seconds, depending on the image receptor used. These exposures exceed some duty cycles and might damage or shorten the tube life.

Manufacturers may not follow the same criteria for deriving a duty cycle. Since some manufacturers may be more liberal than others in defining the duty cycle, a prospective buyer should consult the tube rating charts, the anode cooling curves, and the heat production curves for any particular tube. From these data it is possible to establish 1) the maximum length of an exposure for any given kilovoltage and milliampere setting, 2) the amount of time required between exposures for cooling, and 3) a comparison of these factors with the techniques recommended by the manufacturer for specific procedures.

Since replacement of an x-ray tube is expensive (between $800 and $1200 in 1978), these are not trivial issues. If there is any question about the adequacy of an x-ray machine, have the data analyzed by a qualified physicist.

FILM

For intraoral radiography, only a few significant considerations are involved in the choice of the film. Films have specified speed and contrast characteristics. H&D curves (Figure 1-4) should be available from the manufacturer. These curves provide three important pieces of data. First, they describe contrast; this is determined by looking at the slope of the curve. The more gradual the slope, the lower the contrast; the steeper the slope, the higher the contrast. Second, these curves describe the relative sensitivity or speed of the film. Speed is indicated by the location of the curve on the exposure axis. Curves that lie to the left require less exposure to produce the desired density and are faster films. Curves that lie to the right on the exposure axis require greater exposure for the same density and are slower films. Third, the latitude of a film can be determined by examination of the range of exposures that yield an acceptable density.

The smaller the range of exposures, the lower the latitude; the larger the range of exposures, the greater the latitude. Latitude decreases when contrast increases; therefore, high contrast films may have less latitude than low contrast films in the same speed range.

Other factors of concern in the evaluation of a film include its resolution or its relative ability to distinguish closely approximated structures from one another, its consistency from one batch of film to another, and its packaging. Film also has a finite shelf life, which may vary from one brand to another.

For intraoral techniques, we are usually limited to the use of nonscreen film. In most parts of the United States, regulations require the use of film with a speed or sensitivity above some stipulated minimum. Often this is the fastest film commercially available. Therefore, speed is not a major issue today, and one brand is distinguished from another primarily on grounds of contrast, resolution, reliability, and packaging. There is a dearth of reliable information on the consistency of film coming from different manufacturers. Manufacturers monitor the quality and consistency of their own products as well as the products of competitors, but this information is seldom available to consumers. Again, one must rely to a large extent on personal experience, the experiences of colleagues and suppliers, and the willingness of a manufacturer to provide specific product information.

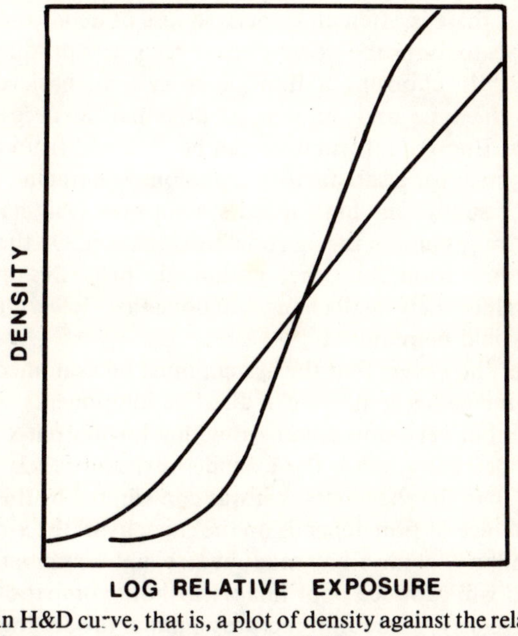

Figure 1-4 An H&D curve, that is, a plot of density against the relative amount of exposure required to produce that density. H&D curves contain important information about the speed, contrast, and latitude of the film.

Extraoral Radiography

In extraoral radiography, the situation is different. Many films are available, and they vary in speed, contrast, latitude, resolution, and processing requirements. They are further classified into those that are used alone and those used in combination with intensifying screens. Essentially the same criteria apply to this category of image receptors, although the number of choices is greater, and product information can often be obtained from the scientific literature. Also, it is possible to purchase extraoral films from medical suppliers as well as from dental dealers.

To a significant extent, an appropriate film or film-screen combination can compensate for the limitations of an x-ray generator. For example, if the output of an x-ray generator is low, a faster image recording system can compensate. Similarly, if the energy spectrum of the x-ray generating system has an excessive tendency toward high contrast imaging, select a recorder with inherently lower contrast or wider latitude. In each instance it is important to keep the diagnostic objective in mind.

Intensifying Screens

Because there is such a variety, speed, as well as contrast and resolution, is a major factor. For example, films or film-screen combinations for extraoral use can vary in speed by a factor of up to 100.[3,4,5] As the speed increases, there is often an associated loss of detail and/or contrast so that in many situations the slowest image recorders produce the highest quality images.[6] In choosing a film-screen system, basic decisions are needed about the type and amount of information necessary for the diagnostic task. Enough information can be obtained from an extremely fast imaging system for a satisfactory cephalometric tracing in orthodontic diagnosis. Visually, the high speed system may lack certain esthetic qualities, yet it may contain the essential information. On the other hand, infection, inflammation, or other pathologic processes in their early stages may produce such small changes in bone that slower, higher resolution systems would be required.

Remember, however, that the system must be examined as a whole, since the final image is a composite of all of its components. An extremely high resolution but very slow film used with a low output x-ray machine would be self-defeating, since the extended exposure time would cause more blurring than the sharpness that was contributed by the film. In this instance, the choice of film depends on the capacity of the x-ray generator and tube. Similarly, some films may require high-temperature machine processing and will produce poor images without compatible processing facilities. Conversely, some film requires manual processing at relatively low temperatures and should not be machine processed.

Extraoral Image Receptors

Extraoral radiographic procedures are being performed in dental offices more and more frequently. Cephalometric views, as well as films of the jaws and facial bones, are routinely used by orthodontists and oral surgeons, and occasionally by other specialists and general practitioners. Panoramic radiology (curved surface tomography) is becoming widely used in surgical as well as in general practices. Other health care trends that are generating interest in temporomandibular joint and salivary gland disease also result in an increase in the use of special procedures, including tomography, sialography, and arthrography. Intraoral x-ray sources with reversed geometry are likely to be reintroduced in the near future and will be discussed elsewhere.

The common denominator in each of these procedures is the extraoral placement of the film or the image recorder. With extraoral placement, many of the constraints of intraoral radiology are removed. Large, inflexible, or heavy devices are practical. Compared to some other types of image systems, film is a relatively inefficient medium for recording x-ray pictures. A significant number of x-ray photons retain enough energy to pass through a film emulsion without interacting and, as a result, fail to contribute to the production of an image. Photons of visible light, on the other hand, are virtually all absorbed by a photographic emulsion. Therefore, the efficiency of the recording of x-rays can be improved by converting the incident x-ray into visible light. This transformation can be accomplished by intensifying screens, which are placed in close contact with the film during its exposure to the x-ray beam.

Intensifying Screens

Intensifying screens are constructed of a semirigid base coated with a fluorescent material. The screens are held in close contact with the film by a cassette (Figure 1-5). The efficiency of the screen is a function of how effectively it absorbs x-rays and converts them to visible light. Most intensifying screens are made with calcium tungstate, zinc sulfide, and/or barium lead sulfate as the fluorescent material or phosphor. The selection of a phosphor depends on its stability and the quality of the visible light that it emits. The most commonly used phosphors emit light in the blue and violet regions of the spectrum, which is readily absorbed by most film emulsions.

Although the absorption of x-rays by an intensifying screen increases with increasing quantities of the phosphor, the gain in efficiency is usually associated with a loss of image quality, which is recognized as grain, noise, or mottle. Therefore, intensifying screens must be made with phosphors that absorb x-rays efficiently even when present in small quantities. Speed or efficiency is increased further if the conversion of x-ray energy into light energy is nearly complete (Figure 1-6).

The phosphors used in color television screens have properties similar to those just described. These phosphors are compounds made of the rare earth elements of the lanthanide series. They readily absorb x-rays over a broad energy range, particularly at high energies where conventional calcium tungstate phosphors lose their effectiveness. The rare

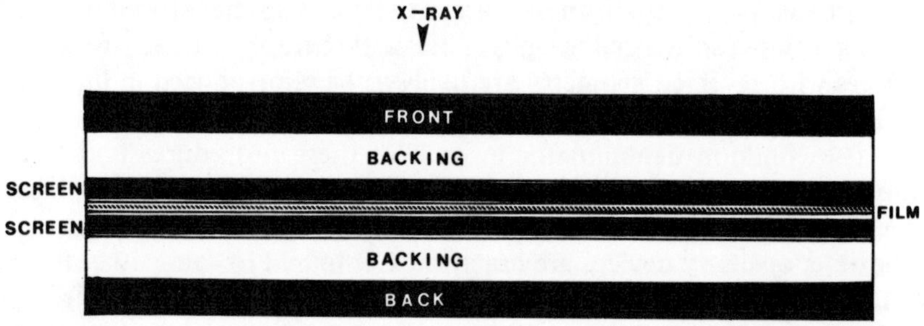

A

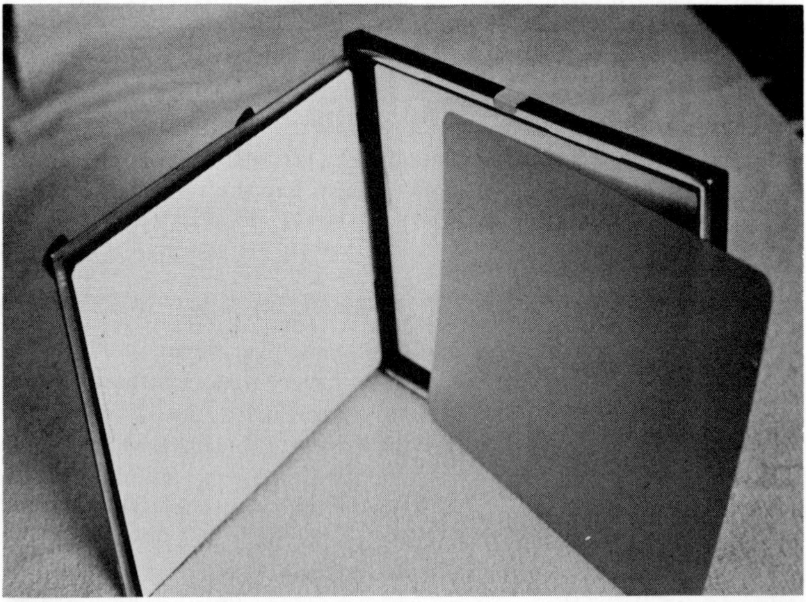

B

Figure 1-5 A. Diagrammatic representation of a cassette with intensifying screens in close contact with x-ray film. The screens are supported by a backing material that allows the screens to be compressed against the film when the cassette is closed. The front of the cassette passes x-rays while the back of the cassette is often coated with lead to block scattered radiation. **B.** This cassette, when closed, places intensifying screens in contact with both front and back surfaces of the film.

earth phosphors also emit more light per unit of absorbed radiation than do their typical calcium and barium counterparts. The light emitted by rare earth phosphors covers a different spectral range. When matched with appropriately sensitized films, this results in a dramatic increase in speed. The increase in speed may be associated with a reduction in exposure latitude and contrast; that is, relatively small changes in x-ray quantity result in relatively large differences in the density seen on a processed film.

The great increase in speed found in the rare earth film-screen combinations is important for many reasons. First, reducing the exposure time lessens motion distortion. Second, the life of the x-ray tube is increased because of the reduction in work load. Most importantly, exposure of the patient can be dramatically reduced. In panoramic examinations patient exposure can be reduced to approximately one-third of that required by conventional imaging systems. In linear tomography and in cephalometric radiography, exposures can be reduced to the level of one-fifth or one-tenth of other imaging systems.[7,8] Finally, the reduced power requirements resulting from the use of rare earth imaging systems make it possible to use x-ray tubes with small focal spots and other physical characteristics which lead to improved image quality.

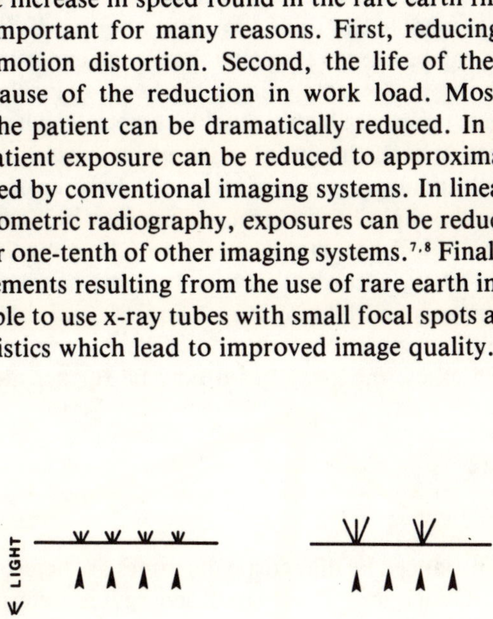

A

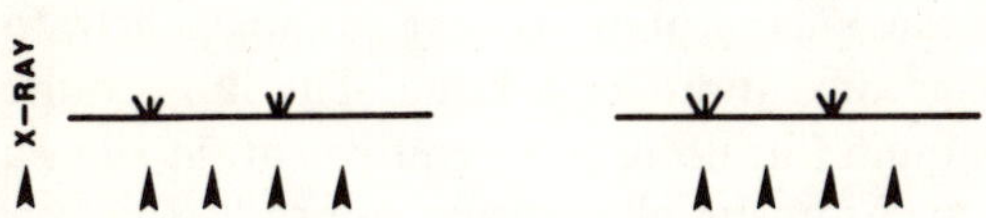

B

Figure 1-6 The effectiveness of intensifying screens can be varied in several ways. **A.** Substitution of a phosphor that absorbs x-rays more efficiently allows four x-ray photons to produce four light photons (right) instead of two (left). **B.** Less efficient phosphors (left) can be replaced with phosphors that emit greater quantities of light (right) for each x-ray photon absorbed.

Intensifying screens must be carefully chosen. Film designed for visible light is different in many ways from film designed for x-rays, and their processing requirements may differ. The choice of intensifying screens must, therefore, take into account the existing or planned processing facility and the choice of film. Also, as in the case of film, the intensifying screens must be compatible with the x-ray equipment, although in this case the potential for noncompatibility is twofold. For example, a film-screen combination may be so slow that it may lack the power to produce an image in a reasonable length of time, but an intensifying screen with compatible film can be chosen that may require an exposure time shorter than that which can be accurately timed by the x-ray machine. Although modern electronic timers are highly reliable, especially when compared to older mechanical devices, the timing of short intervals yields the highest frequency of malfunction or poor performance. In some procedures, such as panoramic radiography, the exposure time may be fixed by other requirements; here it will become necessary to adjust machine output to match the speed of the recording device. In some panoramic units, the range of milliamperes and kilovoltages is limited, and the lowest setting may exceed the exposure requirements of many modern film-screen systems. In such cases, the x-ray beam may be further attenuated with filters.

FILTRATION

The x-rays produced by diagnostic machines are heterochromatic, or have a range of energies. The highest energy is determined by the kilovoltage applied to the tube (Figure 1-7). As x-ray photons leave the target they span a range of energies from near zero to that of the peak kilovoltage. X-rays with low energy have poor penetration, and x-rays of high energy have great penetration. To obtain an energy spectrum that is both safe and compatible with the diagnostic task it is necessary to filter the beam. Some commonly used x-ray filters, such as aluminum and copper, absorb low energy photons that cannot penetrate soft tissue to produce an image of a tooth or a bone. The law requires a minimum amount of aluminum filtration, or its equivalent, in all x-ray machines to reduce patient exposure by eliminating unproductive low-energy x-ray photons. When such a filter is used, a small but significant number of higher energy photons are also absorbed, and the total output of the machine is reduced over the entire energy spectrum.

Some filters exclude high energy photons that needlessly expose the patient and do not contribute significantly to the formation of an image. Several rare earth elements can produce an energy spectrum that matches the sensitivities of the image receptors and/or the image characteristics of the tissues. With appropriate combinations of filters, one can obtain photon energies more ideally suited for either soft tissue or hard tissue diagnosis and minimize exposure of the patient as well.[9,10]

With each addition to the x-ray system, the decision-making process becomes more complex and the desirability of seeking expert advice from a qualified physicist grows. By making appropriate matches among all components of the x-ray system, substantial gains are possible in both image quality and in reduction to radiation exposure.

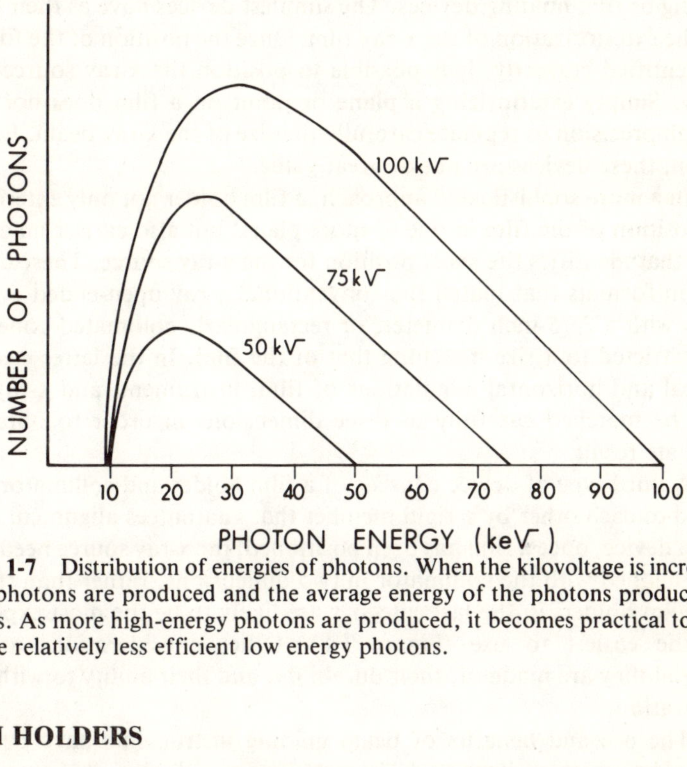

Figure 1-7 Distribution of energies of photons. When the kilovoltage is increased, more photons are produced and the average energy of the photons produced increases. As more high-energy photons are produced, it becomes practical to filter out the relatively less efficient low energy photons.

FILM HOLDERS

X-ray equipment manufactured after August 1974 and used for purposes other than intraoral imaging by law must be provided with devices to guarantee alignment of the x-ray source and image receptor. These regulations also require that the size of the x-ray beam must be either the same as or smaller than the size of its image receptor.

X-ray machines used with intraoral films are exempt from this regulation for reasons that are hard to comprehend. Correct alignment of the x-ray beam, the tooth, and the film is a major difficulty. Many hours are devoted to instruction in the bisecting angle technique and the right angle or paralleling technique to ensure alignment. Because these techniques are ineffective, the x-ray field must be significantly larger than the size of the film. Visual alignment is so inaccurate that an x-ray beam of the same size as the film would inevitably miss all or part of the film during many exposures.

The problem of alignment can be easily solved, however, through the use of a variety of film holders or beam guiding devices that establish correct alignment and make it possible to restrict the size of the beam to the size of the film.

Three general approaches have been used in the design of beam guiding or film holding devices. The simplest devices have as their objective the exteriorization of the x-ray film. Once the position of the film can be identified correctly, it is possible to position the x-ray source accurately. Simply exteriorizing a plane or point on a film does not allow enough precision to regulate carefully the size of the x-ray beam. For this reason, these devices are not of great value.

In a more sophisticated approach, a film holder not only exteriorizes the position of the film in one or more planes but also carries an attachment that identifies the exact position for the x-ray source. These devices exist in formats that match the conventional x-ray open-ended cylinder cones with a 2.75-inch diameter, or rectangularly collimated cones that are restricted to a size matching that of the film. In the latter case, the vertical and horizontal angulations of film, instrument, and x-ray tube must be matched carefully in three dimensions in order to obtain an adequate result.

A third type of device consists of a film holder and collimator, connected to each other by a rigid member that guarantees alignment. With such a device, once a film has been positioned, the x-ray source needs only to be aligned with the collimator in two dimensions, rather than three.

Film holders in the last category are likely to be the most expensive but the easiest to use (Figure 1-8). Other considerations are the material they are made of, their durability, and their ability to withstand sterilization.

The use and benefits of beam guiding instruments have been described by several writers.[11-14] The technique of Gilbert and Hanan[13] is of particular interest. These investigators used compound bite registrations with film holders to facilitate the production of duplicate films in patients who were followed for long periods of time.

EXTRAORAL COLLIMATORS

Collimation in extraoral radiography is rarely a problem. In panoramic machines collimation is fixed, and most general purpose x-ray machines have adjustable shutters made of lead or some other absorber material. All modern general purpose machines also have light fields that

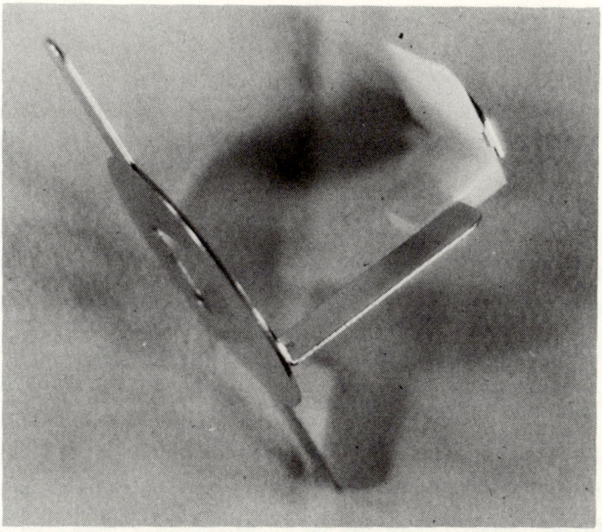

Figure 1-8 This beam guiding device or film holder was designed by Medwedeff[12] (Isaac Masel Company, Philadelphia, Pennsylvania). It permits collimation of the beam at the point of entry, attenuation at the film plate, rigidity, and can withstand sterilization by autoclaving.

correspond with the x-ray fields, so that positioning of the patient and adjustment of the x-ray field size are greatly facilitated.

One problem area is cephalometric radiography. Typical cephalometric units align the x-ray source, a head-positioning device, and the film holder. These units are commonly provided with fixed aperture collimators that can be rotated 90 degrees but cannot be adjusted in size or shape. Accordingly, the same x-ray beam is centered on rods that fit in the ears of the patient positioned in the head holding device, although this rarely constitutes the center of the desired image. As a result, it is often necessary to use x-ray fields that are inappropriate for the patient or the examination being performed. Simple devices can be constructed which provide variable collimation and matched light fields. Substantial reduction in patient exposure can be achieved with such devices, and the quality of the x-ray image is improved because scatter is reduced.[15] Unfortunately, there are no legally certified commercially available devices of this type in the dental marketplace.

IMAGE PROCESSING

All x-ray image receptors require postexposure processing. Fluoroscopic devices also require processing if one wishes to retain the image. Each practitioner has to decide whether to acquire a manual or machine processing system. Every film processing system has requirements for both time and temperature. Overexposure and underprocessing yields a poor quality image and subjects the patient to unnecessary radiation.

There are essentially three types of chemicals for processing x-ray film. One type is designed primarily for rapid results and may entail some sacrifice of image quality. This is most suitable for such working situations as endodontics or emergencies, where a fast result is essential and it is undesirable to leave the patient. The second is intended for manual development with longer processing at specified temperatures and times. If used correctly, this will produce images of extremely high quality that will not deteriorate with time. The third way is machine processing.

Most of the chemicals can be purchased as powders that are dissolved and mixed, or as liquids that are mixed and diluted, or as ready-to-use solutions. Each form has a different level of convenience, but as the convenience level increases the shelf life decreases. Therefore, the choice must be based on accessibility to a supplier and the rate of use. The most stable forms should be considered for rural or low volume practices where shelf life might be an important consideration.

The choice between machine and tank is one of economics and volume. Either method used correctly and carefully produces a good result; either method used carelessly produces films that are not diagnostic. With either system, a quality assurance program should be developed for regular testing. An adequate water supply for rinsing and/or temperature control should be provided. A simple mixing valve that balances hot and cold water to achieve the desired temperature usually is not adequate. Compensation for fluctuations in water pressure on the hot or cold side of the incoming supply is needed. Mixing valves require care and maintenance and are relatively expensive.

IMPROVEMENTS IN X-RAY GENERATOR DESIGN

As already noted, the production of x-rays by traditional generators is inefficient. This inefficiency results from the type of power supply most commonly used—unrectified alternating current. Alternating current allows conversion of low voltage to high voltage power supplies.

A transformer consists of two wire coils wrapped around opposite sides of an iron ring. The electrical circuit supplying current to the first coil, the primary circuit, creates a magnetic field within the iron ring that induces a current in the secondary coil. The voltage in the two circuits of the transformer is proportional to the number of wire turns in each of the two coils. For example, if the primary coil has 10 turns and the secondary coil has 100 turns, then the voltage of the secondary circuit would be 10 times higher than the voltage of the primary.

High Frequency Generators

Alternating current normally supplied for household or industrial use oscillates 60 times per second. If the frequency of these oscillations were increased, several advantages could be achieved in the design of x-ray generators. First, increases in the frequency of the polarity changes increase the efficiency of the transformer and reduce its size. In dental x-ray units, the transformer is normally in the tube housing. Therefore, a smaller transformer means a smaller tube housing. Second, as the tube housing is reduced in size it becomes practical to reposition the target from the front to the back of the tube, which saves space and improves projection geometry.

A further advantage can be gained by rectifying or converting alternating current into direct current. In typical x-ray generators, the x-ray tube acts as the rectifier, producing x-rays only during that half of the cycle when the anode is positive and the cathode is negative. When high frequency current and rectification are combined, a pattern similar to that shown in Figure 1-9 results.

Increased efficiency allows one of two additional advantages. Either the exposure time can be reduced or more effective filtration can be added to the x-ray tube to provide an x-ray beam with a more useful energy range. The GEX, marketed by General Electric, uses the latter option by incorporating a rare earth filter into the x-ray generator. The result is high contrast films. Exposure times are similar to those required by conventional units, but patient exposures are significantly reduced.

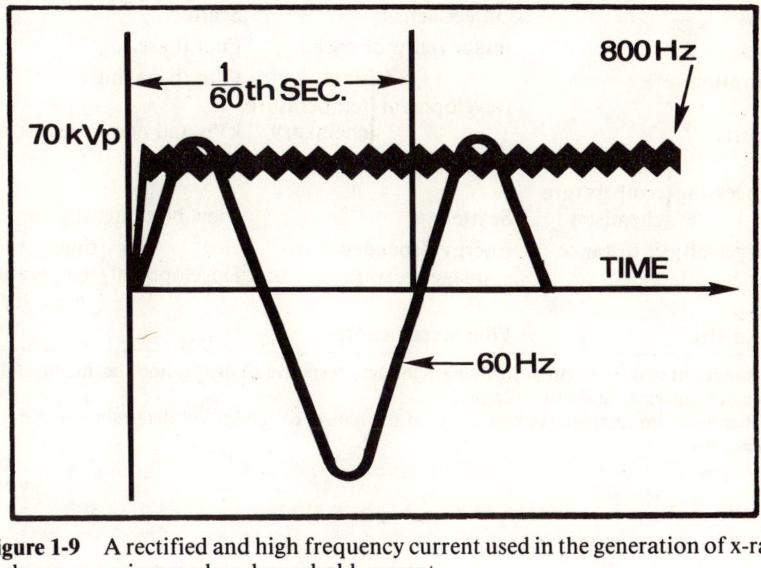

Figure 1-9 A rectified and high frequency current used in the generation of x-rays is shown superimposed on household current.

Voltage Cascade

An x-ray generator using cascading electronic circuits eliminates the use of traditional transformers to produce the high voltages necessary for x-ray generation. X-ray machines using the cascade principle generally have smaller, lighter, and more compact x-ray tubeheads, although at the time of this printing, the author is unaware of an x-ray generator that combines the cascade principle with high frequency current and with full wave rectification.

SUMMARY

New types of generators offer advantages in image contrast, efficiency, dose reduction, and/or size. Prospective buyers should examine these features carefully to determine whether or not they represent significant advantages in a particular practice setting. Some of the factors that affect patient exposure, image contrast, and image density are summarized in Table 1-2.

Table 1-2

Patient exposure	Image density	Image contrast
Patient size and density*	kVp	Subject contrast
Film or image receptor speed	mAs	Film (average gradient)†
mAs	Object density	Scatter
kVp	Image receptor speed	Film (base fog)
Filtration	Development {time, temperature, chemistry}	Film (base tint)
Scatter		kVp and energy spectrum
Processing {time, temperature, chemistry}	Target-film distance	Collimation
	Scatter	View box intensity
Target-object distance	Energy dependence of image receptor	Development {time, temperature, chemistry}
Field size	Film-screen contact	

*Changes in density occur with changes in: age, response to medication, hormonal status, nutrition, disease, and other factors.

†When nonfilm imaging systems are used the nature of the system determines its contrast properties.

REFERENCES

1. Advisory Committee on the Biological Effects of Ionizing Radiations. *The Effects on Populations of Exposure to Low Levels of Ionizing Radiation.* Washington, DC: National Academy of Sciences, National Research Council, 1972.

2. Brecher, R., and Brecher, E. *The Rays.* Baltimore: Williams and Wilkins, 1969.

3. Ardran, G.M., Langmead, W.A., and Crooks, H.E. Exposure reduction using new screen/film combination. *Br J Radiol.* 48:233–234, 1975.

4. Buchanan, R.A., Finkelstein, S.J., and Wickersheim, K.A. X-ray exposure reduction using rare earth oxysulfide intensifying screens. *Radiology* 105:185–190, 1972.

5. Evans, A.L., Davison, M., McLellan, J., and James, W.B. Evaluation of a new screen/film combination. *Br J Radiol.* 48:458–459, 1975.

6. Rossman, K., and Lubberts, G. Some characteristics of the five-spread-function and modulation transfer function of medical radiographic film and screen-film systems. *Radiology* 86:235–241, 1966.

7. Reiskin, A.B., Hummel, E., Kirchhof, S., and Freedman, M.L. Rare earth imaging in dental radiology. *J Prevent Dent.* 4:7–13, 1977.

8. Eddlestrom, B., Moores, B.M., and Walker, A. Eye dose measurements using conventional and rare earth screens during tomography of the paranasal sinuses. *Br J Radiol.* 50:266–270, 1977.

9. Richards, A.G., Barbor, G.L., and Bader, J.D. Sumarium filters for dental radiography. *Oral Surg.* 29:704–715, 1970.

10. Villagran, J.E., Gray, J.E., Hobbs, B.B., and Gillan, G.D. Improvements in the performance of intensifying screens by energy selective x-ray filtration. *Society of Photo Optical Instrumentation Engineers* 96:184–189, 1976.

11. Medwedeff, F.M., Knox, W.H., and Latimer, P. A new device to reduce patient radiation and improve dental film quality. *Oral Surg.* 15:1079–1088, 1962.

12. Medwedeff, F.M., and Elcan, P.D. A precision technique to minimize radiation. *Dent Survey.* Oct. 1967, pp. 45–53.

13. Gilbert, R.R., and Hanan, L. Duplication and quality control for intraoral roentgenographic use in clinical periodontics. *Oral Surg.* 26:31–38, 1968.

14. Eggen, S. Simplification of radiographic technique. *Quintessence Int.* 6:69–71, 1973.

15. Freedman, M.L., and Matteson, S.R. A collimator for reduced radiation dose with improved visualization of soft tissues. *Radiology* 118:226–228, 1976.

2 Microfocus Radiography

The placement of a film or other image receptor in the oral cavity has two important and interrelated consequences. First, relatively soft, flexible, and light-weight image receptors must be used. The exclusion of rigid, screen-containing cassettes means that these imaging systems are necessarily slow. Second, because anatomic constraints prevent ideal placement of the films in relation to dental structures, special procedures, such as bisecting the angle or the paralleling technique, are required to avoid distortion. Particularly in the paralleling technique increased distance between the x-ray source and the image receptor necessitates increased x-ray intensity. As the tube current and kilovolt potential are increased, the size of the target must also be increased to permit adequate heat dissipation.

IMAGE QUALITY

The quality of an x-ray image depends on a great many factors. The size of the focal spot or target is of prime importance. The image produced by a large focal spot is unsharp because the edges of objects in the image are struck by x-rays originating from different parts of the target (Figure 2-1). The result is edge unsharpness or penumbra. Edge unsharpness increases when the object is moved away from the film and toward the tube, as occurs when the paralleling technique is used. This explains the need to increase the target-to-object distance with a long cone so that the relative distances between target, object, and film are more nearly in agreement with the principles of shadow casting.

If the focal spot were extremely small, approaching a point source, edge unsharpness would cease to be a significant problem, and it would be possible to take advantage of the normal divergence of an x-ray beam to magnify images directly on film (Figure 2-2).[1,2] As the size of the focal spot and its heat loading capacity are reduced, the quantity of x-rays that can be generated per unit time is also reduced. Therefore, the use of a small focal spot depends upon a reduction in the distance between the target and the film and/or the use of faster recorder systems.

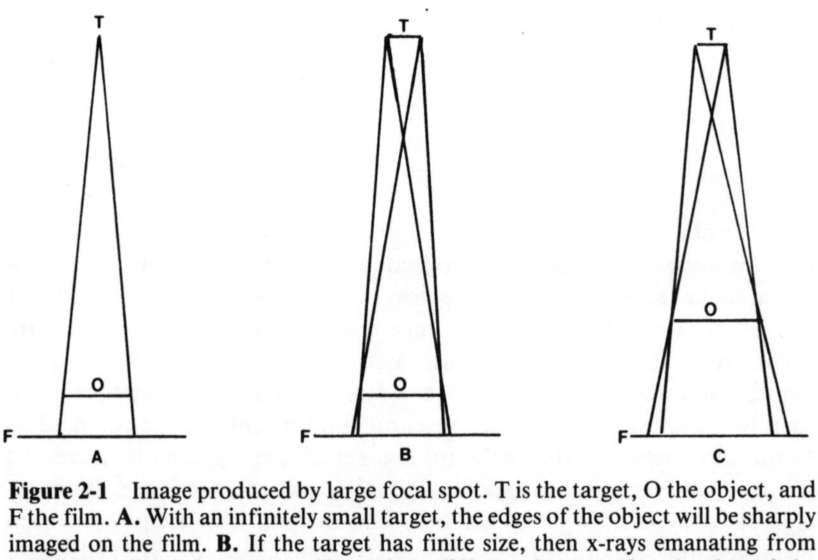

Figure 2-1 Image produced by large focal spot. T is the target, O the object, and F the film. **A.** With an infinitely small target, the edges of the object will be sharply imaged on the film. **B.** If the target has finite size, then x-rays emanating from opposite ends of the target will produce different images of each edge of the object, resulting in unsharpness. **C.** As the object moves farther from the film and closer to the target, this edge unsharpness becomes more pronounced.

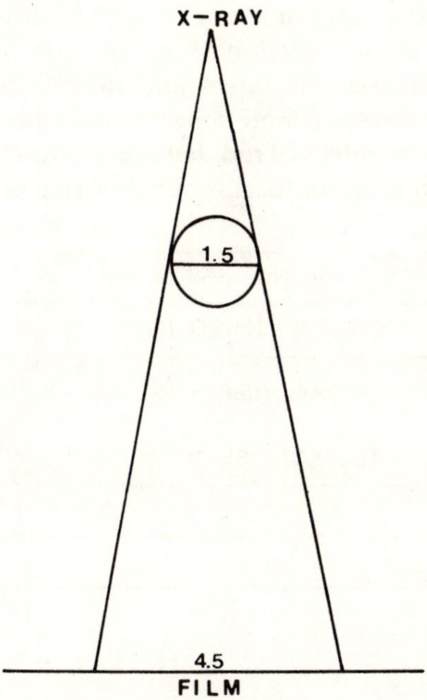

Figure 2-2 With an extremely small x-ray source, an object can be moved close to the source relative to its distance from the film, and magnification of the image occurs.

TYPES OF MICROFOCUS TUBES

Several types of microfocus x-ray tubes with compatible generators have been designed for use in human diagnosis. Some systems depend upon an x-ray tube called an extended rod anode (Figure 2-3). In contrast to conventional x-ray tubes, electrons are accelerated through a narrow tube to a target that is fixed at the opposite end. The shape of the x-ray field is determined in part by the size and shape of the target and in part by the configuration and focusing of the electron beam. The size and shape of the x-ray field can be altered with collimators and/or filters.

Microfocus x-ray units are available in many configurations and designs. Some units use an electron gun and an electromagnetic lens system similar to that found in television tubes. In these units, the focusing device is used to center the electron beam on the target.[3,4] In other microfocus units the configuration and intensity of the electron beam can be altered so that the x-ray tube can be used in different ways.[5] Other microfocus tubes rely less extensively on electron focusing but simply apply a voltage between the target and the filament. Finally, some microfocal systems employ a more conventional x-ray tube configuration as an alternative to the extended rod, but use electron focusing to produce a small circular and uniform focal spot with sharp edges.

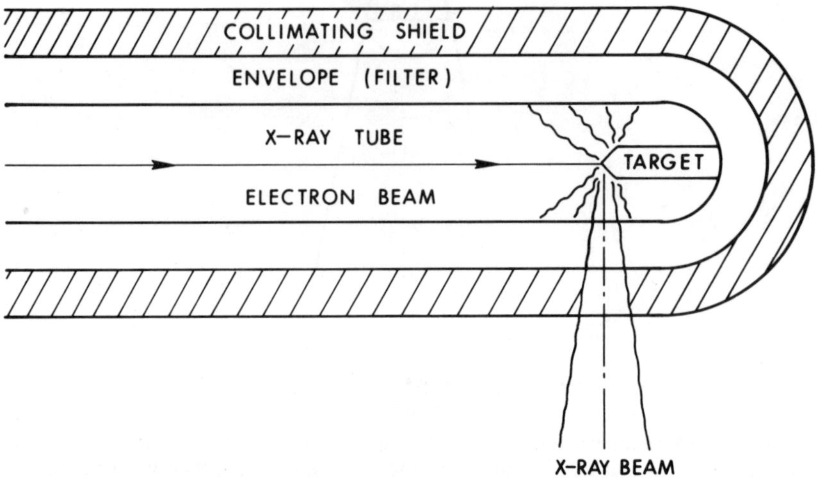

Figure 2-3 Diagrammatic representation of an extended rod anode source. Only that portion of the tube from which x-rays emanate is shown. Electrons accelerated through a hollow tube approximately the same diameter as a pen or pencil strike a target. The size and shape of the x-ray beam is defined by a collimating shield placed around the tube envelope.

Microfocus x-ray units with extended rod anodes (Figure 2-4) have been sold in both this country and in Europe and are likely to return to the American dental marketplace in modified form in the near future. The primary advantage of these devices stems from the small size of the tube, which makes it practical to place the x-ray source within the oral cavity. This "reversed geometry" is associated with several important advantages.[6] First, compared to conventional intraoral radiography, a wide variety of image receptors can be used. These include plain films, film-screen combinations, image intensifiers, and electrostatic or ion systems. Second, it is possible to examine isolated areas, quadrants, or dental arches with a single exposure (Figure 2-5). Third, the small size of the focal spot makes the production of magnified images geometrically reasonable (Figure 2-6).

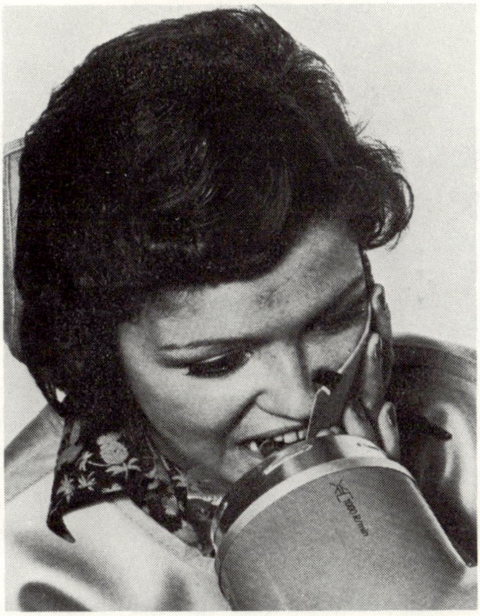

A

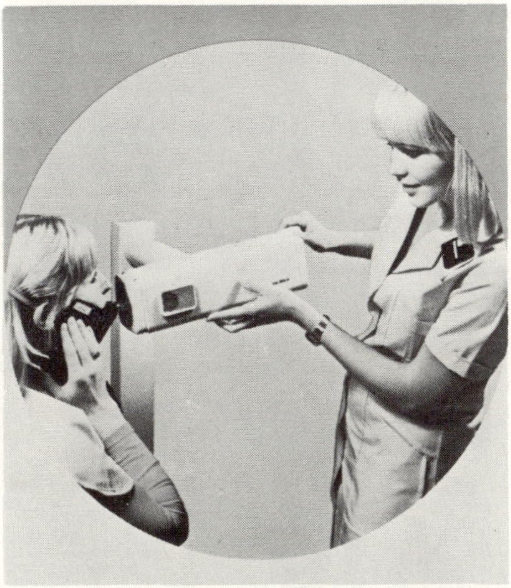

B

Figure 2-4 Microfocus x-ray units with extended rod anodes. **A.** Placement of the x-ray tube within the mouth and external positioning of the film for a half-face projection using the Siemens Status X unit. (Reprinted by permission of the Siemens Corporation. Product specifications are subject to change without notice from the manufacturer.) **B.** System manufactured by the Phillips Corporation is shown with film in position for a full mandibular projection. (Reprinted by courtesy of the Phillips Corporation.)

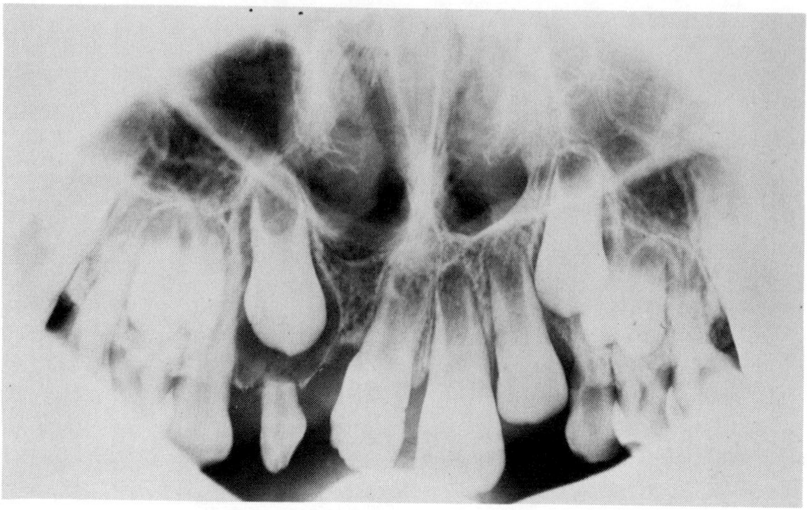

Figure 2-5 These views of the anterior maxillary teeth produced with a Siemens Status X give some indication of the image quality. (Reprinted by permission of the Siemens Corporation. Product specifications are subject to change without notice from the manufacturer.)

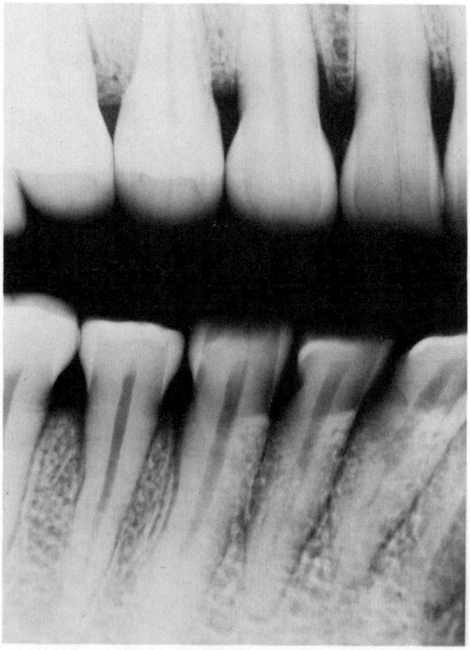

Figure 2-6 This magnified bitewing makes it possible to identify microfractures in the enamel of several teeth and to distinguish between cervical erosion and cervical caries. (Courtesy of Ridge Instruments, Tucker, Georgia.)

RADIATION EXPOSURE

The literature contains limited data on the clinical utility of these devices and on the exposures required for image production. Lieberman and Webber[7] added a fiber optic light indicator and collimator to a Westinghouse Panoramix, which they used in conjunction with an extraoral Polaroid film-screen cassette (Figure 2-7). In vitro and in vivo assays indicated that the detectability of artificially induced enamel defects was significantly lower than with conventional radiographs while larger lesions were readily detectable. In the studies of these investigators, the loss of information content appeared to be related to the use of the high-speed imaging system that reduced patient exposure by as much as 98% and produced positive dry prints in 15 seconds. The authors reported that the system was found to be useful in endodontics and presurgical evaluation of patients.

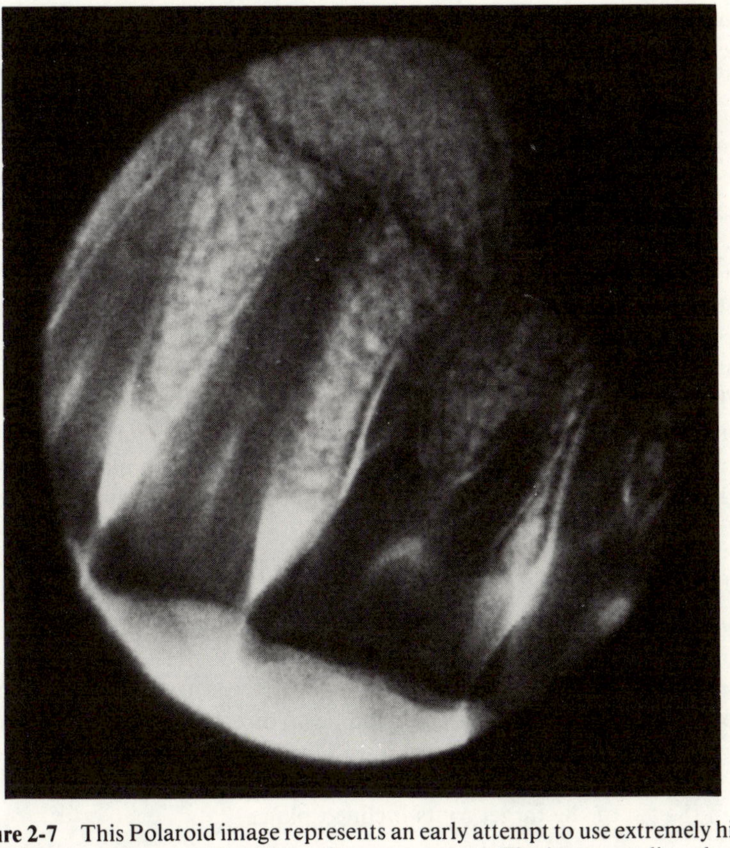

Figure 2-7 This Polaroid image represents an early attempt to use extremely high-speed imaging systems with rod anode x-ray sources. The image quality, though obviously unacceptable for some tasks, may be adequate for selected procedures.

Blomgren, Hollender, and Molander[8] studied radiation doses during radiography with one intraoral unit (Phillips Stat Oralix) and concluded that radiation doses were small except where soft tissue was in contact with the x-ray tube. They suggested modification of collimator design as a method of obtaining further reductions in exposure. Henrickson[9] described a system of intraoral radiography that employed an isotope rather than an x-ray tube as the radiation source. The major advantages of this approach are the convenience and portability that arise from the elimination of the generator and x-ray tube. Henrickson used an isotope of iodine that emits gamma rays in an appropriate energy range. The major disadvantages of the system include the need for a bulky container to house the isotope (placed intraorally), the difficulty of obtaining a source whose size is as small as comparable x-ray sources, and the relatively short half-life of the isotope, which necessitates frequent replacement.

Patient exposures to radiation have also been studied by Kallinger, Canigiani, and Czech[10] using lithium fluoride dosimeters and an Alderson phantom. Two different types of rod anode units were compared (Siemens Status X, Types A and B). As with other systems, the major exposure was found at the point where the tube contacted soft tissue. The Type B unit, which operates at a higher kilovoltage and uses greater filtration, requires significantly less patient exposure for the production of adequate images than does the Type A machine. Exposures with the Type B unit are generally comparable (except at the point of contact) with those encountered in conventional systems. However, these investigators did not use the fastest imaging systems available.

In contrast, Schoenfeld and colleagues[11] evaluated the quality of images produced with a broad range of image receptors. They demonstrated that a slow-speed imaging system provides high quality diagnostic images with nearly ideal contrast while some high-speed systems lack sufficient contrast for some diagnostic tasks. By defining the image quality of specific systems, however, it is theoretically possible to match the speed and other characteristics of the image receptor to the diagnostic task, thereby optimizing the risk/benefit ratio.

Rissi[5] has patented a single device that permits intraoral and extraoral placement of the x-ray tube for dental radiography. In the intraoral mode this tube can be used for projecting images of small areas by moving the screen forward and shielding part of the anode. The unit can also be used for producing images of quadrants or larger areas by removing the anode screen and focusing an electron beam directly on the tip of a conical target. To use the device in its extraoral mode, an adaptor is placed over the rod anode. This automatically moves the focus of the electron beam from the tip of the target to its inclined plane.

CONCLUSION

Although these devices have many theoretical advantages over their traditional counterparts, detailed technical specifications, including focal spot sizes, duty cycles, and other information, have not been readily available. More clinical data are needed that compare the image quality and patient exposures using these units with existing intraoral and curved surface tomographic (panoramic) devices. Specific details of projection geometry and dental applications are also discussed by Bolstorff,[12] Rottke,[13] and Durner.[14]

REFERENCES

1. Sickles, E.A., Goldberg, H.I., and Genant, H.K. Microfocal spot magnification fluoroscopy. *Invest Radiol.* 12:400, 1977.

2. Buckland-Wright, J.C. The micro-focal x-ray unit: a demonstration of its potential. *Med Biol Illus.* 27:163–168, 1977.

3. Fontijn, L.A., and Peugeot, R.S. An operational 150 Kv microfocus rod anode x-ray system for nondestructive testing. Paper presented at the 37th National A.N.N.T. Conference, Detroit, Michigan, Oct. 5, 1977.

4. Foster, B.E., and McClung, R.W. A study of x-ray and isotopic techniques for boreside radiography of tube-to-tube sheet welds. *Materials Evaluation* 35:43–51, 1977.

5. Rissi, W. United States Patent 4,060,731. 1977.

6. Webber, R.L., and Nagel, R.N. Theoretical factors limiting source design. DHEW Publ. No. (NIH) 79-248. Paper presented at the Symposium on Rod Anode Sources, American Dental Association, June 14–16, 1976.

7. Lieberman, J.E., and Webber, R.L. Clinical evaluation of a prototype intraoral x-ray source system. *Oral Surg.* 46:318–327, 1978.

8. Blomgren, P.G., Hollender, L., and Molander, B. Determination of radiation geometry and radiation doses during radiography with an intraoral x-ray tube (Phillips Stat Oralix). *Dentomaxillofac Radiol.* 7:19–26, 1978.

9. Henrickson, C.D. Iodine 125 as a radiation source for odontological roentgenology. *Acta Radiol.* 269(suppl):4–88, 1967.

10. Kallinger, W., Canigiani, G., and Czech, W. Comparative study of exposure to radiation of the patient with Status X, Types A and B. *Electromedica* 2:51–54, 1978.

11. Schoenfeld, C.M., Moore, B.K., Lin, P.J. et al. Image receptor speed versus image quality for intraoral source radiography. *J Dent Res.* 57:304, 1978.

12. Bolstorff, C. Status X projection technique and indication. *Quintessence Int.* 1:1–7, 1971.

13. Rottke, B. Application of the Status X in oral medicine. *Electromedica* 3:1–14, 1971.

14. Durner, H. X-ray diagnosis with the Status X in the dental surgery. *Electromedica* 5:1–3, 1971.

3 Image Intensification

Direct or ''real time'' viewing of x-ray images is uncommon in dentistry for many reasons. The cost of devices that permit instant viewing is high, the units are large, image detail is not as good as on film, and there is no permanent image without additional processing. Furthermore, instant viewing is seldom of great value. Some examples of procedures that can benefit include dynamic studies such as sialography, the evaluation of acute trauma, the placement of instruments during endodontic procedures, and previewing the projection geometry used in conventional radiographic examinations.

Until approximately 30 years ago, instant images were produced by directing x-rays upon a fluorescent screen mounted behind a sheet of lead glass. The resulting image was dim and could be seen only after the fluoroscopist ''dark adapted'' by sitting in a dark room for up to 20 minutes. During the 1950s devices that increased the brightness of fluoroscopic images by electronic amplification were developed (Figure 3-1).[1] X-ray photons interacting with the input phosphor produce light photons that are converted into photoelectrons by a ''photocathode.''

The photoelectrons are focused and accelerated toward an output phosphor. The image at the output phosphor is smaller but brighter. As a practical matter, the size and image quality of these image intensifiers preclude their use in most dental situations (Figure 3-2).

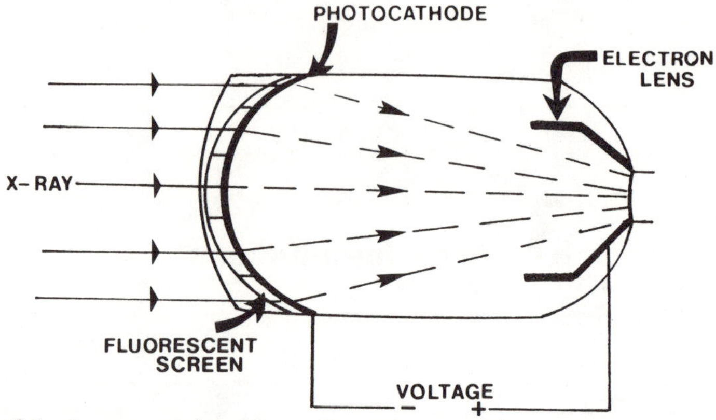

Figure 3-1 In a conventional image intensifier (I.I.) the top surface is coated with a phosphor (cesium iodide) which converts x-ray photons into photons of visible light. A photocathode material on the inner surface of the fluorescent screen converts light photons which are accelerated and focused on an output phosphor.

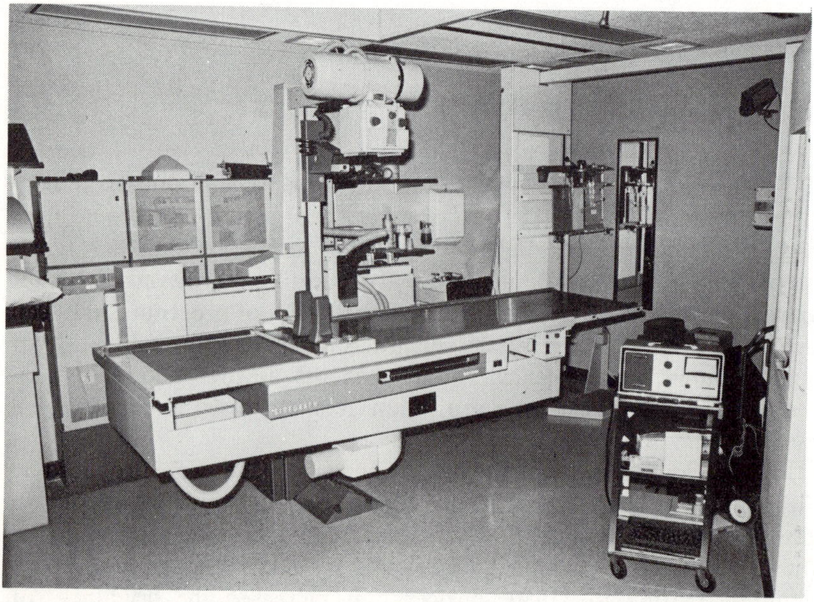

Figure 3-2 Conventional image intensification unit. The cesium iodide screen is located at a position under the table top denoted by the curved arrow. A television camera is placed at the bottom of the image intensifier (straight arrow) to permit indirect viewing.

THE LIXISCOPE

A different approach to image intensification that avoids minification of the image while improving its quality has been described.[2,3] Figure 3-3 shows a schematic representation of a light amplification system that has many applications, including the enhancement of night vision. Light entering a fiber optic plate at one surface is transmitted to a photocathode coating on the inner surface. At this interface, light photons are converted into electrons. A high voltage draws the electrons through a vacuum to a microchannel plate containing closely packed tubes approximately 12 micrometers in diameter. Electrons passing through the channels under the influence of the high voltage strike the walls. With each collision, additional photoelectrons are produced, reaching a gain of approximately 1000 times.[4] Electrons emerging from the far side of the microchannel plate strike a screen coating the fiber optical end of the device through which the incoming light is viewed. The screen converts the photoelectrons back into light photons that can be viewed by eye.

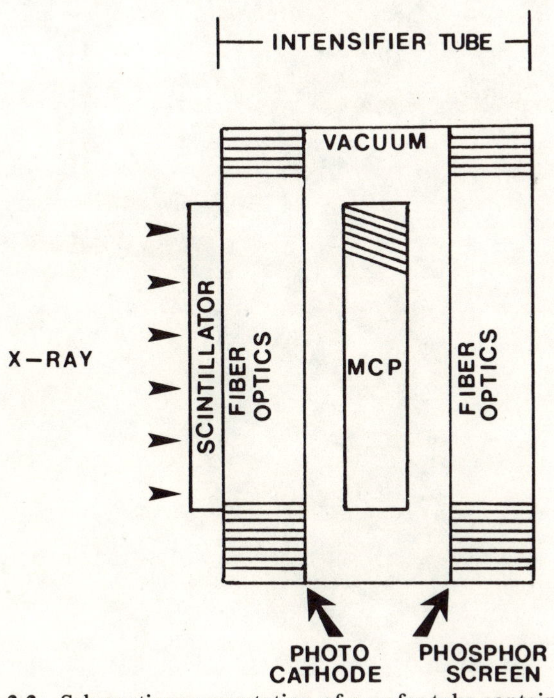

Figure 3-3 Schematic representation of a wafer tube containing a microchannel plate. A scintillator coats the input surface when the device is used for x-ray imaging. Without the scintillator the unit is used to intensify or amplify visible light.

Coating the input side of this light amplification device with an appropriate phosphor, such as that used in an x-ray intensifying screen, makes the device suitable for viewing x-ray images as well as light images. In the configuration designed for use with ionizing radiations, the device has been named Lixiscope for "low intensity x-ray imaging scope." Prototypes have been designed with small radiation sources attached on an extension arm and with a shutter device. The entire unit, including a power supply, is about the size of a small hand-held magnifying glass (Figure 3-4). The exposure rate for objects placed near the Lixiscope is many times lower than that of conventional image intensifiers. Permanent records of objects can be made by attaching a camera to the viewing surface (Figures 3-5 and 3-6). Although the densities are reversed compared to conventional x-ray films, it is possible to recognize small defects.

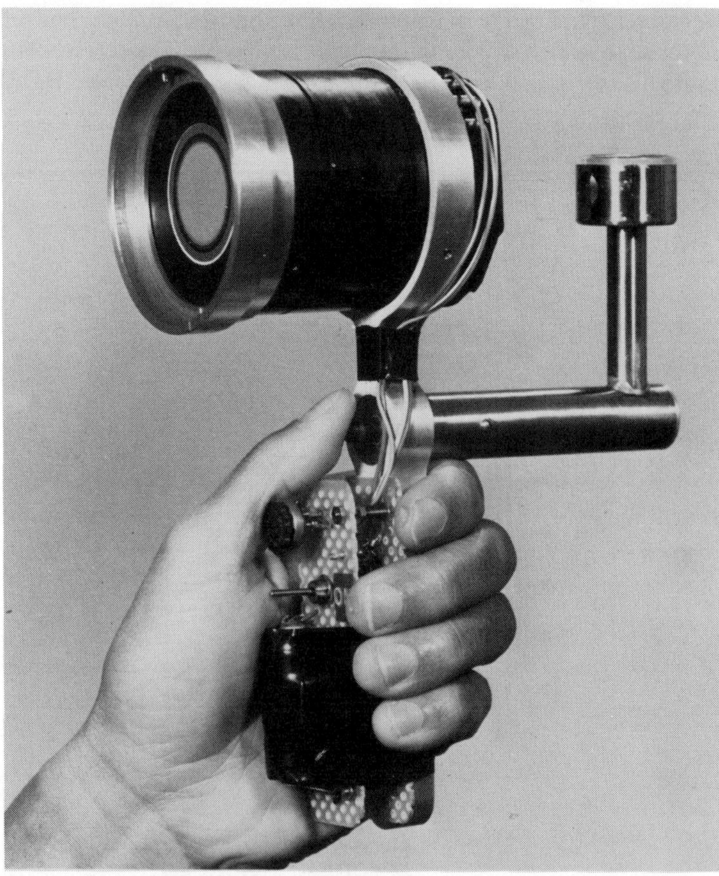

Figure 3-4 The size of a prototype is shown in relation to the size of a hand. This unit contains the radiation source and power supply as well as the image intensifier.

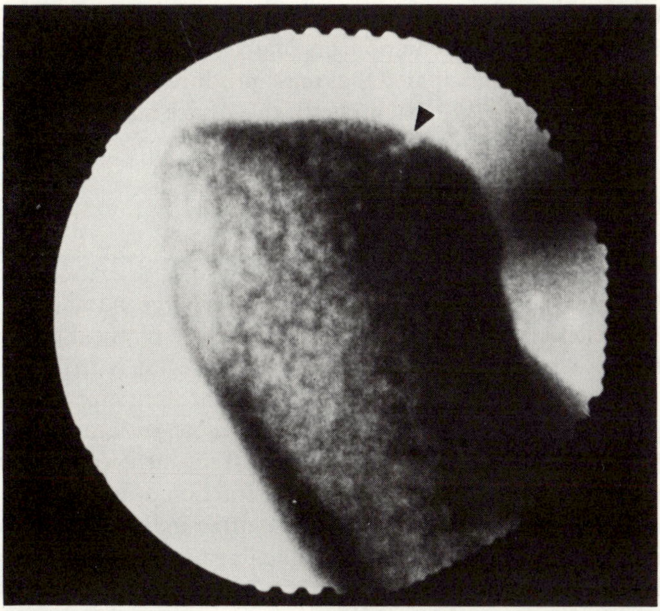

Figure 3-5 This crude Polaroid image was taken from a Lixiscope screen which contained an imperfection seen as a dark spot on the anterior surface of the condyle. However, small lytic defects (arrow) are also evident.

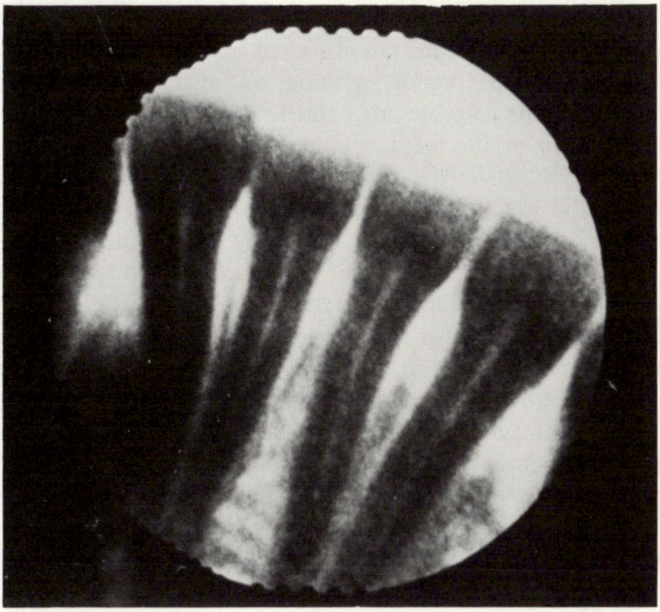

Figure 3-6 This Polaroid image was obtained from the screen of a Lixiscope held in the anterior region of the mandible.

The Lixiscope is being evaluated in government and private institutions. Because it contains components that are already manufactured for other purposes, it is anticipated that mass-produced units would cost less than $5000 apiece. The clinical utility of this device may be demonstrated in the near future.

Potential Applications

The maxillofacial complex consists of a large number of small, irregular, calcified, and paired structures in close physical proximity to each other. Roentgen diagnosis in this anatomic region is difficult because of the need to place films in positions where confusing superimposition is avoided and because important pathologic changes are often dimensionally small. For example, the periodontal ligament space that forms the attachment of tooth to bone is only a fraction of a millimeter wide. Small changes in the size of this structure often indicate the presence of treatable pathology of teeth, bone, or the ligament itself. A doubling of the width of this space represents less than half a millimeter. Radiographs must be capable of resolving such small changes to be of diagnostic value. Similar circumstances apply to other parts of the jaws, to the paranasal sinuses, to the salivary glands, and to the craniomandibular articulation.

The production of adequate images for maxillofacial diagnosis has depended usually on the use of small, fine grain, slow, high resolution films which can be placed inside the mouth. Thick and thin section tomography, magnification, and subtraction radiology are also used. In spite of their sophistication, many of these procedures still have problems.

Examination of the teeth is complicated by the placement of the image receptor intraorally to avoid superimposition of contralateral or adjacent structures. Once the image receptor is in place, however, it ceases to be visible, and orientation of the x-ray source must be estimated through the use of external anatomic landmarks. The difficulty in aiming the x-ray beam at the film has led to the use of an x-ray field that is larger than the film. However, for the radiograph to be of diagnostic value, it must be free from distortion, and adjacent structures cannot be overlapped. The determination of appropriate projection geometry, including the point of entry of the beam and its horizontal and vertical angulation, is of major importance. These problems are sometimes solved by using beam guiding devices (Figure 3-7) that externalize the position of the film and collimate the beam to an appropriate size.

An alternative approach to the imaging of dental structures involves the use of intraoral sources of radiation with extraoral placement of the image receptor. Extended rod anode x-ray sources (Figure 3-8) as well as isotopic sources have been used for these reversed geometry techniques.

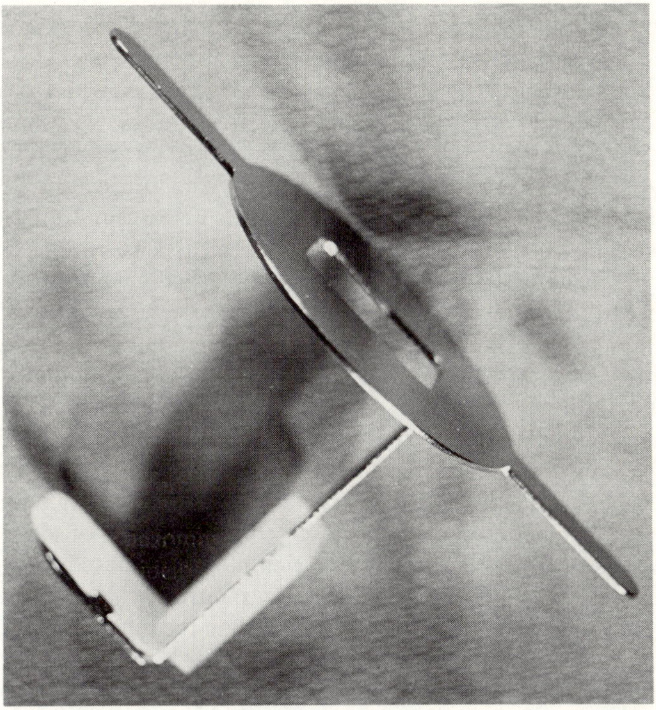

Figure 3-7 This device distributed by the Isaac Masel Company of Philadelphia achieves several desirable objectives. The position of the film is externalized for easy orientation of the x-ray source. The size of the x-ray field is restricted to the size of the image receptor.

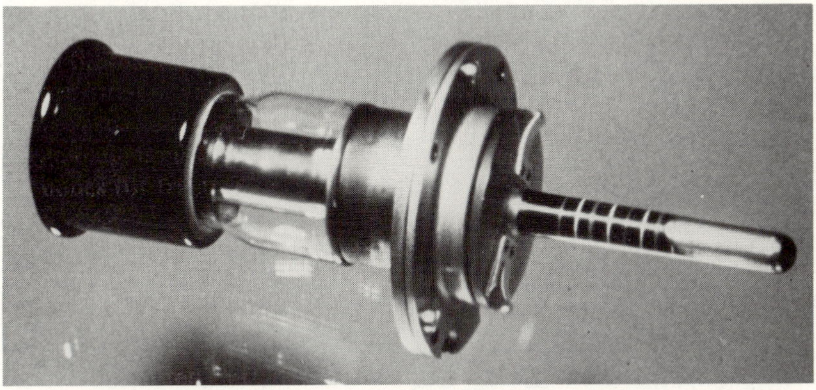

Figure 3-8 Extended rod anode x-ray tube. X-rays are emitted from the tip of the tube, which can be inserted into the oral cavity. (Courtesy of the Siemens Corporation. Product specifications are subject to change without notice from the manufacturer.)

This approach offers increased freedom in the choice of image receptors because the constraint of size imposed by intraoral placement is removed. However, many of the problems of projection geometry persist and may be aggravated by the extremely short source-to-subject distance. This problem might be solved by using the Lixiscope as part of a feedback loop that would allow the operator to correct the projection geometry. Although the Lixiscope does not have adequate resolution for many diagnostic tasks, it does appear to be useful as a scouting or preview device. Once the correct geometry is established, exposures could be made with confidence using higher resolution image receptors. As a result, diagnostic skills should improve, and the number of films rejected because of inadequate technique should decline or be eliminated.

The resolving power of the Lixiscope was examined in several preliminary studies conducted at the University of Connecticut. The objectives were to examine the compatibility of the Lixiscope with several possible radiation sources, and to determine whether or not significant differences in resolution could be observed as a function of source energy or size. Two different Lixiscopes were employed in these investigations. Although both devices had variable gain controls, the range and maximum gain of one was considerably higher than the other. Results of these investigations are shown in Table 3-1.

Table 3-1
Lixiscope Resolution

MCP	Source	Resolution (L.P./mm) Max. G.	Min. G.
H.G.*	70 kVp x-ray	4.0–5.0	5.0
H.G.	36 kVp x-ray	2.2–4.0	
H.G.	Gadolinium 153	3.5	3.0–4.0
L.G.†	36 kVp x-ray	5.5	
L.G.	70 kVp x-ray	4.0–5.5	
L.G.	Iodine 125	4.0–7.0	

*High gain.
†Low gain.
Resolution is stated in line pairs per millimeter as defined by the particular measuring device used. The energies of the radiation sources are indicated by kilovolt peak.

No significant differences in resolution as a function of energy using 36 to 70 kVp x-rays or sources made from iodine 125 and gadolinium 153 were observed. The energy peaks of the x-ray beams were further narrowed with aluminum and samarium filters, without significant effect. Resolution was measured with Siemens' diverging line and bar patterns, and with a United States Air Force test target. The only consistent result was improved resolution in the low gain Lixiscope compared to the high gain device or in either instrument operated in its low gain mode. These studies, though far from definitive, suggest that resolution is limited by the instrument itself rather than by the characteristics of the radiation source or the input phosphor.

In maxillofacial diagnosis, tomography is used for screening or survey purposes in addition to its more traditional applications. Narrow angle curved surface tomographic units (panoramic) are becoming commonplace in dental offices. Their images are relatively low in resolution with moderate amounts of distortion and a relatively high frequency of false negative and false positive recordings. Patient exposure is small but significant and can be reduced by the use of rare earth imaging film and screens. An alternative to curved surface tomography is the reversed geometry obtained with an intraoral source and an extraoral image receptor. With reversed geometry large reductions in patient exposure are possible, but optimal projection geometry remains a problem. For survey purposes, when justified, the Lixiscope might have merit because it can be used selectively and flexibly. However, while the Lixiscope permits manipulation and optimization of the projection geometry of the imaging system, it leaves no permanent record for detailed study or future reference. Although this problem could be solved by coupling the output phosphor of the Lixiscope with a video recorder, the cost and size might become unacceptably large.

Thin-section tomography is used to evaluate facial structures, such as the temporomandibular joints, because it is the only way to demonstrate these structures. Oblique views obscure the articular surfaces and their relationships to each other. Right angle views superimpose the two joints upon each other as well as upon other structures at the base of the skull. The problem of overlap could be reduced by the use of the Lixiscope and an intraoral source. Many of the tomographic systems used for curved surface linear tomography or complex tomography have inherent limits to their resolution in the range of two to six line pairs per millimeter. The Lixiscope, therefore, may be a useful supplement in some instances, although it clearly is not a replacement for thin-section tomography.

Examination of the temporomandibular joint is also difficult because many crucial structures within are radiolucent and cannot be visualized without contrast produced by filling the joint cavities with an opaque substance. This procedure, called arthrography, is easy in large joints such as the knee where conventional image-intensified fluoroscopy can be used to guide the placement of a needle. In the temporomandibular joints, however, the problem of overlap diminishes the value of fluoroscopy in establishing the correct site for an injection of contrast media and in the subsequent evaluation of the joint cavity. Here, the use of an intraoral source with the Lixiscope should provide geometry similar to that which exists in the examination of the extremities. To evaluate the potential of this approach the Lixiscope was used to assess needle placement in the knee joint of a rabbit. The size of this joint is somewhat smaller than the temporomandibular joint of a human but more practical as a test site. A Polaroid image of a Lixiscope view of the knee with the needle in place is shown in Figure 3-9. As previously noted, the most significant problem lies in the recording of the image. Prolonged exposures were required with the available Polaroid system and resulted in higher radiation exposure and occasional blurring. It is not clear that the radiation exposure required for photography was greater than that required for x-ray imaging with conventional film systems. Figure 3-10 shows a Polaroid image taken from a television screen with a system similar to that used with the Lixiscope. Figure 3-11 illustrates a conventional film and a tomogram of a temporomandibular joint injected with opaque dye.

Sialography, the retrograde filling of the salivary glands with radiopaque dyes, is another instance in which reverse geometry and the Lixiscope might be of diagnostic value. Lateral views of the parotid gland

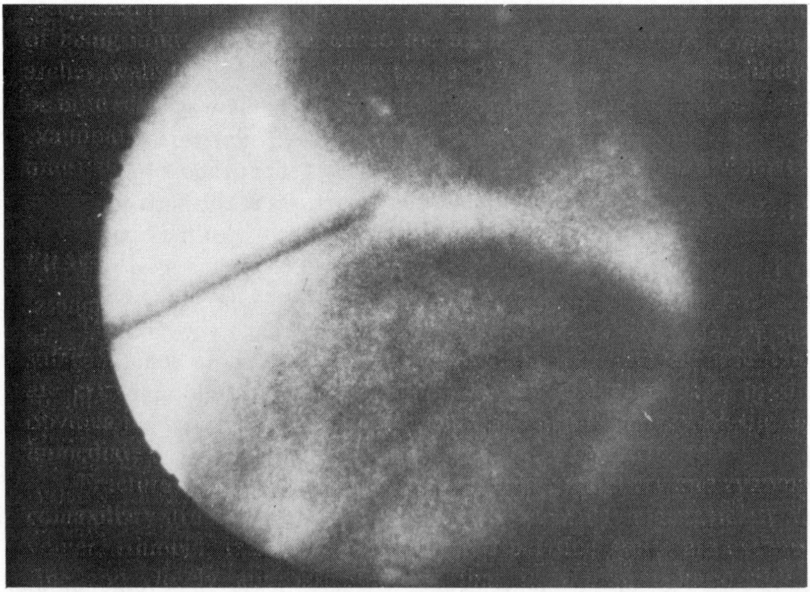

Figure 3-9 The Lixiscope is helpful in identifying the position of a needle placed within a joint.

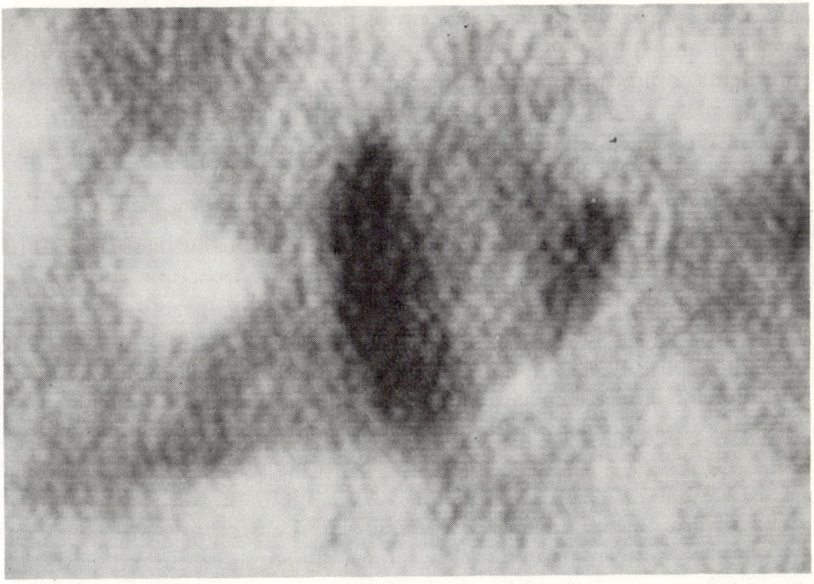

Figure 3-10 Conventional television images with 525 scan lines produce relatively crude pictures.

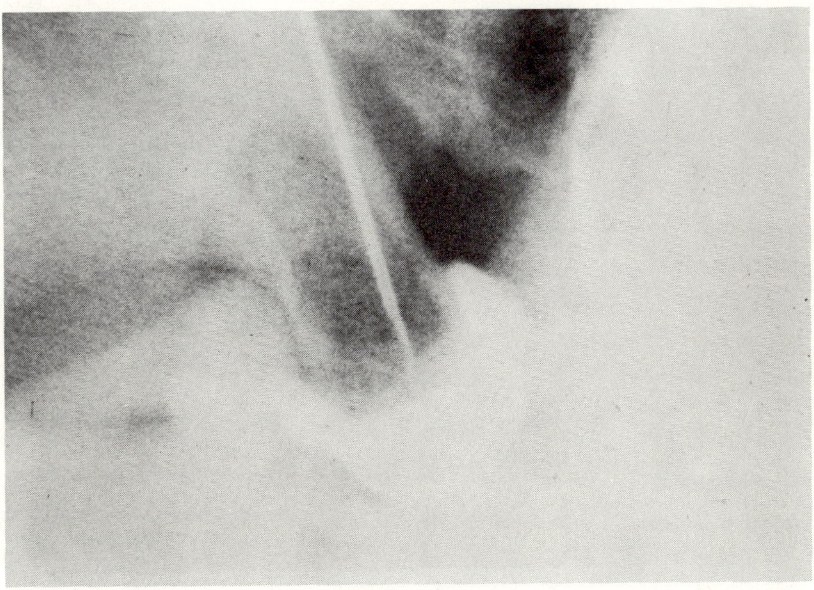

Figure 3-11 Arthrogram obtained by conventional radiographic methods.

are compromised by the oblique projections and the superimposition of the jaws and spine over gland tissue (Figure 3-12). To some extent these problems could be minimized by the Lixiscope, which would also provide a convenient means of monitoring gland filling. This is necessary to detect certain types of obstructions and to prevent inadvertent injection of dye through ductal walls into tissue spaces.

A major concern with the Lixiscope is the lack of any record of exposure time and patient dose. Although the dose rate at the surface of the phosphor is lower than that of conventional fluoroscopic systems, the absence of warning devices and/or metering systems permits inadvertent prolonged use. The ability to manipulate the Lixiscope around many structures has the advantage of providing quantitatively more diagnostic information and the disadvantage of encouraging users to search for pathology in clinical situations that are likely to be unrewarding. We have not computed or measured patient exposures in examinations performed with the Lixiscope, but exposures with existing equipment are small (in the range of 100 milliroentgens per cut for skull tomograms) when fast imaging systems are used. The Lixiscope may not reduce significantly the overall exposure. It may, however, be more convenient and effective.

In summary, the Lixiscope, particularly with intraoral or intracavitary radiation sources and reversed geometry, appears to have many

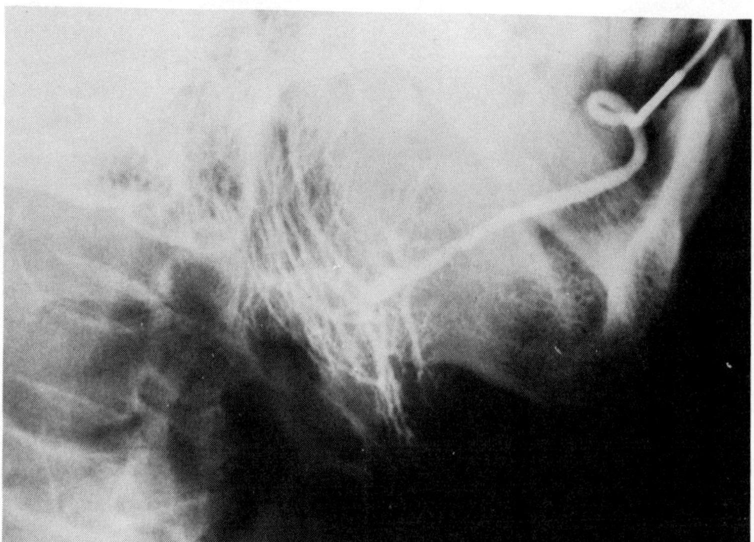

Figure 3-12 Portions of salivary gland structure obscured by overlap and by superimposition.

advantages over conventional approaches to roentgen diagnosis of maxillofacial disease. Preliminary studies, however, suggest that neither the instrument nor the techniques for its use have been optimized. No concrete basis exists now for a comparison of the efficacy of the Lixiscope with currently used roentgen techniques.

ALTERNATIVE METHODS

The primary value of fluoroscopy stems from its ability to provide the observer with an instantaneous and dynamic image. Image intensifiers increase the brightness of the fluoroscopic image, which eliminates the need for dark adaptation and provides substantial reduction in patient exposure.

Nonfluoroscopic types of image intensification, such as intensifying screens, have been discussed elsewhere. Recently, Askins[5] described a new technique for image intensification that requires neither electronic image amplification nor intensifying screens, although the latter could be productively incorporated into the new system.

Radiographs that are regarded by many observers as underexposed are likely to contain most essential diagnostic information. Webber and Stark[6] demonstrated that significant random degradation of x-ray images did not interfere with diagnostic yield. Low density images are, however, visually difficult to interpret. Enhancement of the information contained in underexposed images would facilitate the extraction of information and reduce the amount of patient exposure required for any given examination. Furthermore, reduction in total exposure might minimize the amount of scatter and improve the signal-to-noise ratio of the x-ray beam.

Autoradiographic image intensification, a new method, increases density and contrast to visually manageable levels. The silver in the film image is chemically combined with a radioactive isotope. This combination is then placed in contact with an appropriate photographic emulsion where the density of the autoradiographic film can be controlled by increasing its exposure rather than by increasing the exposure of the patient. Autoradiographs were made with Kodak industrial films and often required exposure times of 2 to 12 hours.

Radiographs that are underexposed by 80% to 90% can produce autoradiographs that compare favorably with films that had been correctly exposed. Although the autoradiographic method of image intensification is in a primitive state, it raises many interesting possibilities for the future (Figure 3-13).

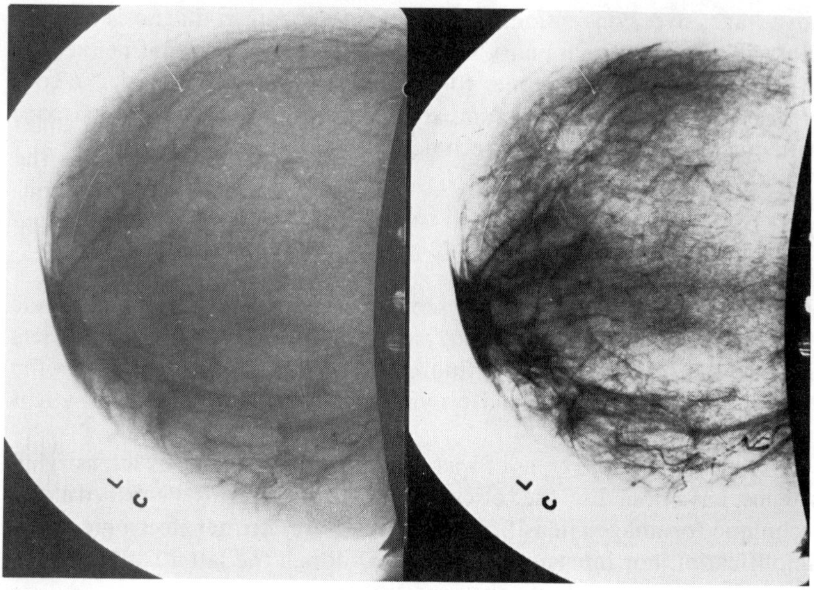

A B

Figure 3-13 Patient exposure can be dramatically reduced by postexposure processing of an image as illustrated above. **A.** Underexposed original. **B.** Postprocessed image. (B.S. Askins. Autoradiographic image intensification: applications in medical radiography. *Science* 199:684–686, 1978. Copyright 1978 by the American Association for the Advancement of Science. Reprinted with permission.)

REFERENCES

1. Teves, M.C., and Tol, T. Reinforcement electronique d'images radioscopiquies. *Philips Techn Rev.* 14:1–11, 1952.
2. Woodhead, A.W., and Eschard, G. Microchannel plates and their applications. *Acta Electronica* 14:181–200, 1971.
3. Yin, L.J., and Seltzer, S.M. *The Lixiscope: A Pocket-Size Imaging System.* Technical Memorandum 78064. Washington, DC: National Aeronautics and Space Administration, 1978.
4. Gould, R.G., Judy, P.F., Klopping, J.C. et al. Quantum detection efficiency of a microchannel plate image intensifier. *Nuclear Instr Meth.* 144:493–500, 1977.
5. Askins, B.S. Autoradiographic image intensification: applications in medical radiography. *Science* 199:684–686, 1978.
6. Webber, R.L., and Stark, L. Influence of fogging radiation and mode of display on the interpretation of dental caries from conventional radiographs. *Invest Radiol.* 7:506–516, 1972.

4 Contrast Agents

Contrast agents are widely used in medicine and in a more limited way in dentistry. A contrast agent or medium is a radiopaque substance used to delineate anatomic structures roentgenographically.[1] Contrast is the difference in density between different structures, and contrast agents are used when the components under examination do not contain sufficient inherent contrast.

In medicine, instillation of barium salts into the gastrointestinal tract delineates structures that would otherwise be roentgenographically invisible. Similarly, a variety of iodinated compounds may be ingested by individuals or injected into their bloodstream to facilitate the radiographic demonstration of kidneys, gallbladders, and other structures. Such agents can be injected into joint cavities to outline the integrity of a capsule or a meniscus (Figure 4-1), and they may be injected into the opening of a fistula or a duct (Figure 4-2) to demonstrate the pathway and architectural characteristics of a pathologic or physiologic structure.

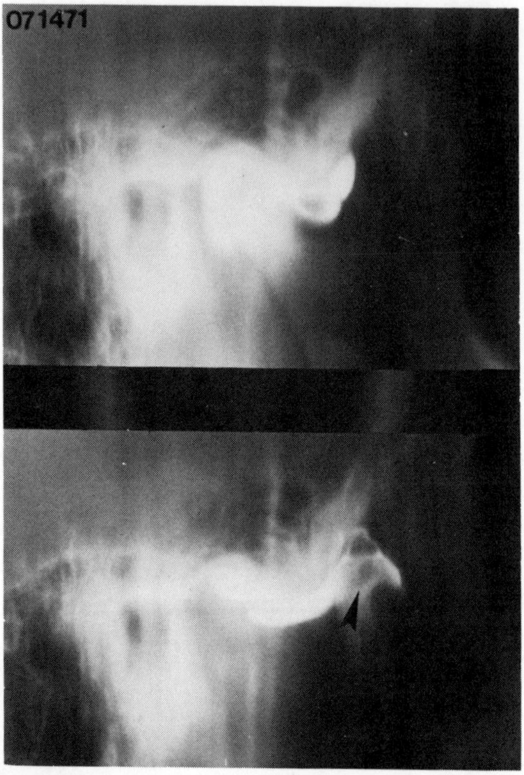

A

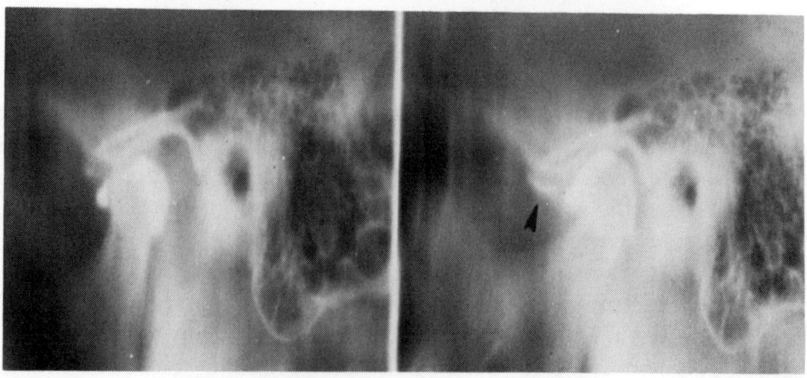

B

Figure 4-1 **A.** Injection of a contrast agent into the upper and lower compartments of the temporomandibular joint allows visualization of a displaced disc. In the top figure, with the mouth closed, the disc is seen to lie anterior to the condyle. In the lower figure, with the mouth open, the disc is seen above the condylar head. A lucent defect in the condyle is denoted by the arrow. **B.** Filling of the lower compartment only. A loss of integrity of the lining of the lower compartment is denoted by the leakage of dye indicated by the arrow.

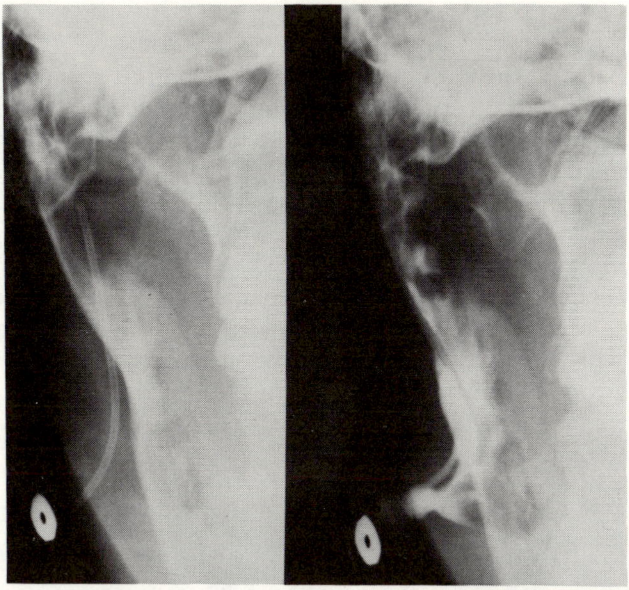

A

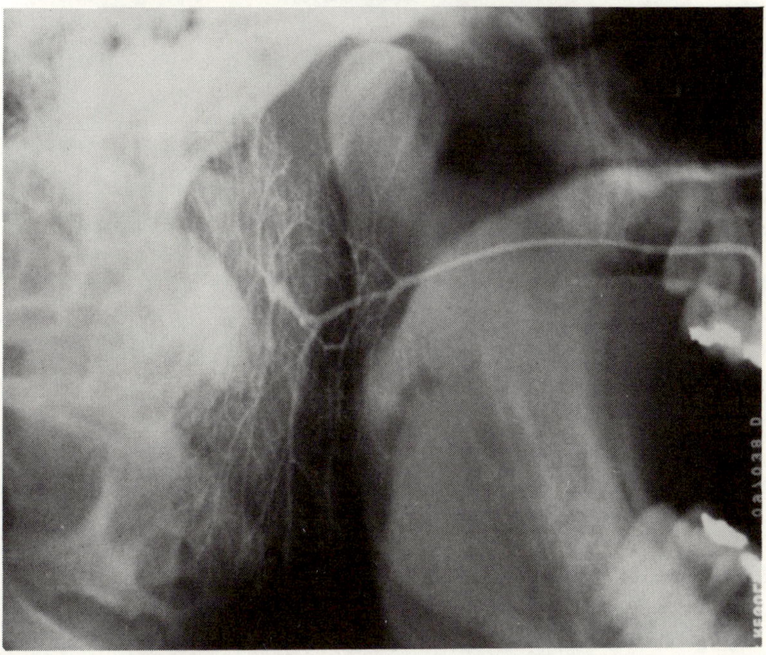

B

Figure 4-2 **A.** Following a mandibular resection, this patient developed a draining fistula. Passage of an opaque tube identified the direction of the fistulous tract, but only the injection of an opaque material defined the nature of the soft tissue defect. **B.** Injection of opaque material through the opening of the parotid duct demonstrated the absence of an obstruction.

USES IN DENTISTRY

In dentistry, the most common use of a contrast agent involves its incorporation into otherwise radiolucent filling materials (Figure 4-3). Although it may be possible to distinguish between a carious lesion and a cavity preparation based on the quality of the hard tissue margins, it is usually impossible to determine radiographically whether or not a cavity preparation has been adequately filled with a plastic or resin material unless that material is opacified.

Less common uses of contrast agents in dentistry include defining periodontal defects with opaque materials,[2] and outlining pulpal morphology with iodinated materials.[3] Additionally, opaque materials such as zircate prophy pastes can be used to outline the floors of gingival pockets, and iodinated compounds are also used to evaluate the salivary glands and temporomandibular joints.

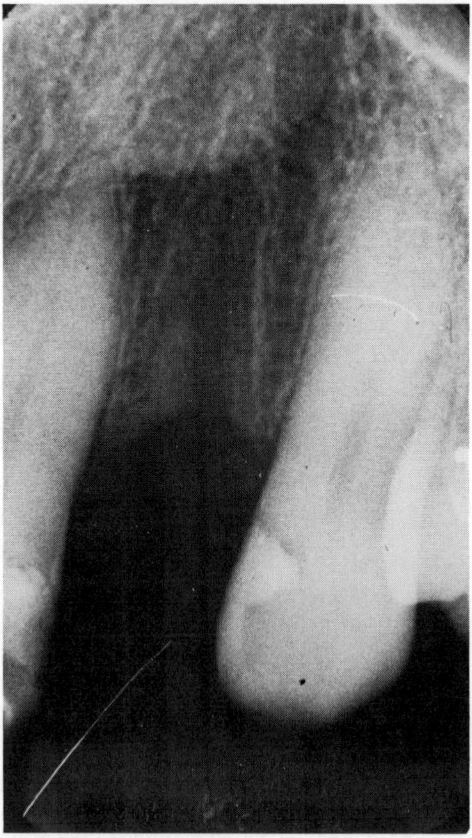

Figure 4-3 The esthetic restoration on the mesial surface of this canine tooth has been opacified by the inclusion of a radiopaque substance.

Restorations

Opaque materials used in restorative preparations have not been well described in the literature, perhaps as the result of proprietary interests. Opaquing compounds used for this purpose are of two types. In some restorative materials, the opaquing substance is evenly distributed (Figure 4-4) while in others it appears as discrete granules (Figure 4-5). It is beyond the scope of this text to comment on the relative advantages of either preparation from the point of view of their adequacy for restorative purposes. However, from a radiographic point of view, it is clear that it is more difficult to evaluate the quality of a restoration filled with a material that is nonuniformly opacified. Since most restorations can be evaluated clinically, this radiographic deficiency may be of little or no clinical consequence.

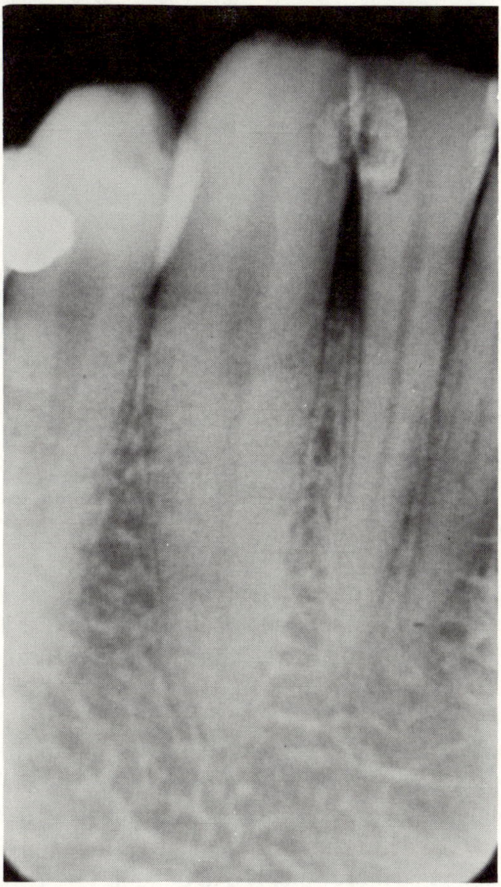

Figure 4-4 Even distribution of the radiopaque additive.

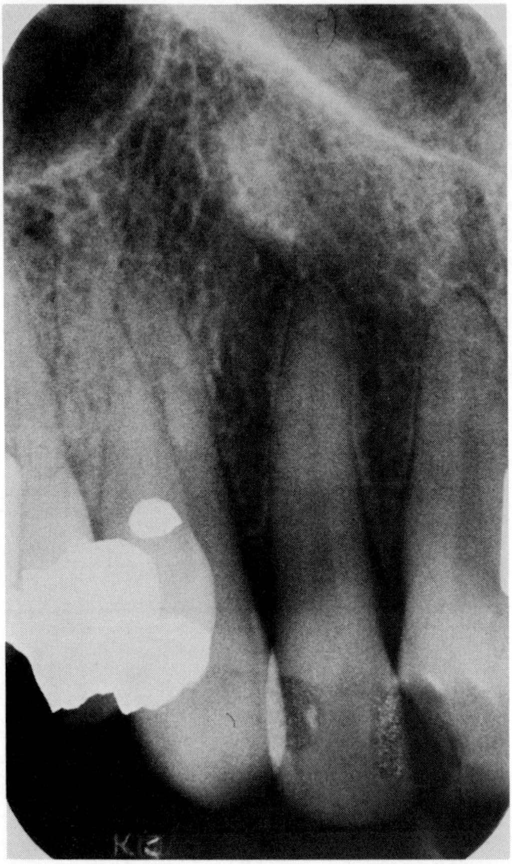

Figure 4-5 Granular and discrete distribution of the radiopaque additive.

Joints and Salivary Glands

Modern contrast agents used for the evaluation of salivary glands and joints are different compounds of iodine that must be evaluated in terms of their toxicity, viscosity, tonicity, and mode of excretion. For the purposes of our discussion, iodinated contrast agents can be divided into two major categories: water soluble, and oily or fat soluble. The water soluble materials are generally intended for intravenous injection while fat soluble contrast agents are more commonly used for other purposes.

Water soluble materials are preferred in the examination of joints. They are adequate to define intra-articular structures and have the advantage of being dissipated more quickly and of being less irritating than their oil based counterparts. In general, water soluble contrast agents have less radiographic density than oil based compounds and therefore produce less contrast on the final radiographic image. For that reason, oil based compounds are often preferred for the study of salivary glands where retention of the contrast agent is less likely to be a problem.

Contrast agents are irritating and may provoke a variety of toxic reactions that can affect virtually all organ systems. For that reason, it is important to assess carefully the physical condition of all patients or candidates for contrast studies and to obtain a careful history of allergies, including prior experiences with iodinated compounds. Furthermore, individuals undertaking contrast studies should have the facilities and the training to deal with emergencies if they should arise. Reviews of contrast agents including their indications, contraindications, and studies of their toxicity are readily available.[4,5]

Periapical Lesions

The use of roentgenographic contrast media as a vehicle for distinguishing among different types of periapical lesions has been studied.[6,7,8] Lilly and colleagues[7] injected 15 different contrast agents into the submaxillary glands of dogs and 0.5 milliliter of each agent subcutaneously into the nipples of the same animals. At autopsy, one to 14 days after injection, salivary glands showed varying degrees of squamous metaplasia or mild sialadenitis characterized by moderate periductal inflammatory infiltrate. Control animals injected with a saline solution showed a mild sialadenitis for three days but were microscopically normal at seven days. In the subcutaneous tissues oil based materials were retained and produced an acute inflammatory reaction while other materials produced a less severe response. Fourteen days after injection there was evidence of chronic granulomatous reactions in animals that had received oily materials whereas there was no trace of tissue reaction with 11 agents that were not retained in the tissues.

Forsberg and Hagglund[6] recognized the difficulty of distinguishing between a cyst and a granuloma on the basis of a conventional radiographic image. These authors also found that puncture of lucent lesions with a small needle occasionally confirmed a diagnosis by demonstrating the typical clear yellowish fluid found in association with a cyst. However, the injection of a radiopaque liquid into an osteolytic lesion through a cleaned root canal proved to be of added diagnostic value.

The differential diagnosis of cyst or granuloma was found to depend upon the filling characteristics of the lesion. Cysts, with preformed cavities, were found to have uniform density and smooth margins.

Granulomas, however, are space-occupying lesions, and the contrast material must be forced into regions of least resistance. As a result, there are irregular boundaries and significant differences in density.

Forsberg and Hagglund also compared the injection of contrast agents through a cleaned root canal and through a tissue puncture. When material was injected through the root canal, it was seen in the periapical region in 23 out of 25 cases. The two lesions that did not show filling with contrast medium proved to be granulomas consisting of dense tissue. The authors concluded that injection was more difficult through tissue even when the lesion proved to be a cyst, although the difficulty in filling the bony defect may have been a function of pressures within the bony cavity.

Cunningham and Penick[8] also injected water soluble contrast agents through prepared root canals into 41 periapical lesions. The resulting roentgenographs were evaluated according to the density and distribution of the contrast medium. Comparison of the roentgenographic pictures with histologic diagnoses failed to demonstrate a clear correlation.

The discrepancy between the findings of these studies is difficult to interpret. On a purely mechanical basis, it is difficult to explain a similar radiographic contrast study resulting from solid- and fluid-filled lesions. However, different contrast agents were used, and one study employed a local anesthetic whereas the second did not. Accordingly, significant differences may have existed in the amount of local vasal constriction, in the forcefulness of the injection, and in the solubility of the injected material. Additional control studies may be of significant value.

REFERENCES

1. Etter, L.E. *Glossary of Words and Phrases Used in Radiology, Nuclear Medicine, and Ultrasound.* 2nd Ed. Springfield, Ill.: Charles C Thomas, 1970.
2. Brown, S.I., and Owings, J.R. A reproducible method for evaluating radiographic changes in periodontal defects. *J Periodont Res.* 8:389–394, 1973.
3. Hasselgren, G., and Stromberg, T. The use of iodine as a contrast medium in endodontic therapy. *Oral Surg.* 41:785–788, 1976.
4. Medical Economics Company. *Physicians' Desk Reference For Radiology and Nuclear Medicine.* Oradell, N.J.: Medical Economics Company, 1975/6.
5. Aspelin, P., and Almen, T. Studies of the acute toxicity of ionic and nonionic contrast media following rapid intravenous injection. *Invest Radiol.* 11:309–314, 1976.
6. Forsberg, A., and Hagglund, G. Differential diagnosis of radicular cysts and granuloma: use of x-ray contrast medium. *Radiogr Photogr.* 33:84–88, 1969.
7. Lilly, G.E., Cutcher, J.L., and Steiner, M. Radiopaque contrast mediums: effect on dog salivary gland and subcutaneous tissues. *J Oral Surg.* 26:94–98, 1968.
8. Cunningham, C.J., and Penick, E.C. Use of a roentgenographic contrast medium in the differential diagnosis of periapical lesions. *Oral Surg.* 26:96–102, 1968.

5 Xeroradiography

Xeroradiography, described extensively in a review by Boag,[1] has been widely used in mammography and other studies that involve body parts with relatively low subject contrast.[2,3] Several features make it an attractive imaging system in specific diagnostic situations. These features include pronounced edge enhancement, high contrast, a choice of positive and negative displays, good detail, and wide latitude. In addition, xeroradiography does not require silver-halide containing films such as those used for intraoral and extraoral radiographic procedures.[4]

PROCESS OF XERORADIOGRAPHY

Conventional x-ray sources are used in the production of xeroradiographs. The film, however, is replaced by a selenium-coated photoreceptor (Xerox plate), which has a uniformly distributed electrostatic charge. The charge is applied by a conditioner that also inserts the charged plate into a light-tight cassette (Figure 5-1). During an

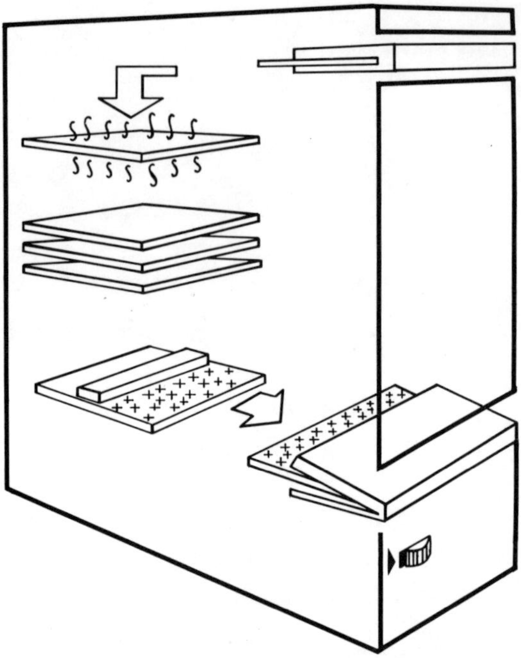

Figure 5-1 Diagrammatic representation of a Xerox conditioner, illustrating how a selenium coated plate is processed prior to exposure. The plate is removed from its cassette and subjected to a process called relaxation, which eliminates old images and artifacts from the surface. Plates are then electrostatically charged and inserted into a cassette at the exit port. A dial allows the operator to adjust contrast by modifying the electrostatic charge.

exposure, x-rays that penetrate a body part or object are absorbed by the surface of the selenium plate causing selective discharging (Figure 5-2A). The distribution and the amount of discharge is related to the distribution and amount of radiation striking the Xerox plate and, therefore, the information in the transmitted x-ray beam is left as a charge pattern on the plate. This pattern of electrical charge, the latent image, is analogous to the latent image produced by the reduction of silver bromide molecules to free silver atoms in the sensitivity specks of a photographic emulsion.

The greatest amount of charge remains beneath the thickest part of the object where most radiation was absorbed (Figure 5-2B). In areas where less absorption occurred, the penetrating radiation dissipates a greater amount of charge from the selenium surface. At the interfaces between areas of greater and lesser absorption, the electrostatic forces are distorted (Figure 5-2C). The resulting electric fields (Figure 5-2D) produce the same effect as the production of mach bands which occur at the boundaries of objects with different densities because of a phenomenon called lateral extinction which occurs in the retina.

The latent image is developed into a visible image. During development a cloud of charged powder particles of toner is exposed to the plate, and the powder particles are attracted to the charge pattern on the surface (Figure 5-2E). The association between the toner and the plate is related to

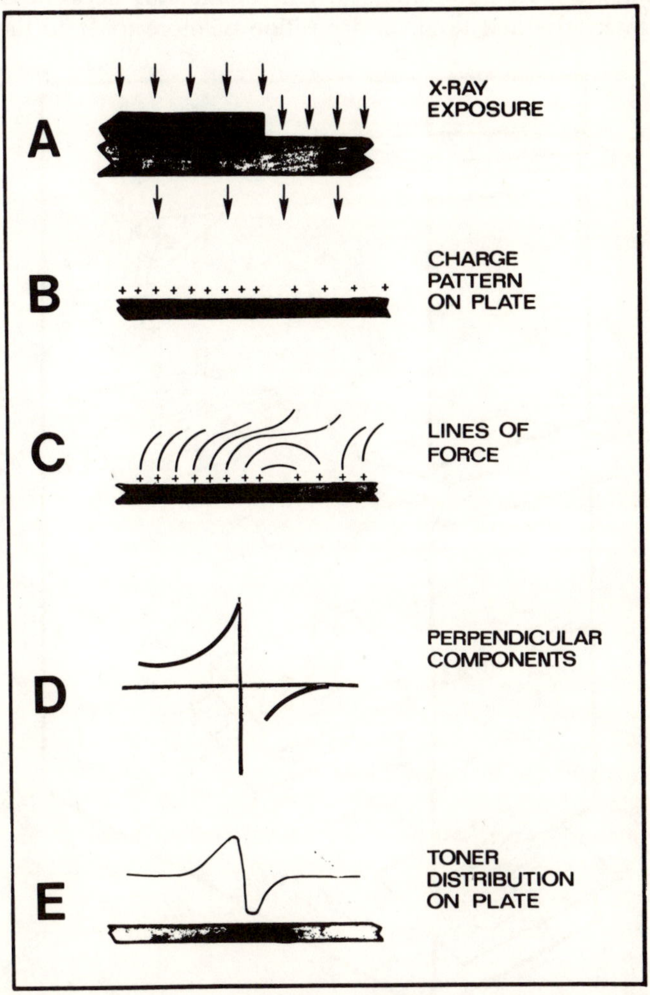

Figure 5-2 **A.** An x-ray beam passing through an object is differentially attenuated according to the absorption characteristics of that object. **B.** The distribution of transmitted x-ray photons alters the charge pattern on a Xerox plate. **C.** Lines of force are produced as the result of the difference in charge densities on the plate surface. **D.** These lines of force have perpendicular components. **E.** These components affect the distribution of toner particles on the plate.

the distribution of charge. When development is complete, the visible image is transferred to paper in a machine referred to as a developer (Figure 5-3).

The electric fields present during development result partly from the voltage applied to the back of the plate for the purpose of delivering toner particles and partly from the differences in charge distribution in the latent image. Nonuniformities exist at boundaries between different charge intensities and result in deposition of more toner to the higher

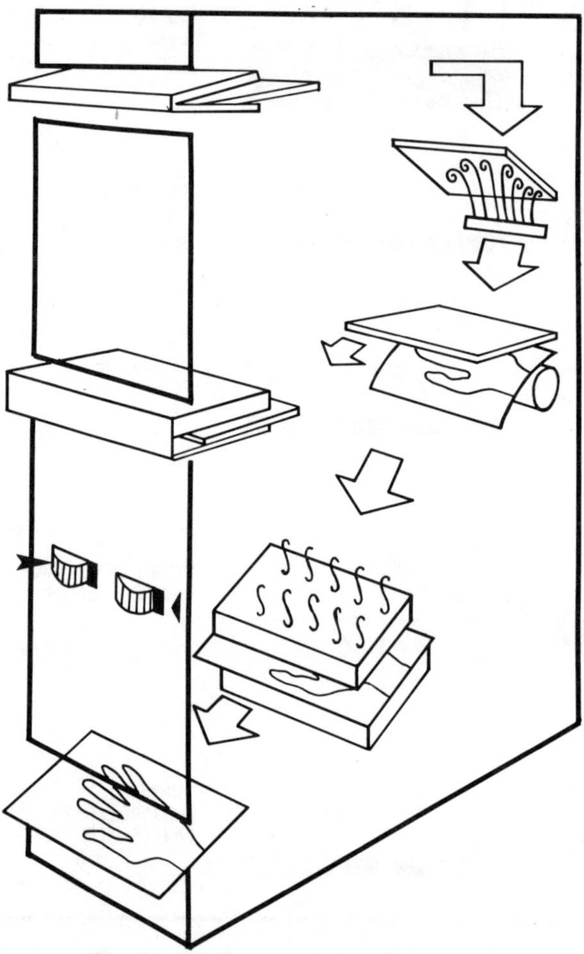

Figure 5-3 The conventional xeroradiographic processor has two controls. The knob indicated by the long arrow allows the operator to select a positive or negative printing mode. The control indicated by the short arrow permits some adjustment in the final density of the image. The exposed plate with its latent image is coated with toner particles. The image is transferred and then permanently fused to paper. The processing cycle requires approximately 90 seconds.

charged side of the boundary and less toner to the lower charged side (Figure 5-4). In the resulting image, the boundaries or edges are enhanced (Figure 5-5).

When a positive voltage is applied to the back of the Xerox plate during development, negative toner particles are attracted to the surface. In this mode, highly charged areas corresponding to the thickest or most dense parts of the body receive more toner than the discharged areas

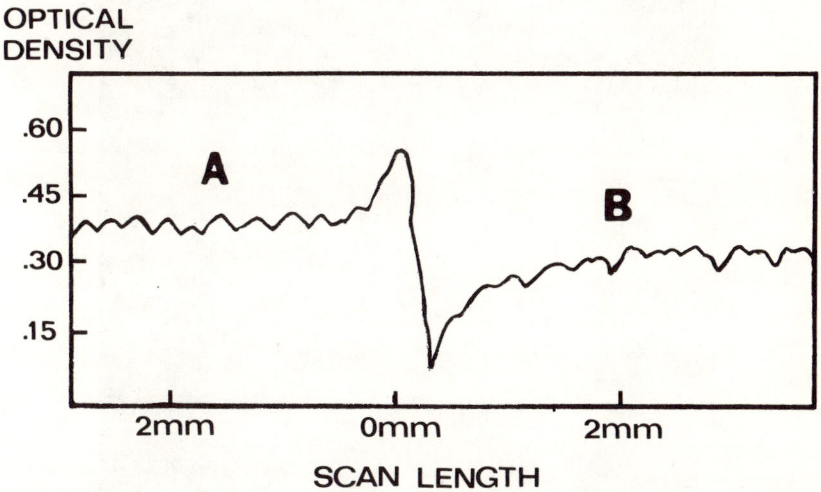

Figure 5-4 An optical density tracing of a xeroradiographic image of paired objects with slightly different densities. Although the optical densities are similar, distortion of electrical fields at their interface alters the distribution of toner to accentuate the boundary.

Figure 5-5 The actual appearance of xeroradiographs described in Figure 5-4. If the interface between the two objects is covered, the density of A and B appear uniform.

covered by thin or low density body parts. This results in a positive image in which the darkest areas of the image correspond to the most dense parts of the anatomy (Figure 5-6).

Negative images can be produced by the application of a negative voltage to the back of the plate, which attracts positive toner particles to the surface. Positively charged particles are preferentially attracted to the

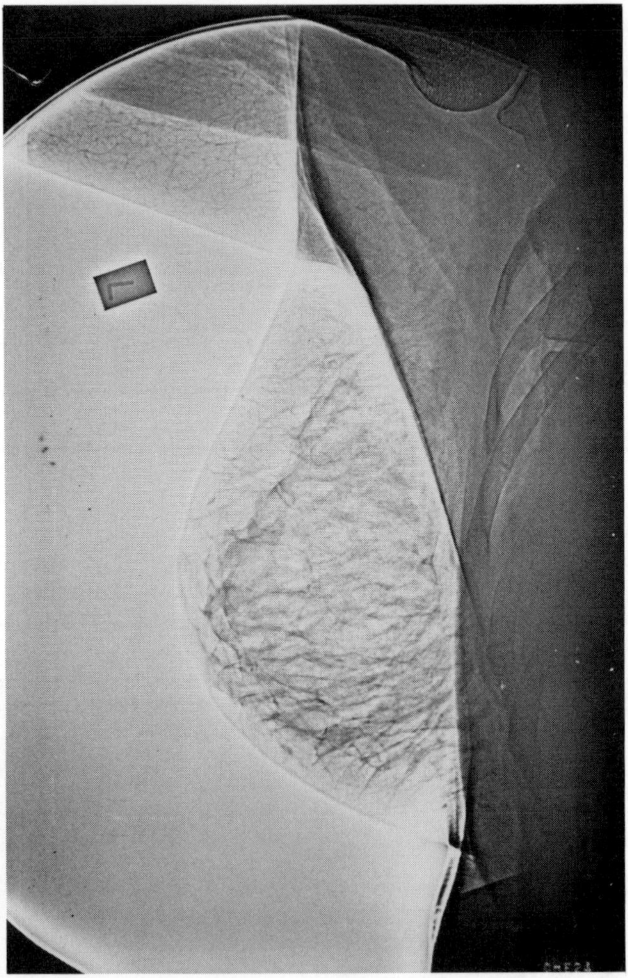

Figure 5-6 In this mammogram, the most dense tissues are dark and the least dense tissues are light. Alternating light and dark bands along the skin surface show the effect of edge enhancement.

discharged parts of the plate, which correspond to the least dense parts of the body. In the final image, dense objects appear white or radiopaque, and less dense objects appear dark or radiolucent (Figure 5-7).

In contrast to conventional films that are viewed with transmitted light, xeroradiographs can be viewed with either reflected or transmitted light. When the latent image is transferred from the plate to paper, the original image is reversed 180 degrees and is seen as a mirror image.

Xeroradiographs have inherently wide latitude; that is, it is possible to image objects having a broad range of densities in a single exposure. The cephalometric radiograph shown in Figure 5-7 demonstrates this wide latitude by showing teeth, bones, and soft tissues in one picture. Wide latitude also means that acceptable images are possible over a relatively

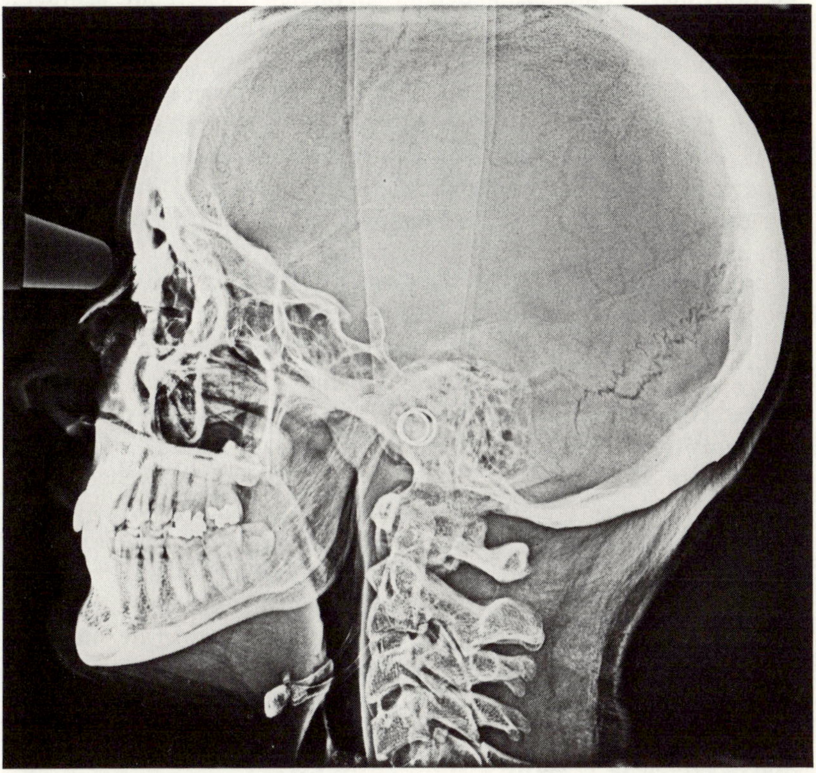

Figure 5-7 In this cephalometric image, the most dense structures are light and the least dense structures are dark. The visibility of both soft tissue and bony structures in a single radiograph illustrates the wide latitude of the xeroradiographic process.

broad range of exposure conditions. This is an obvious advantage because the number of exposures that have to be repeated because of technical inadequacies can be dramatically reduced.

USES OF XERORADIOGRAPHY

In addition to its use in mammography, xeroradiography has also been used for cephalometric analysis,[5,6,7] for the evaluation of bone lesions of the mandible,[8] for sialography,[3] and for study of a variety of dental and nondental structures.[2,9,10]

Xeroradiography is of particular interest in tomography of the temporomandibular joints. A thin-section tomogram is shown in Figure 5-8. Bony margins are seen in detail even though tomographic artifact is imaged as sharply as real anatomic structures. The use of xeroradiographs for recording tomographic images has been studied by Helander and colleagues[11] who recommended special patterns of movement to minimize artifact. Other studies by Castrup and Schutz[12] compared several aspects of image quality in conventional tomography and xeroradiography. They found no difference in resolution in xeroradiographic and film recordings of linear or elliptical thin-section tomograms. Low density borders were more clearly demonstrated in the xeroradiographs even when boundaries or structures lay outside of the focal plane. It was concluded that xeroradiographic representations of structures helps to offset the loss of contrast and definition that often occurs in body section procedures.

The diagnostic value of xeroradiographic images of dental structures has been evaluated by several investigators.[4,9,10,13,14,15] Initial studies used the original Xerox system, which was designed for mammographic and other extraoral examinations. The high contrast and edge enhancement properties of the xeroradiograph appeared to produce artifacts around the margins of metallic restorations. The ability to recognize recurrent decay was reduced compared to conventional radiographs. However, a modified xeroradiographic processing system was designed specifically for dental examinations. The new system uses plates that are similar in size to number one and number two dental films. The contrast is greater than that obtained with conventional films but less than that seen with the original xeroradiographic system. Edge enhancement is also slightly reduced compared to earlier Xerox systems.

Initial studies indicated that fine detail of tooth structure was seen with greater clarity and definition than on conventional films. The same is true of other structures, including trabecular bone, periodontal ligament, and lamina dura.

Intraoral imaging with xeroradiography requires significantly smaller exposures than are necessary with conventional film systems. Gratt and colleagues[13] estimate an exposure level 7 to 14 times lower with

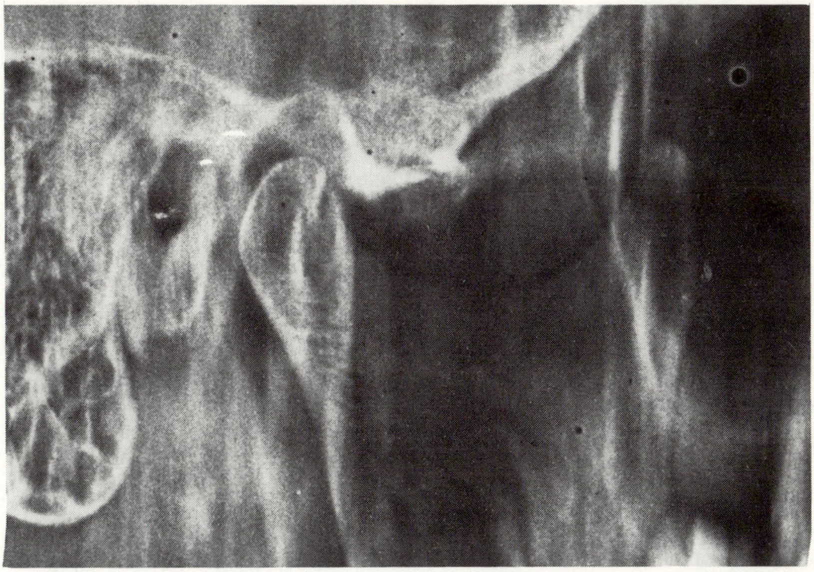

A

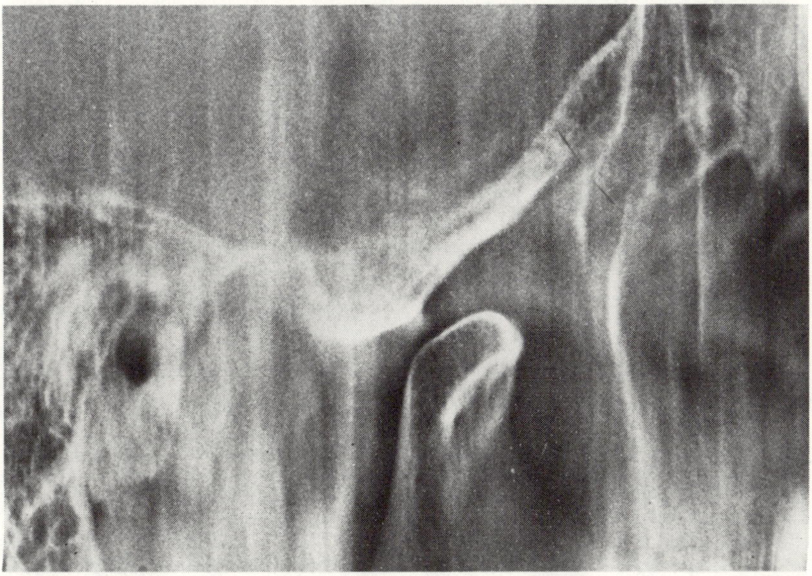

B

Figure 5-8 **A.** A thin-section tomogram of a temporomandibular joint in the closed position. A discontinuity is noted at the anterior surface of the condyle. **B.** This thin-section xerotomogram shows the same joint with mouth in an open position. The condyle is outside of the fossa and slightly rotated.

xeroradiography than with conventional film radiography. Figure 5-9 illustrates xeroradiographic and conventional images of the same anatomic site in a single patient.

The resolution of xeroradiographs has been compared with that of occlusal and screen films by Thunty.[15] His study indicates that xeroradiographs have a maximum measurable resolution of ten line pairs per millimeter (independent of kilovoltage). Resolution on xeroradiographic plates is also independent of milliamperes. The resolution of xeroradiographs is comparable in the positive and negative display modes. Occlusal films are comparable in resolution to xeroradiographs except at low tube currents where the resulting images lack sufficient density. Screen films have less resolving power than either xeroradiographs or occlusal films, but the screen films also require less exposure than either of the other imaging systems.

Nortje and colleagues[8] compared the xeroradiographic image of a simple bone cyst with the image of that lesion on a conventional film. The lesion was clearly demonstrated by both techniques, although the details of bony structure appeared to be most clearly demonstrated by xeroradiography. Hurst and colleagues[7] demonstrated the accuracy of landmark identification in cephalometric studies recorded xeroradiographically. They concluded that Point A, the upper incisal tip, infradentale, and menton, were more accurately visualized on xeroradiographs while Point B and condylion were more accurately seen on conventional cephalograms. Although cephalometric xeroradiograms appear to be superior in many respects, further study is indicated. It must also be recognized that greater exposures are required for the production of xeroradiographic cephalograms.

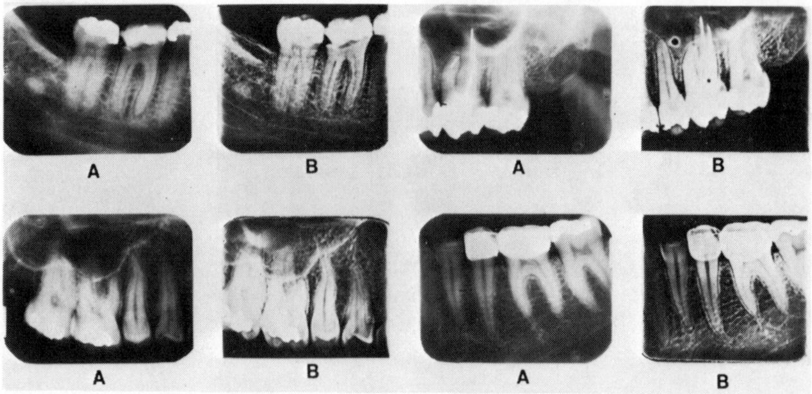

Figure 5-9 Similar radiographic and xeroradiographic views. **A.** Conventional radiographs. **B.** Xeroradiographs. (Images courtesy of Dr. Stuart White, University of California, Los Angeles, and The Xerox Corporation.)

SUMMARY

Xeroradiography appears to have many advantages as an intraoral image receptor in dentistry. These include fine detail, wide latitude, high image contrast, and relatively low exposure requirements. It is also clear that xeroradiographic images may be important as supplements to conventional extraoral examinations, including studies of salivary glands and soft tissues. The value of xeroradiographs in dealing with soft tissue lesions is well documented.

REFERENCES

1. Boag, J.W. Xeroradiography. *Phys Med Biol.* 18:3–37, 1973.

2. Wolfe, J.N. Xeroradiography of the bones, joints, and soft tissues. *Radiology* 93:583–587, 1969.

3. Ferguson, M.M., Davison, A., and Mason, W.N. Application of xeroradiography in sialography. *Int J Oral Surg.* 5:176–179, 1976.

4. Binnie, W.H., Stacey, A.J., Davis, R. et al. Applications of xeroradiography in dentistry. *J Dent.* 3:99–104, 1975.

5. Davis, R., Binnie, W.H., Cawson, R.A. et al. The role of xeroradiography in cephalometric radiology. *J Dent.* 5:32–38, 1977.

6. Johnson, N.A. Xeroradiography for cephalometric analysis. *Am J Orthod.* 69:524–526, 1976.

7. Hurst, R.V.V., Schwannger, B., Shaye, R. et al. Landmark identification accuracy in xeroradiographic cephalometry. *Am J Orthod.* 73:568–574, 1978.

8. Nortje, C.J., Farman, A.G., and de V. Joubert, J.J. The xeroradiographic appearance of simple bone cyst of the mandible. *Oral Surg.* 45:485–487, 1978.

9. Gratt, B.M., Sickles, E.A., and Parks, C.P. Xeroradiography of dental structures. I. Preliminary investigations. *Oral Surg.* 44:148–152, 1977.

10. Snyder, M.B., Stacey, A.J., Davis, R. et al. The advantages of xeroradiography for panoramic examination of the jaws and teeth. *J Periodontol.* 48:467–472, 1977.

11. Helander, C.G., Reichmann, S., and Astrand, K. Xerographic tomography. *Acta Radiol. (Diagn.)* 18:368–382, 1977.

12. Castrup, W., and Schutz, J. Experimental investigations in xeroradiotomography. Edited by L. Oliva and R.J. Berry. In *The New Image in Tomography.* Proceedings of the Symposium Actualitatis Tomographie, Genoa, Italy, 1975. Amsterdam—Oxford: Excerpta Medica, 1976.

13. Gratt, B.M., Sickles, E.A., and Parks, C.R. Xeroradiography of dental structures. II. Image analysis. *Oral Surg.* 46:156–165, 1978.

14. Rawls, R.H., and Owen, D.W. The dental prognosis for xeroradiography. *Oral Surg.* 33:476–480, 1972.

15. Thunty, K.H. Comparison of xeroradiographs with occlusal and screen films. *Oral Surg.* 45:959–964, 1978.

6 Principles of Tomography

The most commonly used radiographs present images that show all objects between the source and the film superimposed (Figure 6-1). The clarity of a radiographic finding depends upon both its visibility (separation from other structures) and the degree to which its density differs from that of surrounding objects. In the diagnosis of caries, periodontal disease, and common forms of periapical pathology, conventional radiographs provide adequate information. In these instances, overlap can be avoided by simple technical maneuvers. Some studies even suggest that periapical radiographs may contain more information than is necessary for routine diagnostic tasks.[1] In some situations, however, superimposition interferes with a clear discernment of the object of interest. In these instances, tomography can be used to eliminate undesirable overlap. Tomographic methods can be divided into two major categories, conventional tomography and computed tomography.

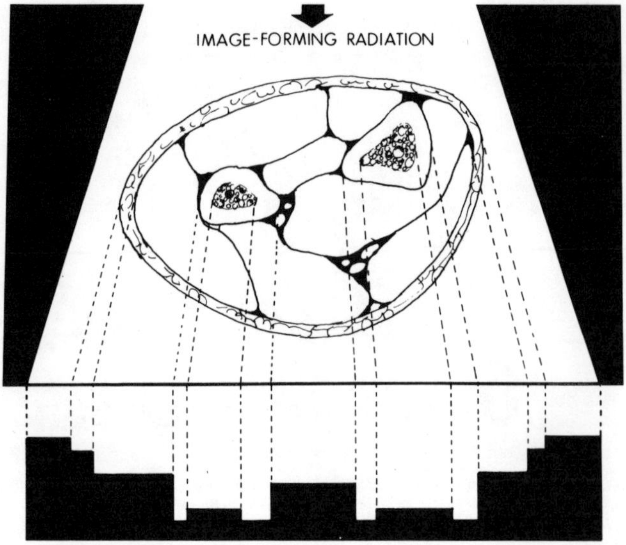

Figure 6-1 Schematic representation of x-ray image formation. It is clear that the density on the film represents the sum total of the absorbers placed between the x-ray source and the film.

CONVENTIONAL TOMOGRAPHY

Tomography or body section radiography produces an image of a layer within a body while images of structures above and below that layer are made invisible by blurring. Mayer, a Polish radiologist, may have been the first to clinically use tomography. Major contributions were also made by Alessandro, Vallebona, Ziedsesdesplantes, and Grossmann. In the United States, Kieffer, an x-ray technician, devised a method for body section radiography of the chest. In 1939 Heckman proposed a method of obtaining an image of a curved plane. Subsequently, Paatero[2] developed a prototype of today's modern panoramic machines.

Sharp photographic images of a moving object require very short exposures (fast films and lenses) or moving the camera at the same speed and in the same path as the object of interest. In the first case, all objects in front of the lens are sharply defined. In the latter case, only the moving object is sharply pictured; everything between the lens and the subject as well as everything beyond the subject is blurred.

In photography, images are produced by incident or reflected light, and the subject of interest can be blocked by objects interposed between the lens and the subject. In x-ray tomography images arise from the differential transmission of x-rays through objects of different densities; and objects between the source and the plane of interest can be penetrated by x-rays of appropriate energy.

The fundamental principle of tomography is illustrated in Figure 6-2. Blurring, or the degradation of images of structures outside of the plane of interest, is accomplished by simultaneous movement of the x-ray tube and the film during the exposure. The tube and the film are connected so that movement occurs around a point or fulcrum. As the distance between the fulcrum and any object increases, the amount by which that object is displaced on the film also increases. To put it another way, as the distance from the point of rotation increases, the amount of image blurring also increases, so that objects closest to the point of rotation are seen most sharply and objects farthest away from the point of rotation are most completely blurred.

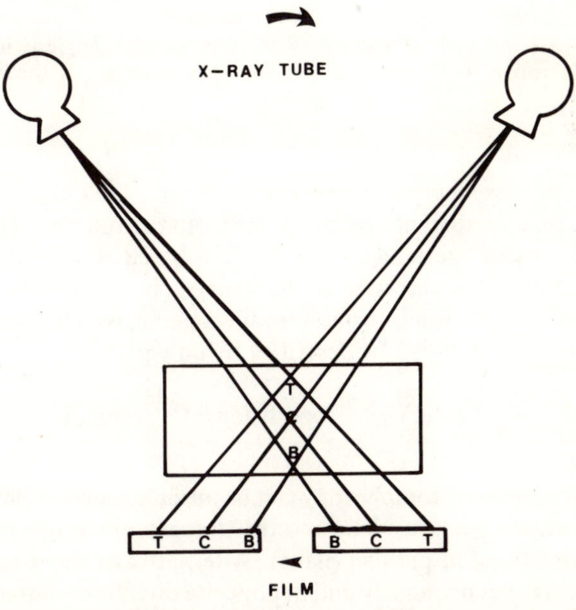

Figure 6-2 The x-ray tube and the film are rotated about a fulcrum (C) during an exposure. When the exposure is initiated, objects at the top of the body being examined (T) are on the right side of the film while objects in the center of the body (C) lie in the center of the film and objects at the bottom of the body (B) lie at the left side of the film. During exposure, the positions of B and T reverse while the position of C remains constant.

The size of the image layer depends on the angle of rotation or the amount of movement. When the path of movement is short and the angle is small, the image layer is relatively thick. As the angle or path of movement increases, the image layer decreases (Figure 6-3). It is important to know, however, that some image degradation or blurring occurs within the image layer in all tomography. The greatest amount of blurring is at the periphery of the image layer, and the sharpest image is at its center.

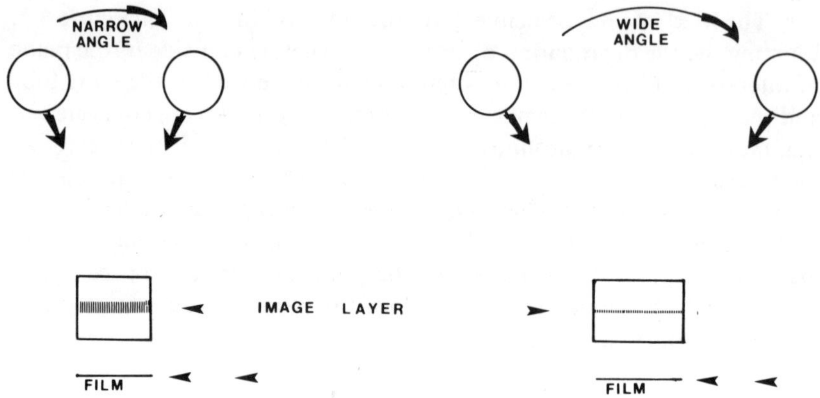

Figure 6-3 As the path of motion or the tomographic angle is increased, the effect of blurring is increased and, therefore, the thickness of the image layer is reduced.

Overall sharpness depends upon many factors, including the angle of movement and the distance of any point from the fulcrum. Definition of the dimensions of the image layer is often based on an allowable blur fringe of 0.5 mm. The thickness of the layer can be described as double the distance between the fulcrum and the object plane, which has a blur of 0.5 mm. The relationship can be described by an equation:

$$\text{B (blur)} = \frac{2\pi}{360} \times \text{(distance)} \times \text{(angle)}$$

The principles of tomography can be mechanically implemented in a variety of ways. The x-ray tube and the film can move synchronously in opposite directions in parallel planes. Alternatively, the x-ray tube and film can move synchronously and in opposite directions in parallel planes but with motions other than straight lines. Circular, cross, spiral, hypocycloidal, trispiral, and other multidirectional movements have been used. It is also possible to have the x-ray tube move in arcs rather than in flat planes or the tube can move in an arc while the film moves in a plane. Common types of tomographic movements are shown in Figure 6-4.

Since x-ray images are the result of an x-ray beam striking materials of different densities or thicknesses, it follows that an x-ray beam striking a density boundary or edge of an object at one point or tangent during a tomographic exposure will produce an image of that object regardless of whether or not it lies close to the point of rotation (law of tangents). Therefore, the blurring of objects outside of a focal plane is accomplished most effectively by compound movements of the x-ray tube and least effectively by simple movements. The choice of tomographic mode and

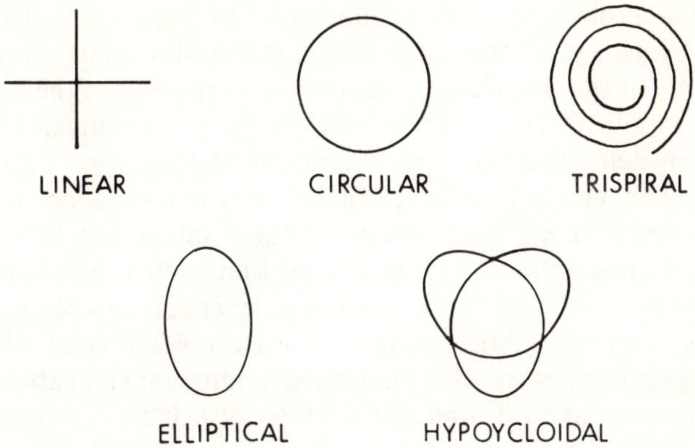

Figure 6-4 Common kinds of tomographic movements. The more complex the motion the smaller the likelihood that the x-ray beam will strike an object of importance at the same tangent through an entire exposure. Therefore, blurring will be less dependent upon the orientation of the object under study.

angle should be determined by the specific diagnostic task and the anatomic site under investigation.

In addition to the choices of simple or compound movements, there are essentially two basic design options used in most units. In one option, the image layer or plane of focus is changed by adjusting the point of rotation, the fulcrum. This is called an adjustable fulcrum system. It has the disadvantage of producing images with different amounts of magnification, depending upon the relative position of the fulcrum between the tube and film.

Alternatively, the film and the x-ray tube can be made to pass in opposite directions through proportional arcs. The distances between the fulcrum and the tube and the fulcrum and the film remain constant. In devices using this principle the object of interest is positioned with reference to the focal plane and all images contain the same degree of magnification.

CURVED SURFACE TOMOGRAPHY (PAN TOMOGRAPHY)

If an apparatus designed to perform linear tomography were rotated around a curved object, it would produce a curved image layer. Using a single point of rotation, the image layer would represent a portion of the circumference of a circle. This assumes, however, that the film is circular or rotated so that the point of film exposure from beginning to end would describe a circle. In panoramic radiography (linear tomography along a curved surface), the x-ray beam is reduced to a narrow slit with collimators at the x-ray source and in front of the x-ray film. The simplest form of panoramic procedure is illustrated in Figure 6-5. The object remains stationary while the x-ray tube and the film rotate around it. It should be noted that the film is also moving in relation to the x-ray tube during the exposure. The distances between the x-ray source, the object, and the film determine the relative amount of magnification, and the position of the center of rotation defines the object layer which is imaged.

The layer with the most sharply defined image can be varied by changing the paths of the x-ray tube and the film from a circle to an ellipse or other similar geometric form. The image layer can also be changed by altering the numbers and the positions of the centers of rotation that are used during each exposure. It is these latter points, that is, path of movement and number and position of the center or centers of rotation, that determine the major differences between different panoramic machines.

The thickness of the image layer is defined by the angle of rotation described during an exposure. Stated another way, the thickness of the image layer is defined by the ratio of film speed to x-ray tube speed. Since the distance traversed by the film remains constant in most simple tomographic systems, increasing the angle of tube travel decreases the ratio of film speed to tube speed and therefore decreases the thickness of the image layer. In panoramic radiography, the relative speeds at which the tube and the film move are often varied to compensate for anatomic variability or to allow for greater or lesser penetration of the x-ray beam. As a result, the thickness of the image layer also varies. Figure 6-6 shows the relative thicknesses and configurations of the image layer produced by three different panoramic machines.

It is important to keep several points in mind. First, since the image layer of a given machine has predetermined boundaries, these boundaries must accommodate the entire range of sizes encountered within a patient

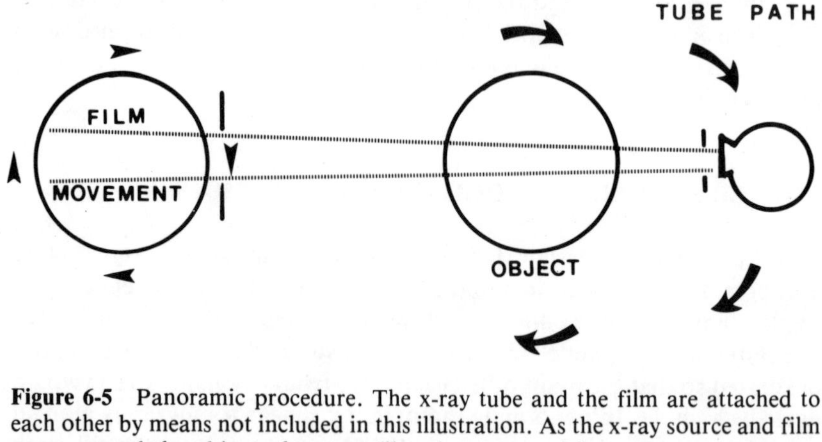

Figure 6-5 Panoramic procedure. The x-ray tube and the film are attached to each other by means not included in this illustration. As the x-ray source and film move around the object, the x-ray film also moves with respect to the source, thereby producing an image layer.

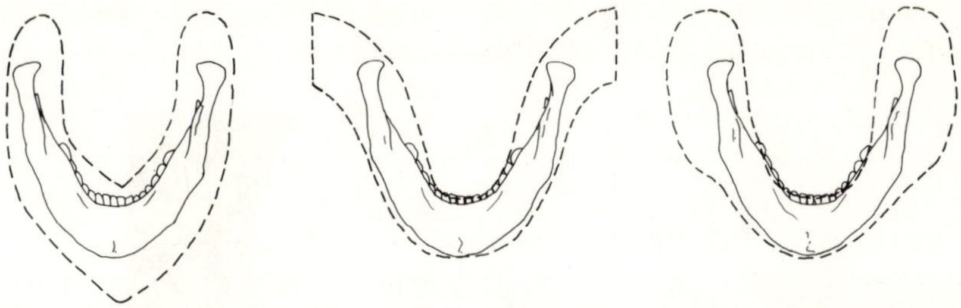

Figure 6-6 The thickness and configuration of the image layer is affected primarily by the number of centers of rotation and the speed of film movement during rotation of the entire apparatus.

population. Lund and Manson-Hing[3] have evaluated the ability of several units to accommodate patients of different sizes and ages. Second, Freedman and Matteson[4] have shown that the quality of the image deteriorates rapidly as one moves from the center of focus outward. Therefore, small errors in patient placement produce substantial loss of image quality and may account for several types of image artifacts. Third, because the tomographic movement is linear in nature, structures that lie in a horizontal plane are blurred less effectively than objects that are vertically oriented. Finally, all of the factors that affect image quality in conventional systems also affect tomography. The introduction of motion and the use of intensifying screens account for a comparatively large loss in overall image quality.

Panoramic Artifacts

Spurious images or artifacts are hazards of any imaging system. As the complexity of the system increases, the possible number and kinds of artifacts also increase. The problem of artifacts in panoramic images has been reported and studied by many individuals.[5–16] Many kinds of artifacts are predictable, based on the characteristics of panoramic systems, and the recognition of their existence can mitigate against misinterpretation.

First, as previously noted, the substitution of a relatively high speed film-screen combination for the more common nonscreen dental film results in a substantial loss in resolution.[17] As a result, the capacity to detect small structures or defects is reduced. Without compensation for this loss of detail, it is unlikely that incipient carious lesions, early periodontal defects, or small periapical lesions will be recognized as often as in conventional intraoral radiographs.

Second, the law of tangents, which applies to all radiographic procedures, enhances the clarity of horizontally placed objects and diminishes that of vertically oriented structures unless they lie close to the center of the image layer (focal trough) (Figure 6-7).

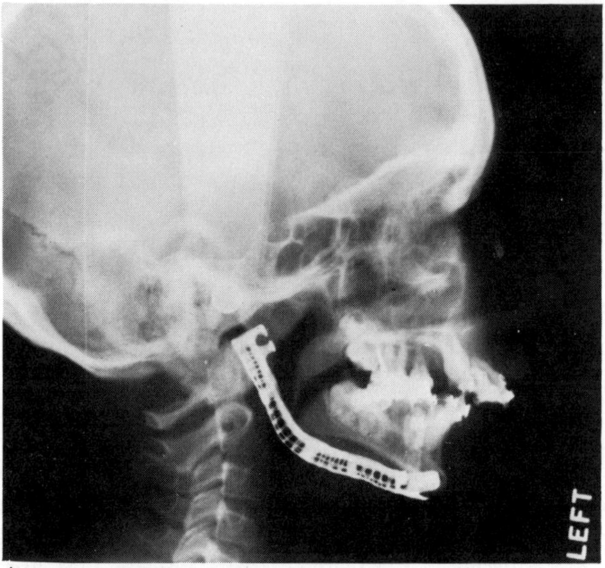

A

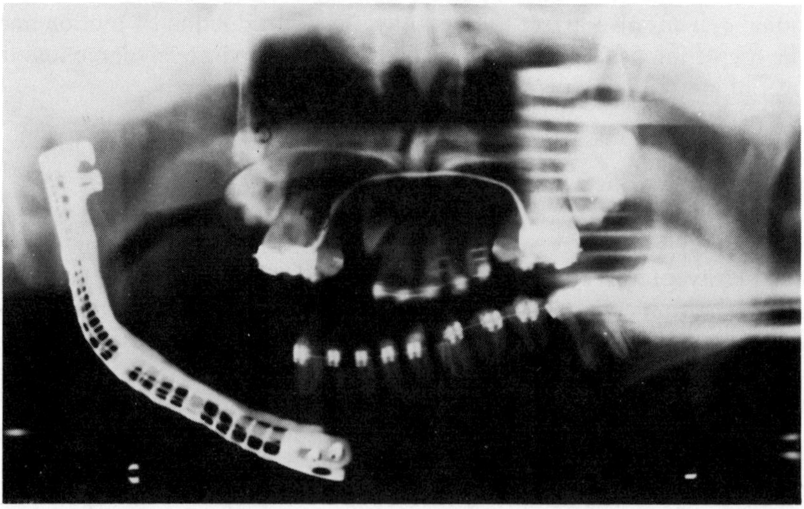

B

Figure 6-7 **A.** A wire mesh implant is shown in a lateral cephalometric view after placement for reconstruction of a surgically resected right ramus and body. **B.** A panoramic film taken at the same time shows the horizontal components of the wire mesh on the opposite side of the patient. Since the x-ray beam struck the edge of these horizontal components (law of tangents) during the entire exposure, they are not blurred.

Third, to minimize exposure requirements, the x-ray tube in panoramic machines is given a slight negative vertical inclination. This reduces the need for penetration, but introduces some geometric distortion.

Fourth, the boundaries of the focal trough or image layer are not sharp but increase gradually with increasing distance from the center of the focal trough or point of rotation. As a result, the partially degraded images of objects lying medial or lateral to the jaws may be unpredictably superimposed (Figure 6-8). Normal anatomic curves such as the mandibular and canine fossae may appear as lytic lesions, while vertically angled structures lying at the periphery of the focal trough may be cropped (Figure 6-9).

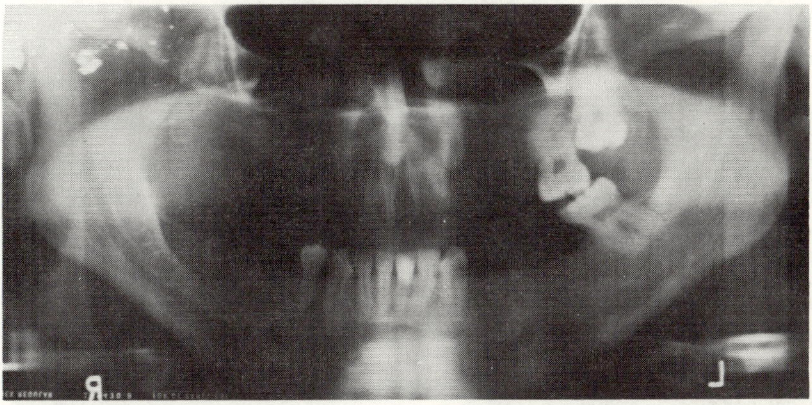

Figure 6-8 Opaque material seen around the mandibular condyle in this panoramic film actually lies within the spinal cord but has been projected during radiographic examination.

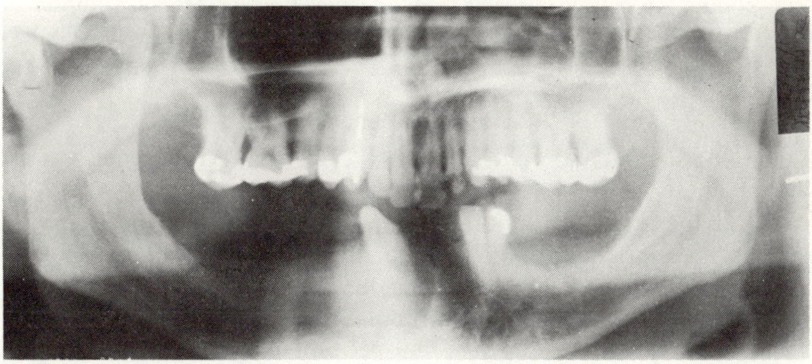

Figure 6-9 Lucent defects in areas of prominent bony curvature are commonplace, as is the amputation of steeply inclined teeth.

Fifth, since the exposure is by scan rather than by composite, motion of the object causes discrete image defects rather than more generalized types of distortions (Figure 6-10).

The recognition of these and other types of artifacts can help to minimize interpretive error. Understanding of the mechanics of panoramic machines can also be useful in defining the most appropriate situations for their use. Some types of artifacts can be overcome by machine modifications, including the use of smaller x-ray sources and magnification to improve detail, better patient positioning devices, and the use of automatic exposure controls.

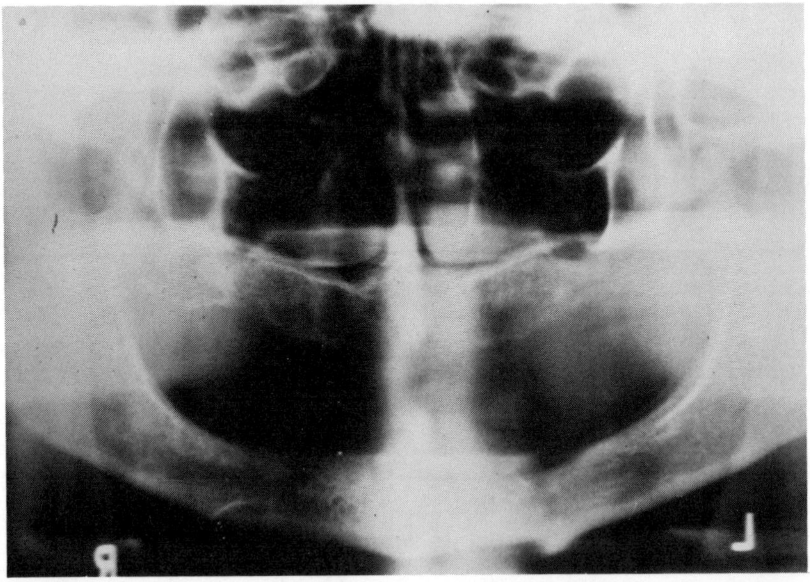

Figure 6-10 This radiograph was produced by slight motion of the patient during the exposure. It is indistinguishable from a genuine fracture. Motion distortion is limited to the particular area being viewed during the interval in which motion occurs.

Panoramic Variants

Until recently, all panoramic units were designed for use with patients in an upright position. Additionally, correct positioning required that the long axis of the patient coincide with the long axis of the stand that supported the x-ray tube and film holder.

In recent years, two devices that permit variations on this requirement have been described in the literature. One unit, the S.S. White Tomorex, resembles conventional panoramic machines, but it is designed for use with the patient in a horizontal position. The primary advantages of the Tomorex are its adaptability to use with unconscious or bedridden patients and a greater flexibility in positioning patients for special examinations of the maxillary sinuses, midface, and temporomandibular joints.

Altonen and colleagues[18] described another unit (the OP-4) developed by Palamex of Helsinki, Finland. Although this panoramic unit is supported on a vertical column, it can be angled through 90 degrees. Accordingly, exposures can be taken with patients in vertical or horizontal positions, and the axis of the tomographic layer can be varied from the vertical axis of the patient. This flexibility permits stereoradiographic images from panoramic examinations by making two exposures of the same patient with a 6 to 7 degree difference in angulation of the central ray. This angle corresponds to the optic axes of an observer standing approximately 6 feet from the films. Initial cadaver studies with the OP-4 confirm the value of stereoscopic views. Furthermore, there appears to be greater flexibility in viewing the middle third of the face and the base of the skull.

COMPUTED TOMOGRAPHY

Conventional and tomographic systems present visual patterns created by specific distributions of silver particles within a photographic emulsion. Images of larger body parts are also commonly obtained in planes running parallel to the long axis of a body. In contrast, computed tomography produces numerical images based on calculations of object density at discrete points across the axis of the object.

Computed tomography was introduced in the 1970s. These systems are often referred to as computed tomography (CT) or computed axial tomography (CAT) scanners.

Computed tomography systems comprise several functional units: an x-ray device that scans the patient, a digital computer, and a device for converting the computed image into a viewable or interpretable format. These systems require magnetic tapes or discs to store data accumulated during examinations and to carry the programs necessary for the computations used in reconstructing an image.

A computed tomographic image is initiated by a process called scanning. Beams from one or several small x-ray sources are passed through the body and intercepted by one or more radiation detectors. These detectors produce electrical impulses that are proportional to the intensity of the x-ray beam emerging from the body. That intensity is determined by several factors: the energy of the x-ray source, the distance between the source and the detector, and, most importantly, the attenuation of the beam by material in the object being scanned. Although a single scan can be produced by one x-ray beam and one detector, the efficiency of the scanning system is greatly increased by using multiple x-ray beams and an equivalent number of detectors. Each scan produces a penetration or absorption profile, and the construction of the image requires profiles obtained at different angles through the subject under study. The x-ray source and detector assembly are rotated around the subject to produce multiple profiles of a particular site (Figure 6-11).

Penetration profiles are stored in the computer, which then calculates the density or absorption at points on a grid formed by the intersections of penetration profiles. The image consists of a raster of individual points or pixels. The size of a pixel is determined by the geometry of the scan, the frequency and spacing of measurements, the number of penetration profiles, and the size of the x-ray source and detector.

Each number or pixel represents a calculation of the actual attenuation of the x-ray beam by materials within the body. The numbers may vary from one machine to another depending upon many factors, such as the energy of the x-ray source. For any particular unit and energy, numbers describing the attenuation of biologic materials with densities lying between hair and bone can be described. Since the numbers represent attenuation or density, the computer constructs an image by printing the numbers or by assigning different degrees of grayness or different colors to each number. A typical image is illustrated in Figure 6-12. In many systems, the numerical values are translated into color or brightness levels that can be displayed on a television screen or printed on paper.

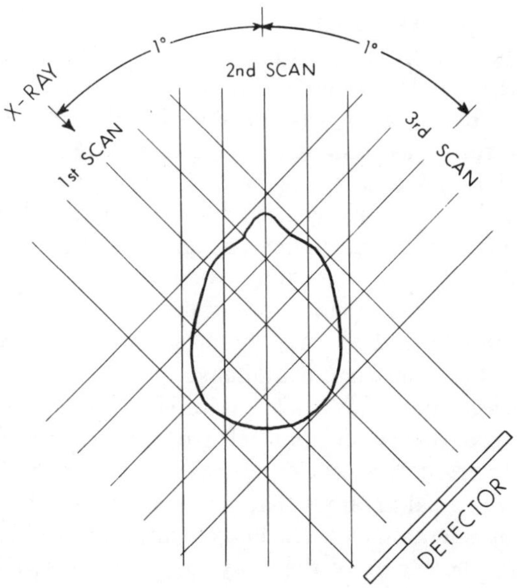

Figure 6-11 The x-ray source may be rotated or moved about an object to produce a pattern of measurement forming a grid.

Since the measurements or pixels that form the image represent discrete subdivisions of space, the effect of blurring is much greater than in conventional radiographic systems. The resolution of the image is, however, also limited by the size represented by a pixel, which is generally greater than the size of silver specks that form the image in conventional radiographs.

Although the detail of a computed tomographic image is not as fine as that obtainable on other radiographs, it has several clear advantages. First, the raster of numbers results in greater geometric precision. Second, the sensitivity of the detector combined with the power of the computer makes it possible to discriminate between objects with small differences in density, such as blood and fat or blood and cerebral spinal fluid. Third, the sensitivity of the detector is so great that a large amount of information can be accumulated with a very small amount of radiation. Figure 6-13 shows a comparison of polytome radiographs and computed tomographic images through the base of the skull of a patient thought to have fibro-osseous disease.

Computed tomography is of particular value in dealing with certain types of pathologies that occur in and around the face. Carter and Karmody[19] summarized their experiences with a number of patients presenting chief complaints related to the head and neck. In the paranasal

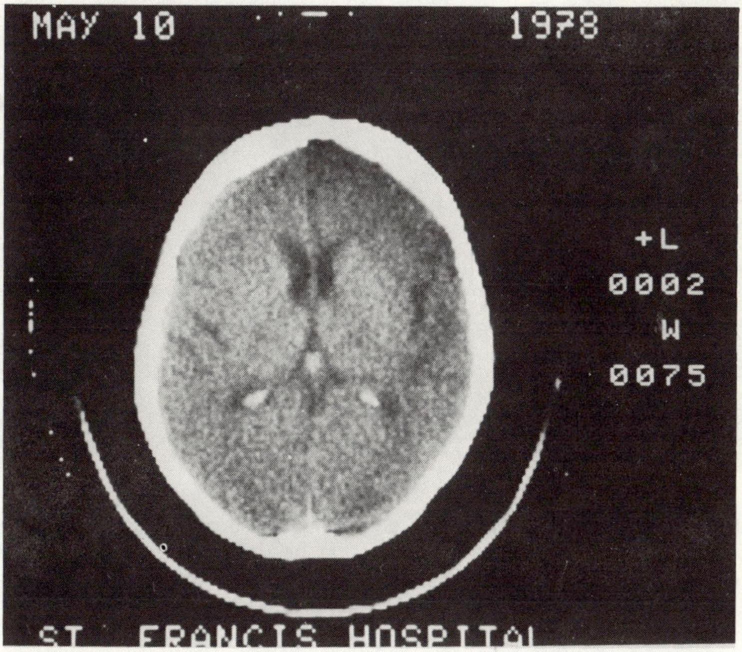

Figure 6-12 Computed tomographic images are commonly displayed as blocks of different density.

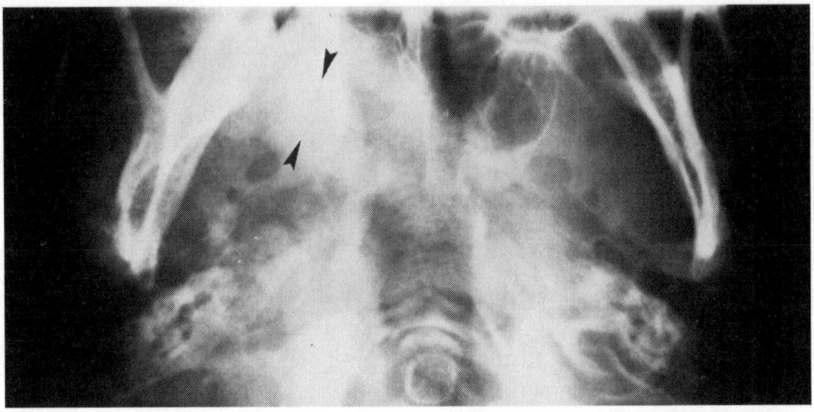

A

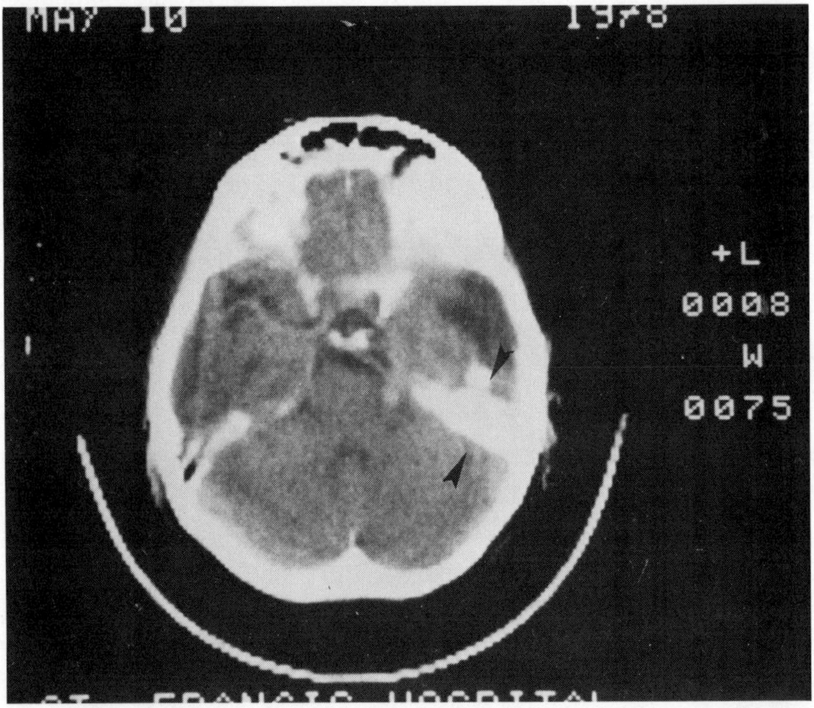

B

Figure 6-13 Although bone lesions defined by the arrows are evident in both views, the accuracy with which the density can be identified as bone is greatest in the computed tomographic image. **A.** Conventional submentovertex view with arrows indicating an area of increased density. Superimposition of adjacent structures prevents a precise definition of the affected structures. **B.** Computed tomographic scan of the same patient showing more sharply the areas of increased density. This image is the result of a reconstruction from x-ray attenuation coefficients.

sinuses computed tomographic scanning was better able to detect extension of disease into the orbit or the base of the skull than either conventional radiography or pluridirectional tomography. Furthermore, when lesions could be identified as malignant, the precise localization that was obtainable with computed tomographic scanning proved to be the most accurate means of deciding whether surgery or radiation therapy was the treatment of choice.

In the case of trauma, Carter and Karmody[19] noted that although pluridirectional tomography is of value in identifying facial fractures, injuries to the midface are commonly associated with subdural or epidural hematomas, which can be demonstrated by computed tomographic scanning but elude conventional tomography.

Computer tomographic scanning has also proven to be valuable in examining the salivary glands, particularly after the injection of contrast agents. In some instances it has been possible to identify masses that lay adjacent to the parotid glands and which could not be recognized during routine sialography.

Thinner bones such as the mandible and cervical spine are adequately evaluated by more routine radiographic approaches, but the potential contribution of computed tomographic scanning should be kept in mind when there are questions about potential soft tissue associations with bony defects.

REFERENCES

1. Webber, R.L., and Stark, L. Influence of fogging radiation and mode of display on the interpretation of dental caries from conventional radiographs. *Invest Radiol.* 7:506–516, 1972.

2. Paatero, Y.V. A new tomographic method for radiographing curved outer surfaces. *Acta Radiol.* 32:177, 1949.

3. Lund, T.M., and Manson-Hing, L.R. Relations between tooth positions and focal troughs of panoramic machines. *J Dent Res.* 53:256, 1974.

4. Freedman, M.L., and Matteson, S.R. Fine structure of the Panorex image. *Oral Surg.* 43:631, 1977.

5. Knight, N. Reverse images and ghosts of Panorex radiography. *J Am Soc Prevent Dent.* 3:53, 1973.

6. Langlais, R., and Mader, C. Radiograph fails to reveal unerupted teeth. *Oral Surg.* 41:541, 1976.

7. Scandrett, F.R., Tebo, H.G., Miller, J.T. et al. Radiographic examination of the edentulous patient. Part I. Review of the literature and preliminary report comparing three methods. *Oral Surg.* 35:266, 1973.

8. McVaney, T.P., and Kalkwarf, K.L. Misdiagnosis of an impacted supernumerary tooth from a panoramic radiograph. *Oral Surg.* 41:678, 1976.

9. Manson-Hing, L.R. *Panoramic Dental Radiography.* Springfield, Ill.: Charles C Thomas, 1976.

10. White, S.C., and Weisman, D.D. Relative discernment of lesions by intraoral and panoramic radiography. *J Am Dent Assoc.* 95:1117, 1977.

11. Davies, E.D., Meister, F., and Lommel, T.J. Panoramic versus periapical surveys—a comparison of findings on freshman dental students. *Dent Radiogr Photogr.* 50:41, 1977.

12. Reiskin, A.B. Panoramic radiography: a reappraisal. Submitted. *J Am Dent Assoc.,* 1978.

13. Stephens, R.G., Kogon, S.L., Reid, J.A. et al. A comparison of Panorex and intraoral surveys for routine dental radiography. *J Can Dent Assoc.* 6:281-286, 1977.

14. Haidar, Z. Diagnostic limitations of orthopantomography with lesions of the antrum. *Oral Surg.* 46:449–453, 1978.

15. Crowley, J.F. Double image in panoramic roentgenographs. *Oral Surg.* 46:463, 1978.

16. Tesini, D.A., and Ficarelli, J.P. Supernumerary tooth? *Oral Surg.* 46:463–464, 1978.

17. Thunty, K.H., and Manson-Hing, L.R. A study of the resolution of dental films and screens. *Oral Surg.* 42:255–266, 1976.

18. Altonen, M., Mattila, K., and Heikinheimo, O. Diagnosis of fractures of the head and neck with the aid of cylindrical pantomograms taken with a new device. *J Maxillofac Surg.* 5:24–31, 1978.

19. Carter, B.F., and Karmody, C.S. Computed tomography of the face and neck. *Semin Roentgenol.* 13:257–266, 1978.

7 Ultrasound

Sound is a mechanical form of energy, unlike light or ionizing radiation. Sound travels in waves produced by the compression of surrounding matter. The human ear is capable of detecting only a small part of the sound spectrum, just as the human eye is sensitive to only a small part of the electromagnetic spectrum, namely, visible light.

Sound used for diagnostic purposes lies above the audible range and is referred to as ultrasound. Human hearing is usually in the range of 30 hertz to 20 kilohertz, but diagnostic ultrasound is of necessity in the range of from 1 to 20 megahertz (one hertz equals one cycle per second). Ultrasonic instruments used for cleaning and scaling teeth operate at about 25 kilohertz.

The properties of sound can be described by a comparison with waves that move across a body of water as the result of some discrete disturbance. The distance between the crests of the waves is their wavelength, and the rate at which successive waves pass a single point is their rate or frequency. The height of the waves or their amplitude depends upon the force of the initial disturbance and is not related to the wavelength or the frequency. Loudness or power in sound is related to the amplitude of the wave and not to the wavelength or frequency.

The effectiveness of sound transmission depends in large part upon the nature of the material through which the transmission occurs. Sound conduction is the result of direct mechanical transmission of vibrations by particles. If particles are fixed or too far apart, conduction is inhibited. Fluids make the best conductors because they are made up of particles that are both movable and close together, while gases are poor conductors because of the large spacing between particles.

Conduction of sound is also related to its frequency. As the frequency goes up, the wavelength becomes shorter. As the wavelength decreases, the likelihood of sound producing vibrations in adjacent particles also decreases. Therefore, long wavelength, low frequency sounds tend to be transmitted most effectively.

Loudness or power also affects conduction or transmission of sound. In air, the distance over which a sound can be heard depends largely upon power or loudness because air is a poor conductor. In water, sound with frequency and power similar to that of the human voice can be detected over a range of miles. If the frequency is greatly reduced and the wavelength increased, sound transmission in water can extend to hundreds of miles.

As sound passes through any material, it encounters a certain level of resistance referred to as acoustic impedance. Sound passing from a material of one acoustic impedance to another is partially reflected. The greater the difference in acoustic impedance, the greater the amount of reflected sound. Acoustic impedance and sound attenuation are not related in any material, so that substances with different levels of acoustic impedance may have similar capacities for attenuation.

DIAGNOSIS

The use of sound for diagnostic purposes depends upon the detection of echoes or reflections from the boundaries between tissues of different acoustic impedance. If fluid is bounded by soft tissue, there is a dramatic change in acoustic impedance and a large echo results. Unfortunately, the acoustic impedance of a tumor within soft tissue may be the same as that of the soft tissue, resulting in echoes that are too small to detect. The interface between air or fluid and bone is also difficult to detect because bone reflects nearly all sound.

In order to measure the distance between materials of different acoustic impedance, the interfaces must be separated by more than half the wavelength of the incident sound. In biological systems many of the interfaces that need to be visualized are less than 0.7 mm apart; therefore, it is necessary to use wavelengths of approximately 1.5 mm or less, that is, one megahertz or more. As noted earlier, however, sound is more easily attenuated at high frequencies and its penetration is limited. Although penetration could be increased with greater amplitude or power, the technical problems in following this approach are extremely difficult. The physical characteristics of dental hard tissues are not well suited to examination by ultrasound, but interfaces between tissues might be evaluated once appropriate equipment is developed.

PRODUCTION AND DISPLAY

Ultrasonic signals are produced and detected by certain types of crystals, including quartz and several other naturally occurring materials. These crystals change their shape when subjected to an electrical voltage. When the voltage is removed, the crystal returns to its former shape (Figure 7-1). The oscillations or vibrations that occur during this interval produce a short pulse of sound, just as a tuning fork produces a sound after it has been struck. The process also works in reverse, with sound causing a deformity in the crystal that results in the production of small oscillating voltages that can be measured or recorded.

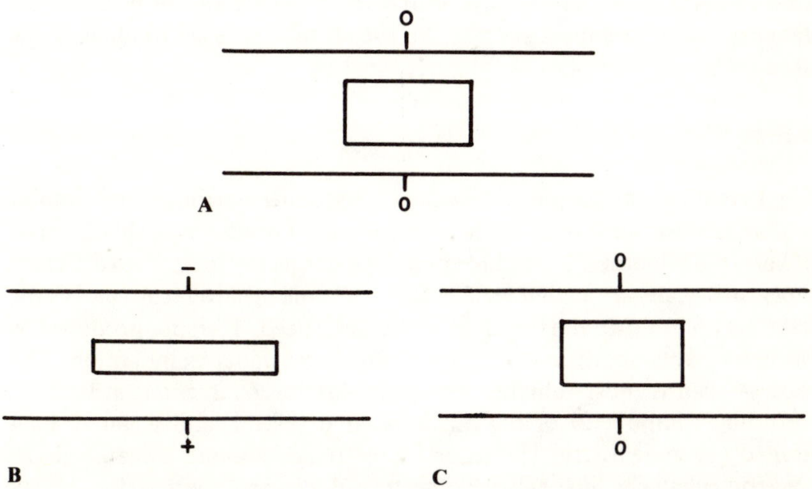

Figure 7-1 Effect of placing a crystal (denoted by rectangle) of quartz or similar material in an electric field. **A.** When there is no voltage applied to the crystal, it maintains its shape. **B.** With the application of a voltage, the crystal deforms. **C.** The crystal returns to its original configuration when the voltage is removed. The process also works in reverse, with deformation of the crystal inducing a potential difference.

Ultrasonic devices can use a transducer to convert sound energy into electrical energy and vice versa. When a single transducer is used, the sound must be pulsed so that returning echoes can be recorded during the intervals between ultrasonic transmissions.

In many devices, pulses lasting about one-millionth of a second are produced at a rate of approximately five hundred per second. This pattern allows the transducer to emit sound for 0.5% of the time while it listens for 99.5% of the time. Pulses travel at a known speed and return only along the original path. Their depth of origin is directly related to the time taken for the echo to return, and therefore, the interfaces producing the echoes can be precisely located.

A-Scan

Pulsed ultrasound can be displayed with modulation of amplitude or brightness. With amplitude modulation (A-scan) outgoing pulses and echoes are displayed on a cathode ray tube. The image appears as spikes extending upward from the baseline. The patient's skin or the point of contact between the skin and the transducer is representative of the baseline on the cathode ray tube. The height of each tracing is related to the intensity of each echo. A-scans, showing the relationship between amplitude and depth, are used for measuring the distances between boundaries of tissues with different acoustic properties. The A-scan is used to distinguish between cystic and solid lesions and to measure the dimensions of structures such as the eye. It may be used to identify the location of the root apex.

B-Scan

Brightness modulation or B-scans are produced in the manner similar to that used for the A-scan. However, instead of producing a spike, a spot of variable brightness is produced on the cathode ray tube. Two different types of B-scans are available. The first, the time position scan, moves the baseline up or down the screen at a constant speed. The spot produced by the echo traces out the movements of structures under examination. This type of scan is most valuable for the evaluation of dynamic structures, including components of the cardiovascular system, and seems to have limited use in dentistry. The second type, the compound B-scan, uses an electromechanical link between the transducer and the baseline of the oscilloscope so that the baseline on the oscilloscope moves with movements of the transducer over the patient's skin. Echoes are stored on the screen, producing a two-dimensional image of the region under examination. This type of scan is most valuable for the evaluation of soft tissue swellings such as those which may be encountered in a salivary gland[1] or thyroid (Figure 7-2).

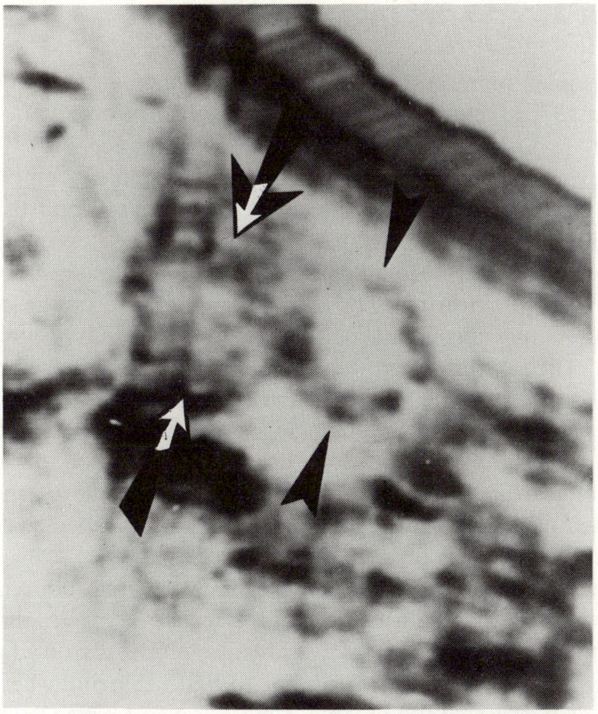

Figure 7-2 Compound B-scan of the neck of a patient with a solid nodule in the thyroid gland. The nodule lies adjacent to the carotid artery which is shown by the black arrows. The nodule, which is solid, is denoted by the white arrows.

Continuous Ultrasound

The use of continuous ultrasound is analogous to an individual standing near a railway line listening to the whistle of a fast-moving train. The pitch of the whistle increases as the train approaches and decreases as it moves away. As the train approaches the individual, each cycle of sound originates from a point nearer the listener than the preceding cycle. The interval between the repetition of successive cycles becomes progressively shorter and the frequency becomes higher. As the train passes, the process is reversed.

In continuous ultrasound techniques, the same change in frequency occurs with echoes that come from a moving interface within the body. However, it is necessary to employ two transducers, one to produce the sound and another for the reception of the echo. This approach is particularly useful for detecting heart sounds and for examining patterns of flow in blood vessels.

Excellent detailed reviews of the principles of ultrasound are readily available.[2–5]

BIOLOGICAL EFFECTS OF ULTRASOUND

Ultrasound represents a mechanical form of energy. Attenuation occurs by several mechanisms, including absorption, scattering, and cavitation.

The exact mechanisms of absorption are extremely complicated. In simple systems, absorption is the result of viscous forces that oppose mechanical movement of the medium, including inter- and intramolecular components. In biological tissues macromolecules are primarily responsible for absorption. The oscillatory pressure of the ultrasound beam causes rearrangement of the hydration shell around protein molecules. The rearrangement requires energy and is followed by a relaxation process during which there is a release of thermal energy.

The scattering of ultrasonic rays is somewhat analogous to the scattering of x-rays. If an ultrasonic beam strikes a boundary between materials of different acoustic impedances, then some of the original beam is transmitted across the boundary and some is reflected away from the surface. During this process energy is released.

Cavitation is a process by which microbubbles are produced in tissue. Oscillations caused by ultrasound pulses cause negative and positive pressure phases. During the negative pressure phase, dissolved gases produce microbubbles in a manner similar to that occurring when deep sea divers are depressurized too quickly. Cavitation appears to have time and energy thresholds and may not occur during many diagnostic procedures.

Biological damage resulting from high energy level ultrasound has been described.[6-9] The disruption of chromosomes by direct physical force and the formation of free radicals during the collapse of cavitation bubbles have been described. However, these effects appear to occur with energy levels higher than those in clinical use. Retrospective clinical studies of obstetric patients[10] have failed to show evidence of injury to mother or fetus. Animal experiments with diagnostic ultrasound have also failed to show any harmful effects.

Because ultrasound deposits energy in tissues, it must have some biological action. The nature and significance are, however, uncertain. Available data suggest that the benefits associated with ultrasound diagnosis outweigh any known risks.

REFERENCES

1. Macridis, C.A., Kouloulas, A., Koutsimbilas, B. et al. Diagnosis of tumors of the salivary glands by ultrasonography. *Electromedica* 4:130–134, 1975.

2. Taylor, J.W. *Atlas of Gray Scale Ultrasonography.* New York: Churchill Livingstone, 1978.

3. King, D.L. *Diagnostic Ultrasound.* St. Louis: C.V. Mosby Company, 1974.

4. Sprawls, P. *The Physical Principles of Diagnostic Radiology.* Baltimore: University Park Press, 1977.

5. Meire, H.B., and Armstrong, P. *Introduction to the Principles of Ultrasound.* Teaching Booklet No. 2. London: British Institute of Radiology, 1976.

6. Hill, C.R. The possibility of hazard in medical and industrial applications of ultrasound. *Br J Radiol.* 41:561–569, 1968.

7. Wells, P.N.T. *Ultrasonics in Clinical Diagnosis.* New York: Churchill Livingstone, 1977.

8. Freimanis, A.K. The biological effects of medically applied ultrasound and their causes. *RC Crit Rev Radiol Sci.* 1:639–652, 1970.

9. Gershoy, A., and Nyborg, W.L. Perturbations of plant-cell contents by ultrasonic microirradiation. *J Acoust Soc Am.* 54:1356–1367, 1973.

10. Hellman, L.M., Duffus, G.M., Donald, I. et al. Safety of diagnostic ultrasound in obstetrics. *Lancet* 1:1133–1134, 1970.

8 Nuclear Medicine: Basic Principles and Dental Applications of Salivary Gland and Bone Scanning

Alan G. Lurie, DDS, PhD

In recent years, procedures used in nuclear medicine have appeared in dental diagnostics. Bone and salivary gland scanning have added substantially to our abilities in the diagnosis and treatment of diseases of the jaws and salivary glands, particularly when borders of bony lesions or salivary gland function are under scrutiny. The objectives of this chapter are 1) to present a brief general description of nuclear medicine, radiopharmaceuticals, and instrumentation, and 2) to discuss the present and future applications of nuclear medicine in the diagnosis and treatment of maxillofacial disease.

BASIC PRINCIPLES

For the purposes of this chapter, nuclear medicine is a diagnostic radiation science in which radiopharmaceuticals, with affinities for particular tissues (target tissues), are administered, concentrate in the target tissues, and then are detected and displayed by a variety of external detector and imaging systems. In this manner, the structure and function of the target tissue may be studied both statistically and dynamically. Nuclear medicine is also involved in the radiation therapy of certain disorders, such as thyroid neoplasms; however, this is not within the domain of this chapter.

Nuclear medicine procedures are similar to those of conventional diagnostic radiology in that ionizing radiation (γ-rays with energies of 20 to 510 kiloelectron volts [keV]) is used to generate an image, and a film looking somewhat like a radiograph is produced. However, there are major differences:

1. The patient, rather than a machine, is the radiation source.
2. The detection instrumentation is different.
3. The sensitivities of the nuclear medicine procedures are very great.
4. The specificities of the nuclear medicine procedures are very low.

In the case of bone, radiology gives a detailed morphologic view of the internal structure of the tissue while the nuclear medicine procedure, a "bone scan," shows areas of altered bone metabolism, without necessarily showing why they are altered. In both radiology and nuclear medicine, the use of computers to analyze the data, either during or after the examination, may considerably enhance the diagnostic yield.

The success of a nuclear medicine procedure depends upon the capacity of a given radiopharmaceutical to concentrate selectively in a particular tissue to a greater degree than in surrounding tissues, allowing a clear image. Thus, the design and preparation of radiopharmaceuticals is a critical step. The requirements for radioactive agents to be used in humans are strict, and they have been described in detail elsewhere.[1]

Some radioactive elements are produced using nuclear reactors or cyclotrons; these elements are then prepared as radiopharmaceuticals. Other radioactive compounds may be prepared using a generator, or "cow."[2] A generator houses at the top of an aseptic chromatography column a parent radioactive element that decays to the desired radioisotope at a temporally constant rate. This decay product can be eluted from the column and used as needed while the parent isotope remains at the top of the column. Two such generators are shown below:

(1)

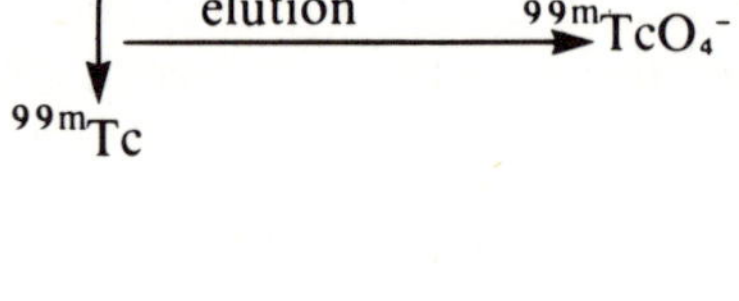

(2)

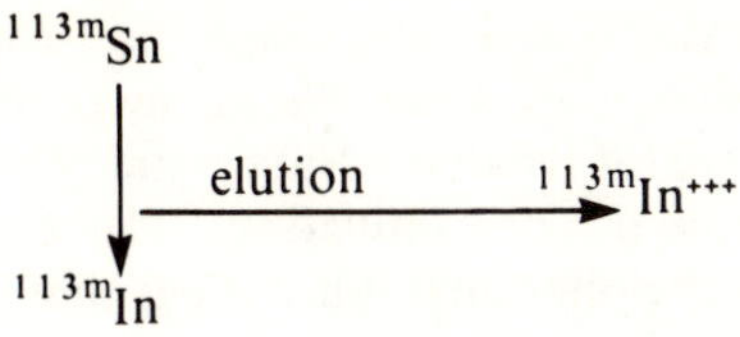

In decay scheme (1), ^{99}Mo is the parent radioisotope and ^{99m}Tc the daughter decay product, while in decay scheme (2), ^{113m}Sn is the parent and ^{113m} In is the daughter. ^{99m}Tc and ^{113m} In are eluted from the column without removing any parent isotope and are ready to be used as needed.

Radiopharmaceuticals may be the radioactive elements or ions such as $^{18}F^-$, $^{113m}In^{+++}$, $^{99m}TcO_4^-$, or may be a nonradioactive carrier compound labeled with the radioisotope, such as ^{67}Ga-labeled citrate, ^{99m}Tc-labeled polyphosphate, or ^{125}I-labeled human serum albumin.

The form in which the agent is administered is determined by the biologic characteristics of the organ to be observed. Three uses of ^{99m}Tc provide a good example. $^{99m}TcO_4^-$, as it comes off of the generator, behaves like I^- and concentrates in the thyroid and salivary glands, providing a salivary gland scan. Labeling a phosphate compound with ^{99m}Tc results in an agent that concentrates in the skeleton and provides a bone scan. Finally, labeling sulphur-colloid with ^{99m}Tc gives an agent that is taken up by reticuloendothelial cells in the liver and spleen, thus providing a liver and spleen scan.

Technetium 99m-labeled compounds and $^{99m}TcO_4^-$ are the most widely used agents in nuclear medicine. They have a short half-life of 6.5 hours, which minimizes patient radiation exposure; they are easily and inexpensively produced using the $^{99}Mo/^{99m}Tc$ generator; and they give off 141 keV gamma rays, which are ideal for gamma camera imaging. These agents are essentially the only ones used for dental procedures.

Following administration of the radiopharmaceutical, a detector measures the radioactive emissions and produces the image. One of the more common types of detector currently used in nuclear medicine is the rectilinear scanner, which moves back and forth and produces an image composed of discrete dots, each taken at a given point in time (scan). Gamma cameras, which are stationary, produce an image composed of small dots (scintiphotos). Gamma cameras, developed recently, produce images with greater definition and are generally used in salivary gland scans and bone scans of the maxillofacial complex.

The production of an image or scintiphoto by a gamma camera is schematically shown in Figure 8-1. The patient is placed on a motorized movable table top (A) with the area to be imaged as close as possible to the imaging head (B). Within the imaging head is a collimator (b_1), a sodium iodide crystal (b_2), and photomultiplier tubes (b_3). The collimator functions in a manner similar to that of a grid in plane radiology, absorbing scatter radiation and allowing only photons useful in image production to pass through and strike the crystal. The gamma emissions that are not absorbed by the collimator strike the NaI crystal. Their energy is converted into fluorescent emissions or scintillations. The scintillations are detected and magnified by the photomultiplier tubes that relay the information into the console (C) via electric signals proportional to the incident light intensity. This information may now be processed through the console in a variety of ways. The image may be displayed on an oscilliscope (D), which allows precise patient positioning prior to obtaining images. The images may then be produced either by exposing Polaroid film, which produces a somewhat low resolution image composed of white dots on a black background (E), or by exposing mammography x-ray film with a "microdot" system, which produces a higher resolution image composed

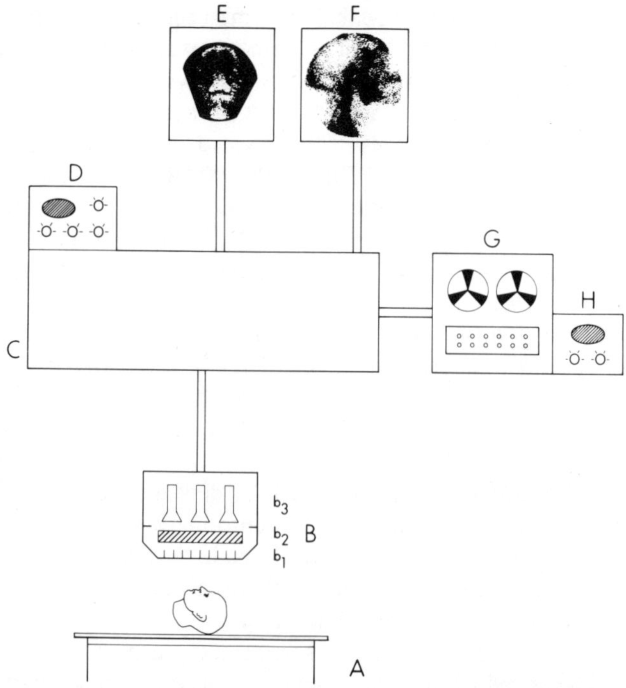

Figure 8-1 Schematic representation of bone scan of the head using a gamma camera. A. Movable table with region of interest (face) located nearest to the imaging head. B. Imaging head (b_1: collimator; b_2: NaI crystal; b_3: photomultiplier tubes). C. Console, where energies to be detected and film exposure factors are controlled. D. Oscilloscope, used for positioning patient prior to obtaining static images. E. Anterior bone scan of skull produced on Polaroid film (white image, black background). F. Lateral bone scan of skull produced on mammography film (black image, clear background). G. Computer for recording selected parts of examinations. H. Console with oscilloscope for viewing material in the computer and performing computer analysis of the material.

of black dots on a clear background (F). The Polaroid system allows one image per Polaroid film, while the microdot mammography film system allows up to nine images to be made on one sheet of film. A final treatment of the data is to enter it through the console into a computer (G) during the examination. All or parts of the examination may be recalled and displayed on an oscilloscope (H) and can then be subjected to a variety of quantitative analytical techniques. This approach appears to be particularly useful in the analysis of functional salivary gland disturbances. Images may be produced rapidly during the injection of the radiopharmaceutical—a flow study—to demonstrate the vascularity of the region of interest, or images may be produced after the radiopharmaceutical has concentrated in the target organ—static images—to demonstrate the organ of interest.

This is admittedly an extremely brief description of radiopharmaceuticals and instrumentation. For more comprehensive discussions, the reader is referred to textbooks of nuclear medicine.[1,3]

RADIOBIOLOGIC CONSIDERATIONS

A major difference between radiographic and nuclear medicine procedures lies in the distribution of the radiation dose to the patient. Radiographs are collimated and expose only the area being examined. Radiopharmaceuticals circulate and concentrate, to varying degrees, in different organs throughout the body. The tissue distributions and the speed and routes of elimination of radiopharmaceuticals make the determinations of organ doses during such procedures complex. Dosimetric studies have led to the concept of critical organs, those receiving the greatest exposures during a procedure. In a bone scan, the bladder is a critical organ since the epithelium is radiosensitive and the radiopharmaceutical is excreted via the genitourinary system. The skeleton and marrow are also critical organs due to the concentration of the radiopharmaceutical in bone and the high radiosensitivity of bone marrow. In a salivary gland scan, the thyroid may receive a substantial radiation dose. Due to the known sensitivity of thyroid tissue to external radiation carcinogenesis and to a lesser extent isotopic radiation carcinogenesis,[4,5] the thyroid is thus a critical organ. The stomach, mammary glands, and salivary glands also receive measurable radiation doses; however, their radiation sensitivities are presently unclear. Estimated doses to critical organs during bone and salivary gland scans as well as conventional head and neck radiologic procedures are shown in Table 8-1.

It is clear that the radiation exposures to patients undergoing these procedures are not insignificant, and that these procedures carry small but definable risks. However, there are substantial potential benefits to be

Table 8-1
Absorbed Radiation Doses (Rads) to Critical Organs During Bone and Salivary Gland Scanning Procedures* and Dental Radiographic Procedures†

Examination	Radiopharmaceutical	Skeleton	Marrow	Thyroid
Bone scan‡	^{99m}Tc-phosphate	0.45 rad	0.10 rad	—
Salivary gland scan§	$^{99m}TcO_4^-$	—	0.19	1.5 rad
Lateral skull radiograph		0.10 (conventional screen) 0.05 (rare earth screen)	—	—
Molar periapical radiograph		0.50 (bisecting angle, long cone, 90 kVp) 0.25 (precision instruments, long cone, 90 kVp)	—	—

*From Subramanian and McAfie,[6] Hine and Johnston,[7] Syed, Hosain, Dugal et al,[8] and Hosain, personal communication.
†The x-ray doses were determined using LiF thermoluminescent dosimetry in the Oral Radiology Department of the University of Connecticut Health Center. The doses are skin entry doses.
‡Total organ doses assuming a 10 mCi administration and skeletal retention of 50% injected activity.
§Total organ doses assuming a 10 mCi administration.

gained from scanning. Thus, as with any diagnostic procedure involving the radiation exposure of a patient, salivary gland and bone scans should be undertaken only when there is a clear and definable patient-care-related need for the information they would provide.

SALIVARY GLAND SCANNING

General Principles

When $^{99m}TcO_4^-$ is eluted from the generator and injected into the patient, it behaves quite similarly to the iodide ion (I^-) and is concentrated and excreted by several glandular tissues, including mammary, thyroid, and salivary glands. This agent provides an excellent vehicle for the study of salivary gland function and pathophysiology.

A salivary gland scan usually consists of a dynamic study followed by a static study, and takes approximately 60 minutes to perform. Five to ten millicuries of $^{99m}TcO_4^-$ are injected intravenously while the patient's face is against the imaging head. This is called the anterior position and results in a "head on" view. Multiple images taken during the first 30 to 120 seconds show the flow of blood first into the arterial and venous systems of the head and neck and then into the organs of the region. This constitutes the flow study and yields information on the vascular architecture of the area and on any functional or anatomic vascular abnormalities that may be associated with the salivary glands. During the next 30 to 45 minutes, several static images are taken with the patient's head in left and right lateral, anterior, and sometimes posterior (posterior skull against imaging head) positions that demonstrate the anatomy of the major salivary glands and their ability to produce and secrete saliva (Figure 8-2).

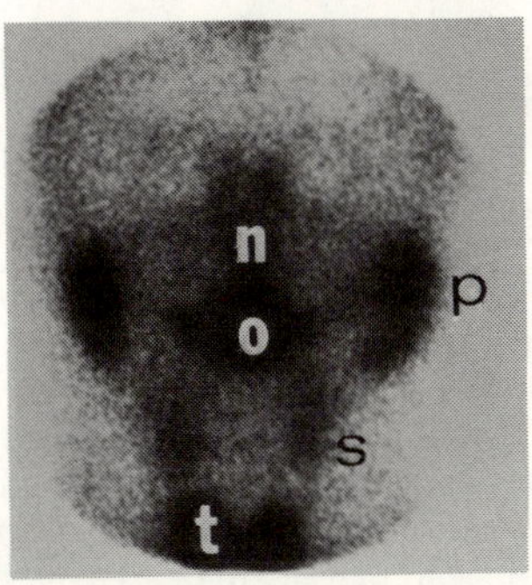

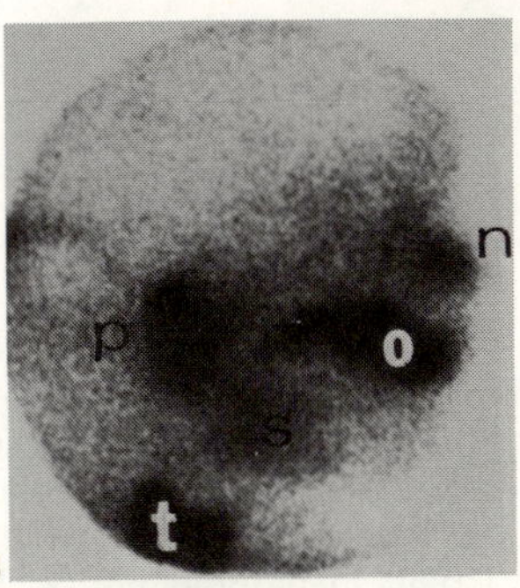

Figure 8-2 Normal anterior (**A**) and lateral (**B**) static images from a salivary gland scan, taken 20 and 25 minutes after administration of 10 mCi $^{99m}TcO_4^-$. p = parotid gland; s = submandibular gland; o = oral cavity; n = nasal cavity; t = thyroid gland.

Finally, the patient is challenged with a sialagogue, such as lemon juice or citric acid, and a series of static images is taken to demonstrate the stimulated secretory capabilities of the glands.

The static images from a typical salivary gland scan on a normal patient are shown in Figure 8-3. The $^{99m}TcO_4^-$ steadily accumulates in the major glands during the first 10 to 25 minutes and also begins moving into the oral cavity at this time. Peak activity usually occurs in normal glands

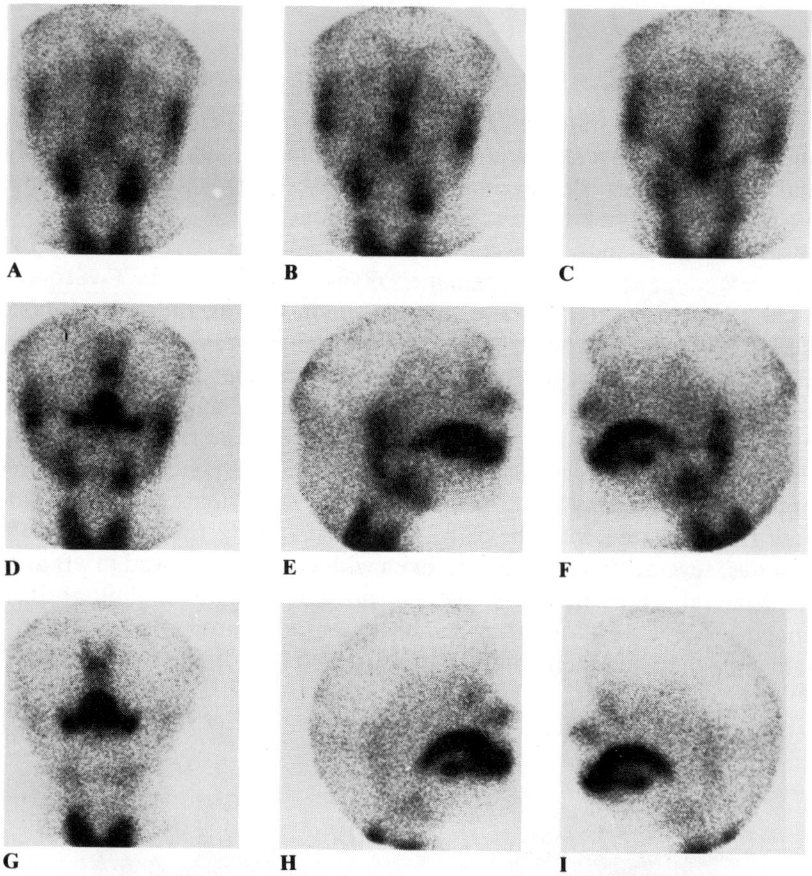

Figure 8-3 Sequential static images of a patient with normal salivary gland function during a salivary gland scan. **A, B, C,** and **D** are anterior views taken 3, 6, 9, and 12 minutes after $^{99m}TcO_4^-$ administration. **E** and **F** are lateral views at 15 and 20 minutes in which the Stensen ducts are easily visualized. **G, H,** and **I** are anterior and lateral views taken after citric acid stimulation. Note early accumulation of activity in major glands **(A, B)**; appearance of activity in oral cavity due to saliva and minor salivary glands **(C, D)**; symmetrical and complete delineation of oral and salivary gland structures within 30 minutes **(D, E, F)**; and functional elimination of activity from major salivary glands upon sialagogue challenge **(G, H, I)** with retention of activity in minor salivary glands of oral cavity.

from 20 to 40 minutes after tracer administration. After this time, activity in the glands steadily decreases until it is indistinguishable from background soft tissue activity in about 90 to 120 minutes after tracer administration or following citric acid stimulation. Since salivary gland scans may be evaluated visually and may also be quantitated through the use of a computer, a strong baseline of normal studies can be generated. Subsequent scans often provide useful information in the diagnosis of a variety of pathophysiologic conditions.

There are substantial differences between salivary gland scanning and contrast sialography, the conventional radiographic technique most frequently used to examine the major salivary glands. These techniques are compared in Table 8-2. A sialogram is primarily an anatomic study using conventional contrast radiology techniques while a salivary gland scan is primarily a functional study using a tissue-specific radioactive tracer. A critical feature emerges: the techniques complement each other significantly and, when used together, render more complete information on the salivary glands than either technique used alone. If they are to be used together, it is important to perform the scan first. Sialography causes a mild diffuse inflammation of the gland examined, thus causing increased uptake of $^{99m}TcO_4^-$, and a spurious scan result.

Infectious and Inflammatory Diseases of the Salivary Glands

Primary infections of the major salivary glands are mediated by a variety of organisms, including bacteria, viruses, and fungi. Additionally, the infection may be primary or it may be secondary to an obstruction, such as a sialolith or ductal stricture. Reports of salivary scanning on patients with salivary gland infections are scarce because the diagnosis is usually made on the basis of history and clinical observation. Nevertheless, scans are potentially useful in acute inflammation because sialography is generally contraindicated. Acute inflammation generally results in increased tracer uptake and a visually "hot" or dense salivary gland image. This is thought to be due to hyperemia and vascular stasis in the gland. Chronic recurrent infections often lead to progressive fibrotic obliteration of functional parenchyma. This results in glandular atrophy and decreased tracer uptake by the gland, giving a visually nondense or "cold" salivary gland image.

Figure 8-4 shows an anterior salivary gland scan taken on a patient with chronic recurrent parotitis. The ability of the left parotid to produce saliva and concentrate the tracer is substantially reduced compared to the right.

Table 8-2
Similarities and Contrasts Between Salivary Gland Scanning and Sialography

Parameter	Salivary gland scan	Sialography
Agent used	$^{99m}TcO_4^-$	Iodinated contrast media; x-rays
Administration	Intravenous	Retrograde pressure placement of contrast media into major duct
Detector	Gamma camera; Polaroid or x-ray film	Fluoroscope; x-ray film
Structures visualized	Glandular parenchyma; oral cavity; all salivary glands visualized simultaneously. Vascular supplies of gland areas shown in flow study	Ductal system; one major salivary gland visualized at a time
Advantages	Shows glandular function; bilateral comparisons; high sensitivity; availability of computer analysis; lack of medical contraindications; can be performed on patient with acute inflammation or known tumor	High resolution of duct system; controlled, localized radiation dose; much existing information on appearances of specific disease states
Disadvantages	Lack of specificity in agent concentration; demonstrates little morphology; generalized, higher radiation dose; lack of substantial baseline information on appearances of specific disease states; cannot be performed shortly after sialography	Parenchymal changes must be inferred from changes in ductal morphology and function; medical contraindications (allergy to iodine, known tumor, acute inflammation, improper equipment)

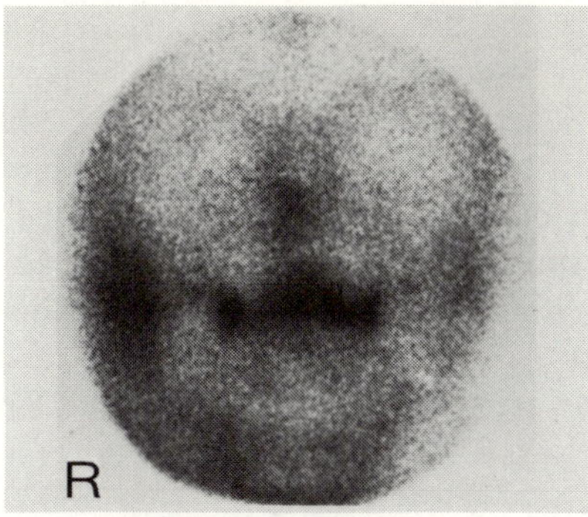

Figure 8-4 Anterior static image from salivary gland scan of patient with recurrent infectious sialoadenitis of the left parotid gland, taken 30 minutes after $^{99m}TcO_4^-$ administration. Right parotid shows normal activity while fibrotic left parotid has minimal activity. The patient had partial xerostomia and frequent painful episodes, due to fibroatrophy, repeated infection, and periodic obstruction of the left parotid gland.

Figures 8-5 and 8-6 show the results of two sequential examinations on a young woman who was successfully treated for multiple sialoliths and functional deficit in the tail of the left parotid gland. Although there is greater activity visually in the left parotid tail five months after treatment (Figure 8-5), the differences between scans are subtle and difficult to appreciate. However, computer analysis of the data from the static images (Figure 8-6) convincingly shows the return of function to the lower lobe of the left parotid five months after treatment. It should be evident from this case that computer-analyzed sequential salivary gland scans have great potential in the clinical follow-up of certain salivary gland disorders.

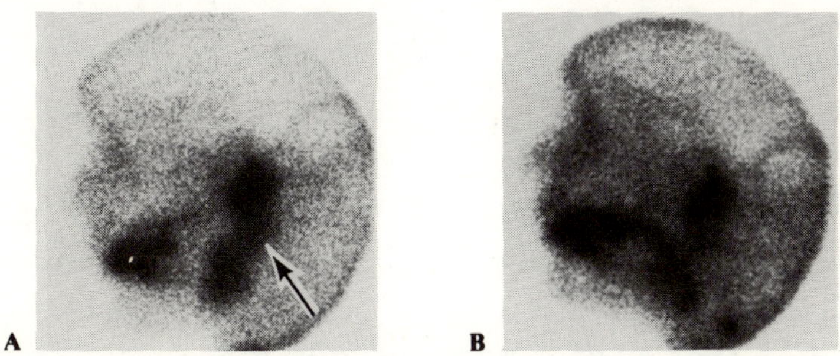

Figure 8-5 Twenty-minute left lateral static images from posttreatment (**A**) and pretreatment (**B**) salivary gland scans on a patient with partial obstruction of the left parotid gland due to multiple small sialoliths. Posttreatment was taken five months after treatment (surgical shortening of parotid duct, repeated NaCl rinsing of ducts, home use of sialagogues). Note increased tracer uptake in tail region of parotid after treatment (arrow). Patient symptoms (pain, mild swelling behind mandibular angle) were eliminated by treatment.

Sjögren's syndrome, an autoimmune disease in which salivary gland function is partially to completely destroyed, is particularly suitable for evaluation by salivary gland scanning. Because of the progressive nature of the loss of salivary function, salivary gland scans have proven to be useful not only in determining the severity of the disease but also in following the response of salivary function to anti-inflammatory chemotherapy.[9,10] Static salivary gland scan examinations performed on patients with early, mild Sjögren's syndrome and advanced, severe Sjögren's syndrome are shown in Figures 8-7 and 8-8.

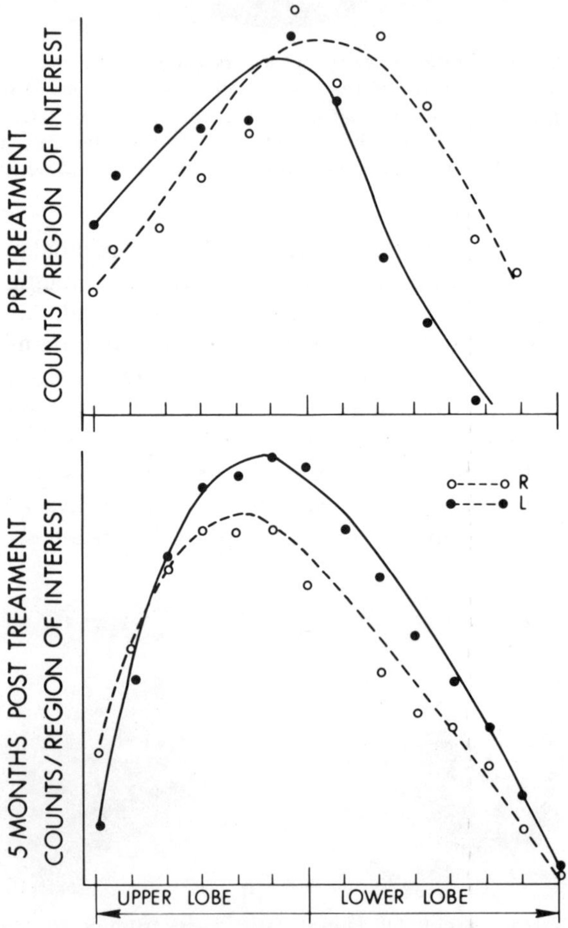

Figure 8-6 Computer analysis of right and left parotid $^{99m}TcO_4^-$ uptake in the sequential salivary gland scans from the patient in Figure 8-5. Pretreatment (above) graphs of right (○) vs left (●) parotid gland $^{99m}TcO_4^-$ uptakes show below normal activity in lower lobe of left affected parotid. Posttreatment (below) graphs of right and left parotid uptakes show normal $^{99m}TcO_4^-$ activity in both parotid glands.

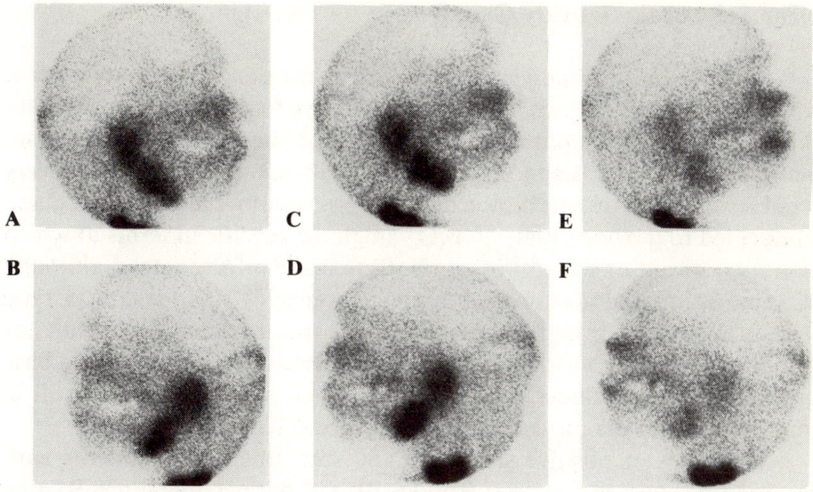

Figure 8-7 Lateral static images taken during a salivary gland scan on a patient with early, mild Sjögren's syndrome. **A, B.** 25 minutes. **C, D.** 45 minutes. **E, F.** Postcitric acid stimulation, 90 minutes after $^{99m}TcO_4^-$ administration. There is no activity in the oral cavity, probably due to autoallergic destruction of the minor salivary glands. The uptake of the major glands is not yet substantially affected; however, there is some retained activity in both parotid and submandibular glands after citric acid stimulation, suggesting obstruction and/or partial parenchymal damage.

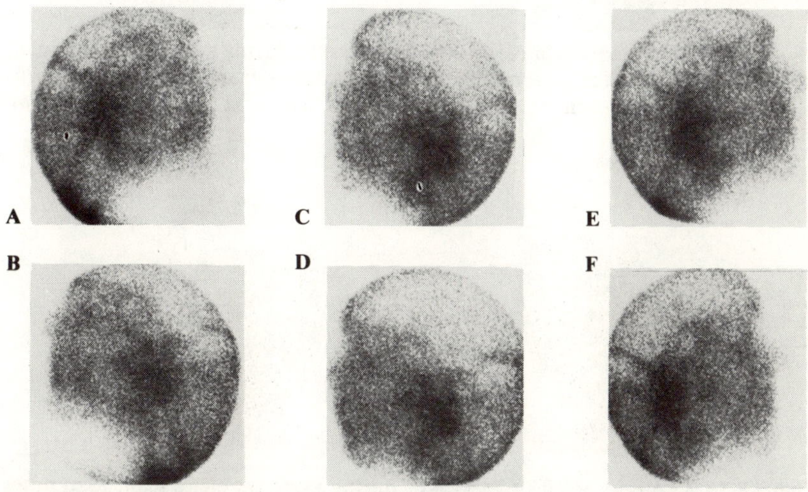

Figure 8-8 Lateral static images taken during a salivary gland scan on a patient with advanced Sjögren's syndrome and accompanying complete xerostomia. **A, B.** 30 minutes. **C, D.** 60 minutes. **E, F.** Post-citric acid stimulation, 90 minutes after $^{99m}TcO_4^-$ administration. There is little if any significant activity in either the oral cavity or in the major salivary glands at any time, thus demonstrating destruction of salivary gland function.

Neoplasms of the Salivary Glands

The difficulty of salivary gland biopsy, the dangers to cranial nerve VII from parotid surgery, the high incidence of malignancy in submandibular gland tumors (greater than 50%), and the shortcomings of conventional radiologic diagnosis have made salivary gland neoplasms very troublesome. The unique biologic characteristics of various salivary gland tumors led to the hope that $^{99m}TcO_4^-$ might be specific in terms of which tumors it would or would not concentrate in.[11] Unfortunately, although Warthin's tumor almost invariably concentrates $^{99m}TcO_4^-$ and metastatic lesions are almost invariably devoid of the tracer, the overall results of tumor scans have been inconsistent. It is expected that a greater data base and improved techniques, such as tomographic scanning,[12] will result in improved tumor diagnosis using salivary gland scanning.

Examples of positive salivary gland scan findings in patients with tumors are shown in Figures 8-9 and 8-10. The patient in Figure 8-9 had a

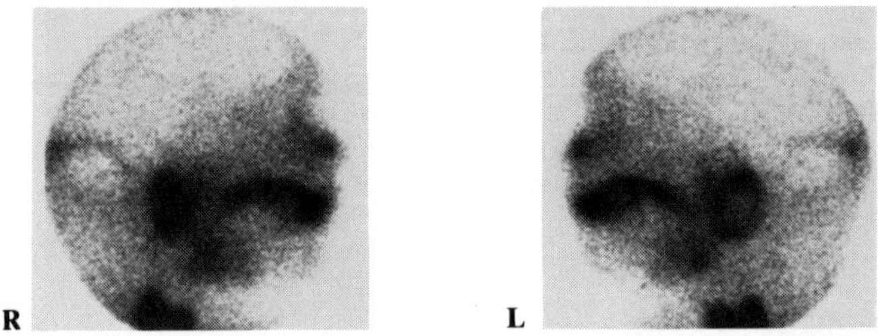

Figure 8-9 Right and left lateral static images taken during a salivary gland scan, 30 minutes after $^{99m}TcO_4^-$ administration. A sharply demarcated area of diminished tracer uptake is seen in the left parotid gland. This area proved to be a benign mixed tumor.

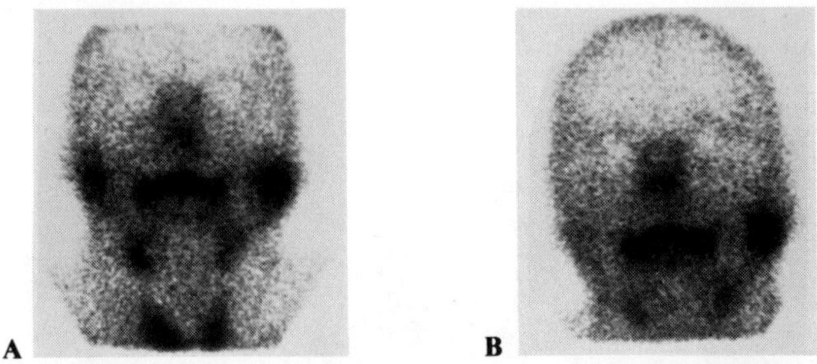

Figure 8-10 Anterior static images taken during a salivary gland scan, 25 minutes after $^{99m}TcO_4^-$ administration (**A**) and 45 minutes after $^{99m}TcO_4^-$ administration (**B**) following citric acid stimulation. The left parotid gland appears larger and "hotter" than the right in the 25-minute image, and most activity remains in the left parotid after citric acid stimulation. This area was subsequently found to be a benign papillary cystadenoma lymphomatosum (Warthin's tumor). [Courtesy of Dr. John Szicklas, Nuclear Medicine, Hartford Hospital, Hartford, Connecticut.]

benign mixed tumor of the left parotid gland that did not concentrate $^{99m}TcO_4^-$, thus leaving an area of reduced activity, or a "cold" spot. The patient in Figure 8-10 had a Warthin's tumor of the left parotid gland that concentrated $^{99m}TcO_4^-$. The involved gland has increased activity (a "hot" lesion), and activity is retained in the lesion even after citric acid stimulation.

BONE SCANNING

General Principles

Imaging of the skeleton using radiopharmaceuticals has been performed with a wide variety of bone-seeking radiopharmaceuticals since the early 1940s.[13] Although diverse agents, such as ^{89}Sr and ^{18}F, have been used for skeletal imaging, the ^{99m}Tc-labeled phosphate compounds, with their low radiation dose, short half-life, and high yield of photons with an energy suited to a gamma camera, are the primary agents used in bone scanning today. This chapter will deal exclusively with bone scanning using ^{99m}Tc-labeled phosphate compounds. The principal use of bone scanning has been and is in the detection of occult metastatic disease in the skeleton.

In contrast to a radiograph, a bone scan gives almost no information on the morphology of a lesion, either internally or in areas of bone adjacent to the lesion. The scan does demonstrate, however, areas of altered bone metabolism within and around a lesion, thus allowing a reasonably accurate assessment of the growth of a lesion and the extent of its borders. Bone scanning also allows one to view the entire skeleton with no additional radiation burden to the patient. Positive findings usually lead to conventional radiographs of the suspicious areas, allowing morphologic study of regions with altered bone metabolism.

The preparation of a bone scanning radiopharmaceutical involves the elution of $^{99m}TcO_4^-$ from the generator and the subsequent reaction of the $^{99m}TcO_4^-$ with a phosphate compound in the presence of tin. The agent is freshly prepared daily. The phosphate compounds, usually polyphosphate, diphosphonate, or imidodiphosphate, are readily available commercially as bone scanning kits, thus simplifying and streamlining the procedure. The resulting ^{99m}Tc-Sn-phosphate compounds are complex, and the exact structures are presently unknown. The phosphate group is taken up by the skeleton; thus, it acts as a carrier for the ^{99m}Tc. Its uptake in a given area of the skeleton is proportional to the quantity and rate of bone deposition in that area.

A bone scan takes longer to perform than a salivary gland scan. Ten to fifteen millicuries of ^{99m}Tc-labeled compound are injected intravenously. If inflammation or infection in the area of interest is suspected, a flow study during the first 30 to 180 seconds may be useful in quantitating the vascularity of the area. A waiting period of two to three hours permits the radiopharmaceutical to accumulate in the skeleton and to be removed from vascular and soft tissues via the urinary system. At that time, static images of the entire skeleton and/or individual bones may be obtained using a variety of collimators. The kidneys and bladder are also visualized in the bone scan since they are the route of excretion for the imaging agents.

Existing and Potential Clinical Applications

Scans of the facial bones are shown in Figures 8-11 and 8-12. A gamma camera produced the images in Figure 8-11, while a rectilinear scanner was used in Figure 8-12. The increased resolution of gamma camera images is easily appreciated, and this is the instrument of choice in a bone scan of the maxillofacial complex.

Unfortunately, several common dental diseases, including marginal periodontitis and periapical pathology, frequently lead to reactive bone formation in the jaws. This almost invariably results in localized areas of increased radiopharmaceutical uptake in the jaws.[14] Since numerous patients have such disease, nuclear medicine physicians generally regard such "hot" spots in the jaws as dental disease of uncertain significance. There has been little study of bone scanning of the human maxillofacial skeleton, and there is a dearth of information on the bone scan appearances of most lesions in the jaws.

At present, the two best indications for a bone scan of the jaws appear to be in evaluating the take of a bone graft in the jaws and in

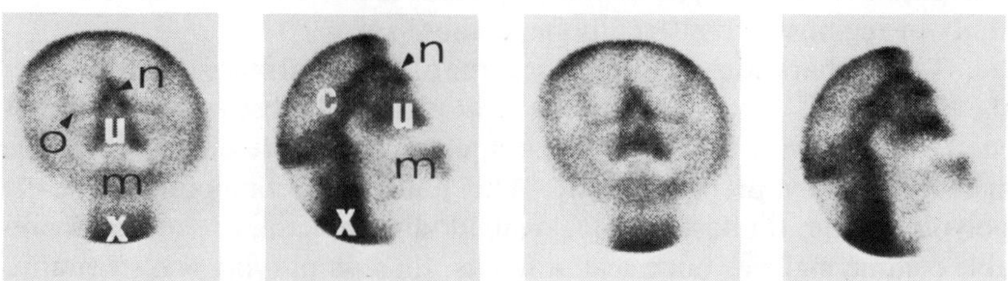

A **B** **C** **D**

Figure 8-11 Normal anterior (**A, C**) and lateral (**B, D**) static images of the facial bones from a bone scan taken using a gamma camera 2.5 hours after ^{99m}Tc-diphosphonate administration. x = cervical spine; u = maxilla/palate; m = mandible; o = orbital floor; c = cranial base; n = nasal complex.

defining the extent of a lesion or area of infection as an aid in treatment planning. Extensive studies have been performed on dogs receiving mandibular bone grafts[15,16]; the results strongly indicate that bone scanning will predict the success or failure of a graft significantly sooner than conventional radiology. Bone scanning appears to be particularly useful in defining the extent of locally aggressive lesions in the jaws to aid in the planning of surgical margins. Such a case is shown in Figure 8-13, where a recurrent odontogenic keratocyst was found on scan to have a more anteriorly placed margin than had been suspected from the radiographs.[17]

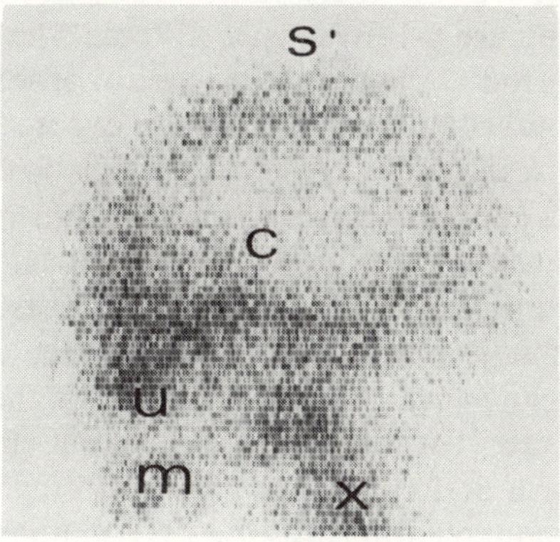

Figure 8-12 Normal lateral static images of the skull and facial bones from a bone scan taken using a rectilinear scanner 2.5 hours after ^{99m}Tc-polyphosphonate administration. x = cervical spine; u = maxilla; m = mandible; s = calvarium; c = cranial base.

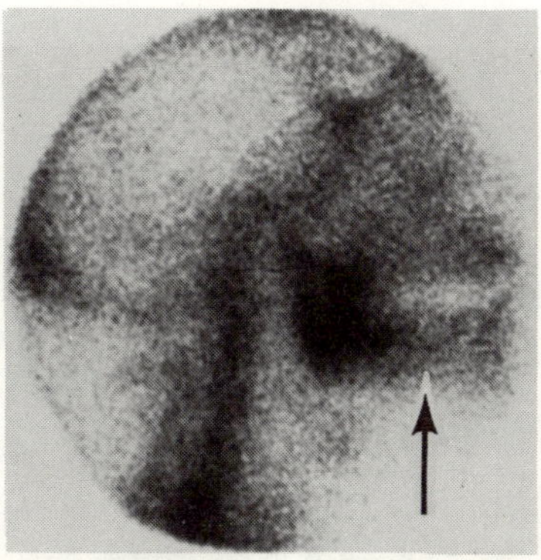

Figure 8-13 Lateral static image of the facial bones taken using a gamma camera 3 hours after ^{99m}Tc-diphosphonate administration. There is an area of considerably increased uptake occupying the entire ramus and extending anteriorly in the mandibular body to the area indicated by the arrow. The patient had a recurrent odontogenic keratocyst with superimposed infection and was successfully treated by partial right mandibular resection and replacement with an autograft of marrow and cancellous bone.[17]

The difficulties in interpreting bone scans of the jaws are shown in Figures 8-14 and 8-15. The patient in Figure 8-14 had long-standing bilateral mandibular osteomyelitis and undiagnosed aleukemic leukemia that was fatal one year later. As one would expect, the attempts at involucrum formation, coupled with inflammation, accompanying hyperemia and vascular stasis, resulted in a substantial uptake of radiopharmaceutical. This, unfortunately, obscured any leukemia-related osseous abnormalities that might have been revealed by the scan. The patient in Figure 8-15 was a 14-year-old girl with a cystic-appearing lesion that later proved to have a mural ameloblastoma at its base (Figure 8-15A). The scan (Figure 8-15B) reveals a "cold" lesion, with increased uptake around its borders, an appearance typical of some intrabony cysts. There is heavy uptake at the base of the lesion. However, a large periapical lesion is seen involving the first molar with greatly increased tracer uptake in the entire posterior mandible, thus making conclusions about the cystic-appearing area on the scan tenuous.

Obviously, a considerably greater number of cases need to be examined to draw conclusions on the scan appearance of specific lesions. Several individual scan patients with bone disease of the jaws were recently discussed by Alexander.[18] A variety of arthropathies have been studied in peripheral joints with bone scanning.[19] Considering the diagnostic difficulty presently encountered in working up a temporomandibular joint patient, the systematic application of bone scanning, specifically to evaluate joint inflammation, might prove to be productive.

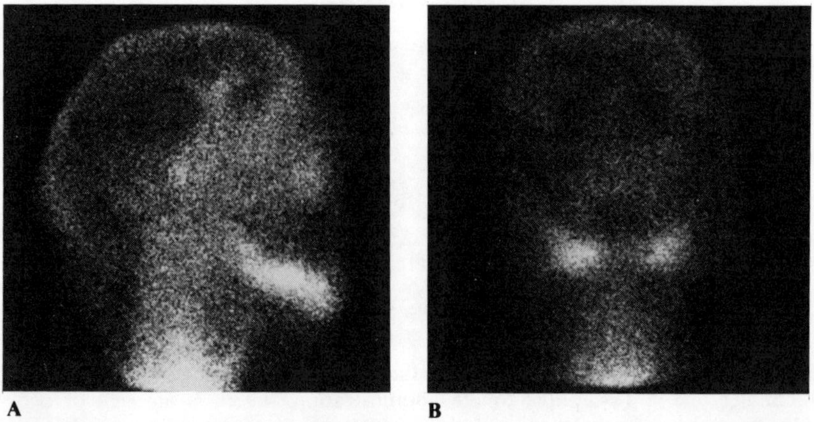

A B

Figure 8-14 Lateral (**A**) and anterior (**B**) images of the facial bones using a gamma camera and Polaroid film recorder. This patient shows greatly increased tracer uptake bilaterally in the mandibular body. He had chronic osteomyelitis of 2 years' duration and aleukemic leukemia.

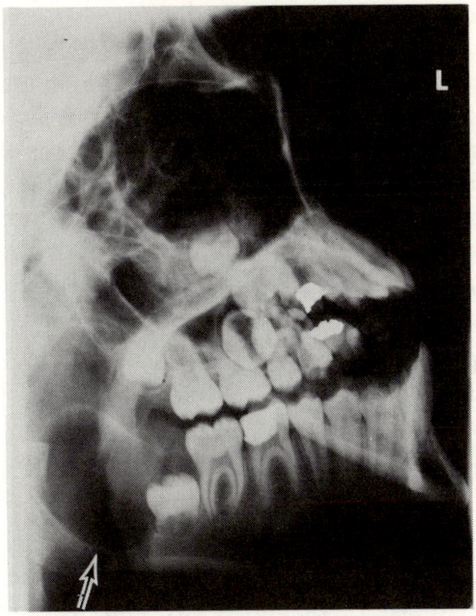

A

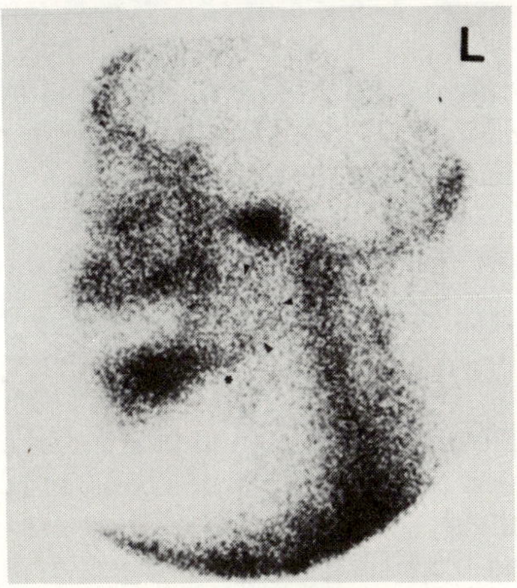

B

Figure 8-15 A 14-year-old female patient who presented with a large asymptomatic cyst-like lesion in the left mandibular ramus associated with an impacted third molar. **A.** Lateral oblique radiograph of the left mandible. **B.** Left lateral bone scan static image. Note the slight indication of undulation at inferior border of the lesion on the radiograph (arrow). Also note the substantial periapical pathology of the first molar. The scan shows an area of increased uptake in the mandibular body, probably reactive bone formation associated with the periapical pathology. An ill-defined area of diminished tracer uptake is seen in the ramus possibly surrounded, in part, by a thin border of increased uptake (arrows), a somewhat typical appearance for a bony cyst on a bone scan. Uptake is greatest at inferior aspect (*), but this may be associated with the periapical pathology. The lesion proved to be a dentigerous cyst with a mural ameloblastoma at the inferior aspect.

Experimental Applications

Bone scanning provides an interesting and potentially precise quantitative means for studying bone changes in the jaws of experimental animals. Several categories of dental pathology have been studied in animals using both imaging and quantitative uptake of bone-seeking radiolabeled tracers. These studies include osseous graft healing[15,16]; osseous wound healing[14,20]; periodontitis[21]; orthodontic tooth movement[22]; and tooth eruption.[23] Research is certainly one of the most evident and productive dental applications of bone scanning.

TUMOR SCANNING

In recent years, there has been an intensive search for radiopharmaceuticals that will localize specifically in tumors. Such agents would be extremely powerful, both diagnostically and therapeutically. Among several agents presently being utilized, ^{67}Ga-citrate has been the most useful, particularly in cancer of the head and neck. Examinations with ^{67}Ga-citrate not only define the size of head and neck tumors, but also show areas of infection.[24,25] This and similar agents may provide a useful means of tumor diagnosis in the years to come.

CONCLUSION

Bone and salivary gland scanning are diagnostic techniques in nuclear medicine that can be useful in detection and definition of diseases of the jaws and salivary glands. However, there are limitations on the information obtained from such scans. Furthermore, the radiation burden to the patient is not inconsequential. Consequently, these procedures, like all procedures involving radiation exposure, should be undertaken only when a clear diagnostic or therapeutic rationale exists. Properly used, these procedures can be of considerable value in the diagnosis and treatment of many types of dental, osseous, and salivary gland pathology.

The author is especially grateful to Dr. Richard Spencer, Chairman, Department of Nuclear Medicine, University of Connecticut Health Center, for making all nuclear medicine patient records available for illustrations, as well as for his helpful comments in reviewing the manuscript.

REFERENCES

1. Subramanian, G., Rhodes, B.A., Copper, J.F., et al. *Radiopharmaceuticals.* New York: The Society of Nuclear Medicine, 1975.

2. Doering, R.F., Tucker, W.D., and Stang, L.G., Jr. A simple device for milking high-purity yttrium-90 from strontium-90. *J Nucl Med.* 4:54–59, 1963.

3. Blahd, W.H. *Nuclear Medicine.* 2nd Ed. New York: McGraw-Hill, 1971.

4. Advisory Committee on the Biological Effects of Ionizing Radiations. *The Effects on Populations of Exposure to Low Levels of Ionizing Radiation.* Washington, DC: National Academy of Sciences, National Research Council, 1972, pp. 120–125.

5. Hempelmann, L., Hall, W., Phillips, M. et al. Neoplasms in persons treated with x-rays in infancy: fourth study in 20 years. *J Natl Cancer Inst.* 55:519–530, 1975.

6. Subramanian, G., and McAfie, J.G. A new complex of ^{99m}Tc for skeletal imaging. *Radiology* 99:192–196, 1971.

7. Hine, G.J., and Johnston, R.E. Absorbed dose from radionuclides. *J Nucl Med.* 11:468–469, 1970.

8. Syed, I.B., Hosain, F., Dugal, P. et al. Bone scanning agents: present status and choice. *Indian J Cancer.* 10:280–284, 1973.

9. Schall, G.L., Anderson, L.G., Wolf, R.O. et al. Xerostomia in Sjögren's syndrome. Evaluation by sequential salivary scintigraphy. *JAMA.* 216:2109–2116, 1971.

10. Lurie, A.G. Applications of nuclear medicine in dentistry. Edited by D. Seligson. In *CRC Handbook Series in Clinical Laboratory Science. Section A. Nuclear Medicine.* Cleveland: CRC Press, 1977.

11. Gates, G.A., and Work, W.P. Radioisotope scanning of the salivary glands. A preliminary report. *Laryngoscope* 77:861–875, 1967.

12. Gates, G.A. Current status of radiosialography in tumor diagnosis. *Trans Am Acad Opthalmol Otolaryngol.* 74:1183–1195, 1970.

13. Merrick, M.V. Bone scanning. *Br J Radiol.* 48:327–351, 1975.

14. Lurie, A.G., and Matteson, S.R. ^{99m}Tc-diphosphonate bone imaging and uptake in healing rat extraction sockets. *J Nucl Med.* 17:688–692, 1976.

15. Kelly, J.F., Cagle, J.D., Stevenson, J.S., and Adler, G.J. Technetium-99m radionuclide bone imaging for evaluating mandibular osseous allografts. *J Oral Surg.* 33:11–17, 1975.

16. Kelly, J.F., Cagle, J.D., Adler, G.J., and Donovan, R.L. Sequential quantitative radionuclide evaluation of mandibular bone graft repair. *J Dent Res.* 55:1111–1117, 1976.

17. Lurie, A.G., Puri, S., James, R.B., and Jensen, T.W. Radionuclide bone imaging in the surgical treatment planning of odontogenic keratocysts. *Oral Surg.* 42:726–730, 1976.

18. Alexander, J.M. Radionuclide bone scanning in the diagnosis of lesions of the maxillofacial region. *J Oral Surg.* 34:249–256, 1976.

19. McCarty, D.J., Polcyn, R.E., Collins, P.A., and Gottschalk, A. ^{99m}Technetium scintiphotography in arthritis. I. Technique and interpretation. *Arthritis Rheum.* 13:11–32, 1970.

20. Green, L.J., Gong, J.K., and Neiders, M.E. Relationship between Sr^{85} uptake and histological changes during healing in dental extraction wounds in rats. *Arch Oral Biol.* 14:865–872, 1969.

21. Kaplan, M.L., Garcia, D.A., Goldhaber, P. et al. Uptake of ^{99m}Tc-Sn-EHDP in beagles with advanced periodontal disease. *Calcif Tissue Res.* 19:91–98, 1975.

22. Garcia, D.A., Higginbotham, D.J., House, J.E., and Kapur, K.K. Tc-99m-polyphosphate bone imaging of orthodontically treated dog teeth. *Am J Orthod.* 66:665–674, 1974.

23. Garcia, D.A., Davis, M.A., Kapur, K.K., and Goldhaber, P. Detection of local changes of mineral metabolism within the jaws of rabbits by bone scanning. *J Dent Res.* 53:447–452, 1974.

24. Higashi, T., Kashima, I., Shimura, K. et al. Gallium-67 scanning in the evaluation of therapy of malignant tumors of the head and neck. *J Nucl Med.* 18:243–249, 1977.

25. Higashi, T., Aoyama, W., Mori, Y., and Everhart, F.R., Jr. Gallium-67 scanning in the differentiation of maxillary sinus carcinoma from chronic maxillary sinusitis. *Radiology* 123:117–122, 1977.

9 Photographic Copying of Radiographs

Michael L. Freedman, PhD

Several techniques are available for the photographic copying of radiographs. Ratios of image to subject sizes may range downward from 1:1 with small intraoral films. These procedures can provide 1) projectable positive images (slides) for illustrating lectures or for data bulk reduction, 2) negative intermediate images for production of paper prints to illustrate manuscripts, poster presentations, and the like, and 3) same size (1:1) duplicates of original radiographs.[1,2] While there is no substitute for a high quality original, some flexibility exists in these techniques, and modest adjustments of overall density, length of grey scale, and composition may be made in the copy.[3-7] Lack of image sharpness in the original radiograph cannot be overcome; instead, it will increase as the copy of an inferior original is enlarged for viewing or photographic printing. This is usually true also for artifacts introduced in the processing of the original, such as static discharge, air bubbles, fingerprints, and chemical stains.

THE CAMERA

Slides and negatives of large-size extraoral radiographic projections (such as Towne's view, TMJ study, sialogram, and cephalometric series) and negatives of small intraoral films (periapical, bitewing, occlusal) are conveniently made with a 35 mm camera. The popularity of the single lens reflex (SLR) has grown dramatically, and it is reasonable to expect that most individuals disposed to copy radiographs own or have access to this type of camera. The SLR has several advantages.[8] First, the photographer sees the image that will be recorded on the film, although depending upon the make of camera the viewed image may be slightly reduced in size compared to the 35 mm film frame. There is no parallax or lack of congruity between the viewed radiograph and its recorded image (Figure 9-1A). This is important because parallax is most troublesome at the short subject-to-film distances encountered in copy work,[9] and, if uncorrected, results in deletion of the top of the original (Figure 9-1B). Second, modern SLR cameras invariably afford lens interchangeability and have built-in exposure meters.

Frequently, the built-in light meter of the 35 mm SLR is center-weighted; that is, the portion of the subject measured for exposure is biased toward or comprises only a portion of the center of the field of view. Different manufacturers have larger metered areas and/or smaller spot meters. For radiographs in which the area of interest is readily

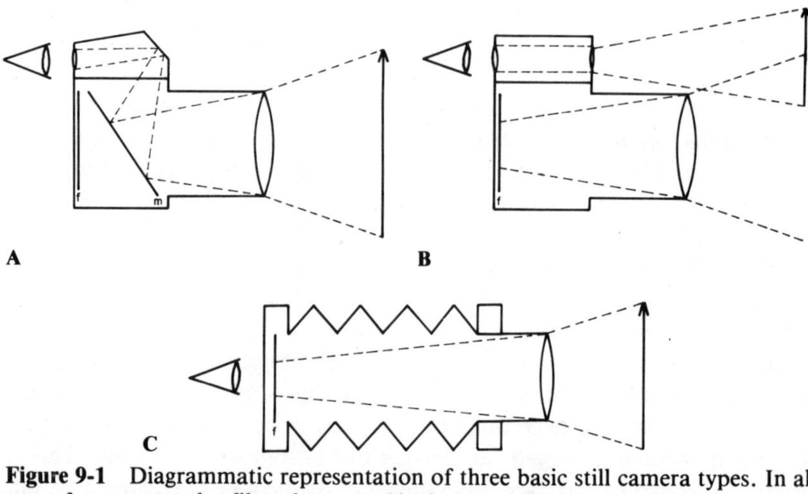

Figure 9-1 Diagrammatic representation of three basic still camera types. In all cases f represents the film plane. A. Single lens reflex: the movable mirror, m, reflects the image to the viewer during composition, thereby overcoming parallax. B. Range finder: there is a lack of congruity between the viewed and recorded images at close focusing ranges (parallax). C. View camera: the image may be composed and focused on a screen at the film plane prior to inserting the sheet of film.

apparent by virtue of the difference between its density and the density of its surroundings, a center-weighted or large metered area is adequate. However, a spot meter has advantages: 1) for basing photographic exposure on a small region of the x-ray film; 2) for basing exposure on a region of atypical density; or 3) when most of the radiograph has a uniform density different from that of a small region of interest. Its use prevents the exposure determination from being biased by less important features of the radiograph, the inclusion of which would lead to an average exposure for the entire film with over- or underexposure of the structures of concern. Also, as the lens is extended for close-up work by bellows, extension tube, or other device, the light intensity reaching the film diminishes. A built-in meter allows simple exposure correction.

There are high quality SLRs with film formats larger than 24 × 36 mm. A larger film image requires less magnification to fill a projection screen or to produce a photographic print and, therefore, preserves more detail and shows less of the film's grain. However, such cameras frequently are in the realm of professional photography. Their cost and the lack of commonly available equipment for projecting large slides limit their usefulness. The same is true for the view camera with its single sheet film packs (Figure 9-1C). For greatest copy fidelity, however, a view camera with a specially designed copy or process lens that is designed to reproduce faithfully a two-dimensional subject, may be indicated. Because of the parallax problem, already discussed, and some difficulty in determining exposure, the 35 mm range-finder camera is not generally suited to copy work. The supplementary reflex adapters that fit between the range finder camera's body and lens or bellows assembly are cumbersome and obsolescent.

THE LENS

The ability to fit, for copy work, an extended-focusing-range macro lens of about 50 mm focal length with large (f/2.8) maximum aperture satisfies three requirements. 1) The 35 mm film frame, which is 24 × 36 mm, can be filled with a single radiograph or part of a large radiograph. 2) Fall-off of image quality in the corners of the film frame and curvilinear (barrel or pin cushion) distortion, sometimes a problem with a nonmacro lens at the near limit of its distance range (0.5–1 m), is reduced. 3) The use of supplementary close-up lenses, extension tubes, or a bellows is obviated. Close-up lenses have positive diopter values of +1, +2, and so forth, and effectively shorten the focal length of the camera's normal lens, and extension tubes come in sets of several lengths. For a particular distance setting on the camera lens' barrel, these devices allow only one film-to-subject distance and hence one image size for which the subject will be in focus. Thus, the useful range of any close-up lens or extension tube is quite narrow. Close-up lenses and extension tubes limit the range of subject-to-film distances and hence image sizes attainable and introduce extra manipulations. In addition, close-up lenses frequently lack the quality of the camera lens to which they are added. Their tendency to reduce image quality may be tolerable in copying a three-dimensional subject but not in copying a two-dimensional radiograph. The expedient of combining close-up lenses (with the stronger lens closer to the camera) to attain a short subject-to-film distance degrades image sharpness. The use of small aperture (f-stop) to combat this problem is not feasible with some slow copy films. Figure 9-2 is a copy of a grid of 1 cm squares photographed with a 50 mm nonmacro lens at the near limit of its working range, < 0.5 m. The lens was fully extended and the aperture fully open. There is some pincushion, shape distortion, but the image is tolerably sharp. Figure 9-3 is the same grid photographed with a macro lens at its nearest working distance, which provides a 1:1 image:subject size ratio. In Figure 9-4 extension tubes have been added to the normal lens to permit close-up work. Compared to Figure 9-3, there is considerable fall-off of image quality and some flare.

The focal length of the normal lens for a 35 mm camera is about 50 mm, this being the diagonal length of the 35 mm film frame. As the distance from the front surface of the lens to the subject decreases in copy work, the lens must be focused outward, away from the film plane, to

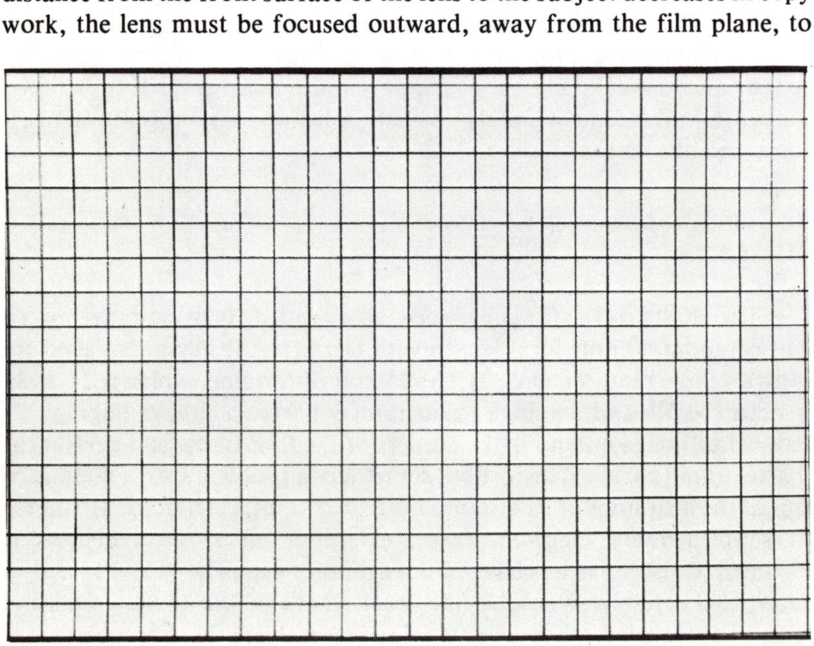

Figure 9-2 Grid of 1 cm squares photographed by a normal 50 mm focal length (nonmacro) lens at the near limit of its working range.

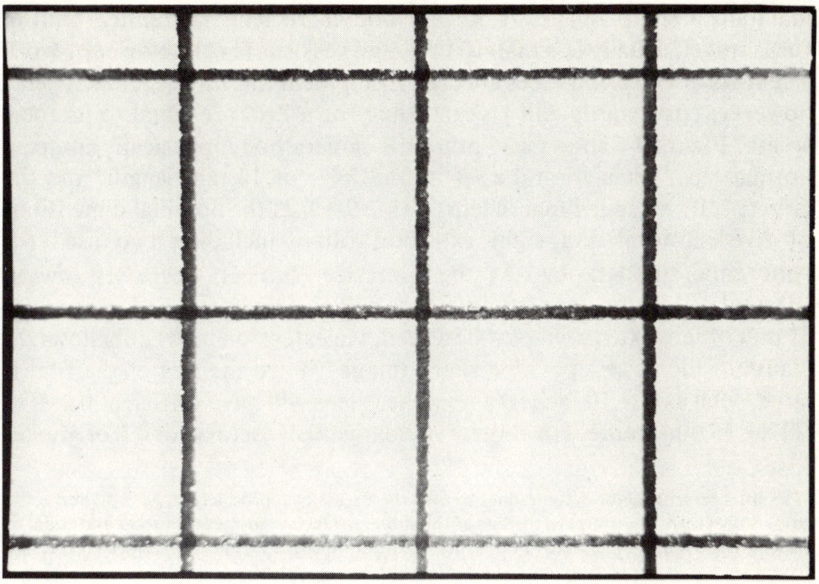

Figure 9-3 Grid of 1 cm squares photographed with a 60 mm focal length macro lens illustrating a 1:1 subject:image size ratio.

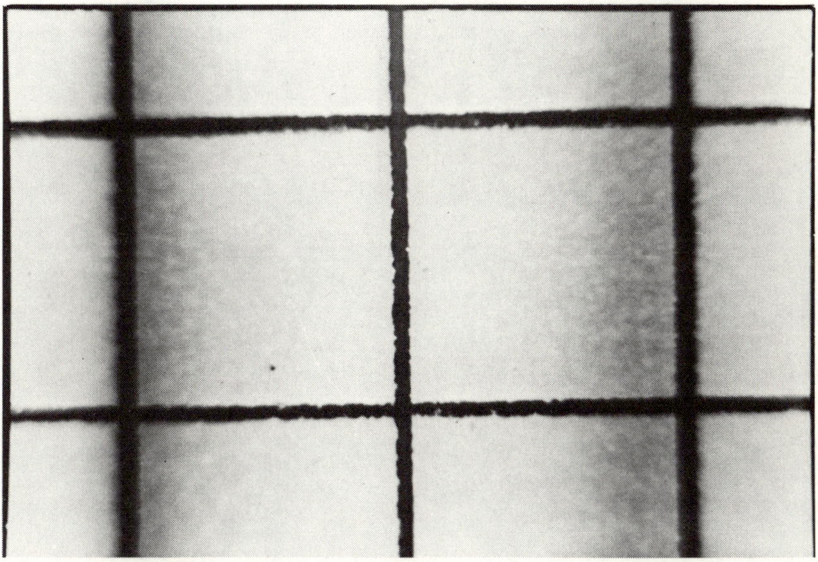

Figure 9-4 Grid of 1 cm squares photographed with the 50 mm lens used in Figure 9-2 but with 51 mm of added extension in the form of tubes. Although the field size is smaller than Figure 9-3, image quality is lower.

maintain a sharp image. A 50 mm nonmacro lens has limited built-in focus travel, usually less than 10 mm, and to focus for close-up copy work a bellows or extension tubes are used to augment this travel. A macro lens, however, customarily will be extensible for a distance equal to its focal length. Figure 9-5 shows a 35 mm SLR camera body, physically compact normal lens, extension tube set in multiples of 10 mm length, and the larger, fully extended macro lens. Table 9-1 lists the nominal dimensions of five intraoral and eight extraoral films, including two used for panoramic tomography. As the film size (subject) decreases toward "Dental 0," its distance from the lens will also decrease, and as much as 51 mm of lens extension must be added, via extension tubes or bellows, to maintain the largest possible sharp image. When the size of the film is large, such as 8 × 10 inches, a nonmacro lens will have sufficient travel to fill the 35 mm frame. However, for enlargement factors* of 0.2 or greater

*The enlargement factor is sometimes termed the "scale of reproduction, M"[10-13] and is the ratio of the size of the image to the size of the subject. The image size is constant and equal to the length (36 mm) or height (24 mm) of the 35 mm film frame, while the subject's respective dimension varies depending upon the radiograph being copied.

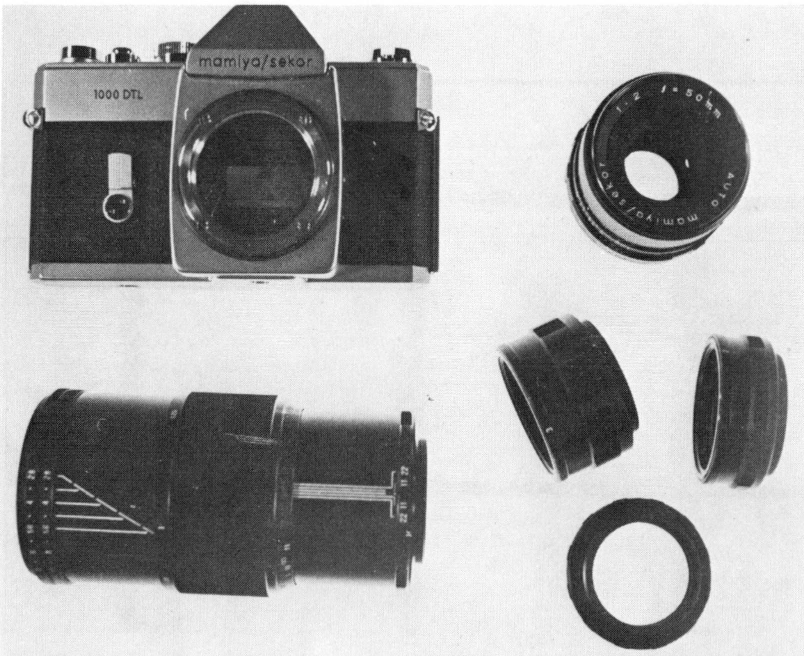

Figure 9-5 Clockwise from top left: typical single lens reflex camera body, normal lens, automatic extension tube set, and fully extended 60 mm macro lens.

Table 9-1
Subject-to-Lens Distances for Copying Radiographs with Normal 50 mm Lens

Type	Nominal film dimensions: *Inches* a	*Inches* b	*Millimeters** a	*Millimeters** b	Distance from subject to front of lens, mm	Added extension, mm (bellows or tubes), lens set at ∞	Enlargement factor† Size image:size subject
Dental 0	7/8	1 3/8	22	35	99	51	1.03
Dental 1	15/16	1 9/16	23	39	104	46	.92
Dental 2	1 3/16	1 19/32	30	40	113	40	.8
Dental 3	1 1/16	2 3/32	27	53	124	34	.68
Occlusal	2 1/4	3	57	76	169	21	.42
Extraoral	5	7	127	178	313	9.5	.19
Extraoral	8	10	203	254	467	‡	.12
Panoramic	5	12	127	305	467		.12
Panoramic	6	12	152	305	467		.12
Extraoral	9 1/2	11 3/4	240	300	550		.1
Extraoral	10	12	254	305	581		.094
Extraoral	11	14	279	356	631		.086
Extraoral	14	17	356	432	796		.067

*Field adjusted to accommodate underlined dimension, light spillover from remaining dimension masked; a = width; b = height.
†Sometimes denoted "Scale of reproduction, M."
‡Sufficient lens extension without use of extension tubes or bellows.

to fill the 35 mm frame with a subject less than 8 × 10 inches, a macro lens is the most convenient.

Figure 9-6 graphically displays, for a 50 mm lens, the correlation between lens extension, resultant enlargement factor, and the subject size that would completely fill the 35 mm frame. Lens extension of 50 mm allows a 1:1 image:subject size ratio with a 50 mm focal length lens. Less extension reduces enlargement and allows accommodation of larger subjects, while extension by a distance more than the lens' focal length enlarges the subject to fill the 24 × 36 mm frame.

Depending upon the manufacturer, a macro lens may have a focal length greater than 50 mm. However, for 1:1 image: subject size ratio, extension† will always be equal to focal length. This is expressed by the formula:

$$\text{Enlargement factor} = \frac{\text{Lens extension, mm}}{\text{Focal length of lens, mm}}$$

†When set at infinity (∞), a lens is fully collapsed. Lens extension to focus on close-up subjects, therefore, is affected by moving the lens away from the film plane with bellows, tubes, or the lens' own focusing control.

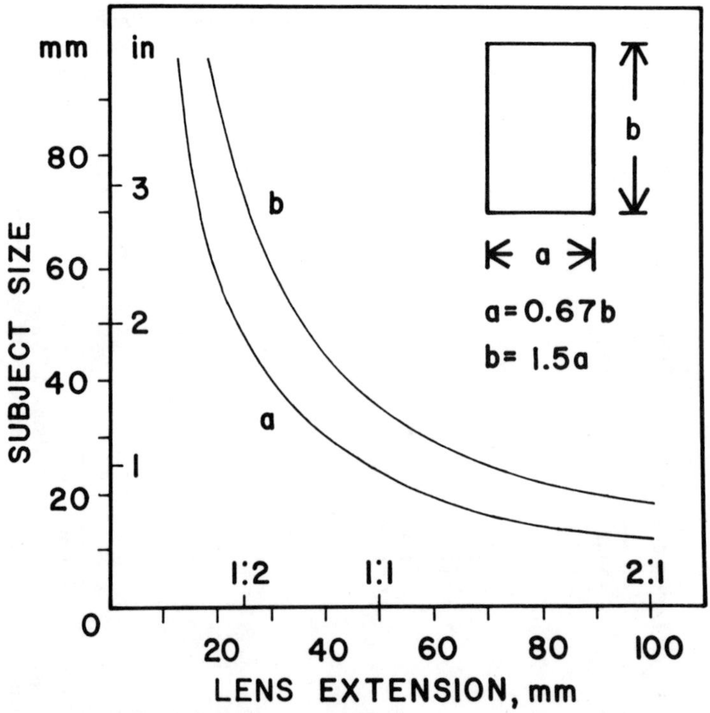

Figure 9-6 The relationship between subject dimension (a = width, b = height) and the amount of lens extension beyond the infinity setting. For the 50 mm lens illustrated here, 50 mm of extension permits 1:1 copying and a subject size equal to the 35 mm film frame size.

and is shown graphically in Figure 9-7. As lenses of shorter focal lengths are used, less extension of the lens provides greater close-up potential.

This may also be seen in Figure 9-8, in which 50 mm and 100 mm lenses are compared for distance from the subject to the front surface of the lens and the resultant enlargement factor. As the subject distance from lens increases, the degree of enlargement decreases; that is, larger subjects can be accommodated but at lower enlargement factors. This was seen in Table 9-1 as well. The formula:

$$\text{Enlargement factor} = \frac{\text{Focal length of lens, mm}}{\text{Subject distance from lens, mm} - \text{Focal length of lens, mm}}$$

demonstrates that for an enlargement factor of one (1:1 image:subject size ratio) the distance from lens to subject is two times the focal length. For this same enlargement factor, the lens is extended an amount equal to its focal length. Most radiographs are copied within the range of distances given in Figure 9-8 and have sizes as in Figure 9-3.

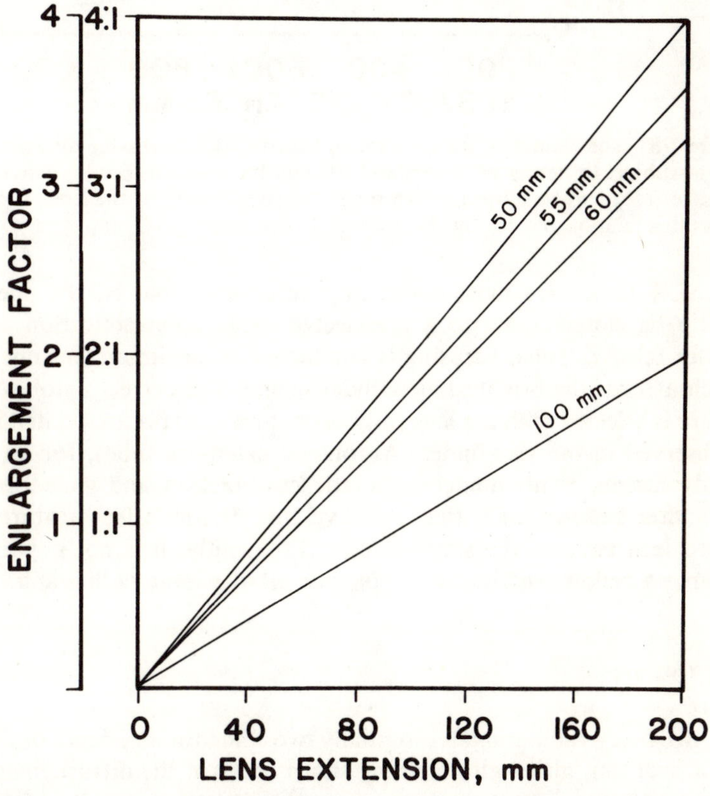

Figure 9-7 The relationship between lens extension and resultant enlargement of subject (enlargement factors > 1) for lenses of different focal length.

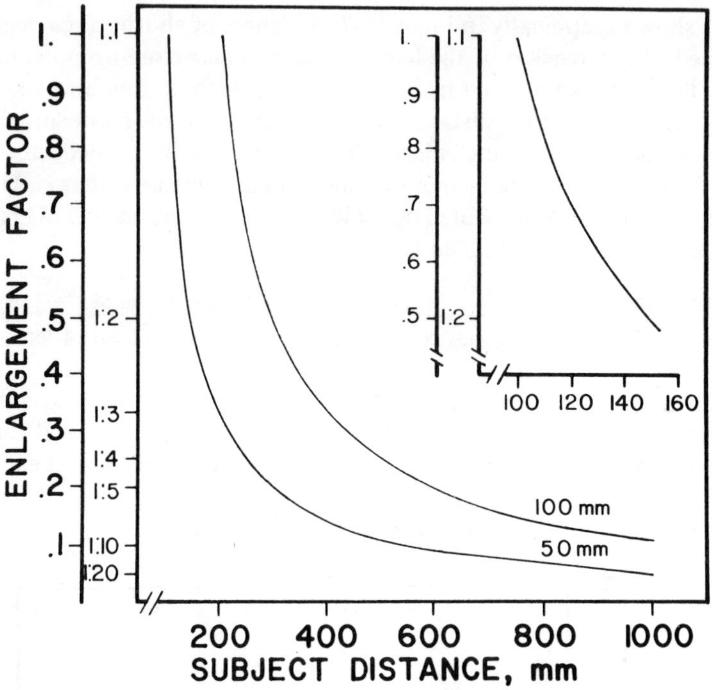

Figure 9-8 The change in the enlargement factor with increasing distance from lens-to-subject for lenses of 50 mm and 100 mm focal length. For 1:1 copying the distance from lens-to-subject is two times the focal length of the lens. The inset shows this relationship for the 50 mm lens at distances < 200 mm.

SLR lenses are most commonly automatic; that is, the aperture (f-stop) is closed down to a preselected value upon activation of the shutter release. Thus, focusing is conducted at maximum lens opening, which affords the brightest viewfinder image. The correct f-stop for exposure is selected with the lens fully open, and an exposure-related index is observed in the viewfinder. Automatic extension tubes, for all their disadvantages, do not hinder automatic lens function, and while there are automatic bellows units that preserve this desirable lens feature, the macro lens remains the simplest unit. Frequently, it is not possible to collapse a bellows sufficiently to include all of a large radiograph.

FOCUSING

Because a radiograph is essentially two-dimensional, depth of field is not a problem, although obtaining sharp focus of the diffuse image on grainy x-ray film is. A simple focusing aid is the use of a piece of fully exposed x-ray film placed in the field of view. The edge of this film is flexed against the radiograph to be copied and is brought into sharp focus (Figure 9-9). The radiograph below the focusing aid will also be in focus. Some SLR cameras have interchangeable prisms and viewing screens as well as supplementary magnifiers and angled extensions for the viewfinder. Where available, fine grain focusing screens are a help, although the choice is quite subjective and depends much upon the user's visual acuity. The importance of precise focusing, however, cannot be overemphasized.

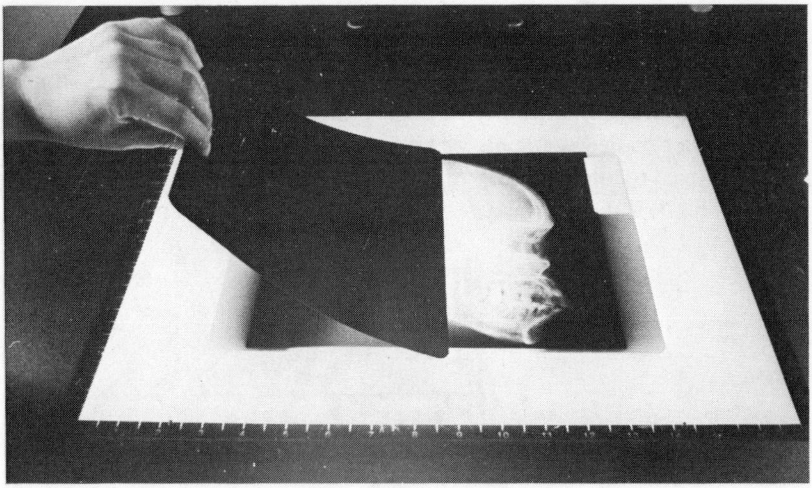

Figure 9-9 Use of focusing aid in copying radiographs.

ILLUMINATION AND CAMERA SUPPORT

Generally, the brightest, most uniform (white) light source available is the best. This is because film for producing fine grain negatives, such as Kodak Panatomic-X, has a modest speed of ASA 32, while film for producing black-and-white slides for projection, such as Kodak SO-185, is extremely slow and requires lengthy exposures. The camera's shutter and lens aperture are available to reduce film exposure if required. Consequently, the low light intensity of the radiograph view box imposes the most severe limitation. Uniform illumination, in which the fluorescent tubes are matched and of similar age and manufacture and the opal light diffuser is clean, will prevent bands of subtly different densities from appearing in the copy.

There is some latitude in the selection of a camera mount for radiograph copying. If the view box is normally mounted vertically, a tripod is suitable for the lengthy exposures required by SO-185 copy film.

However, for the shorter exposures with faster films that yield negative intermediates for prints, a shutter speed of at least 1/125 sec, released while standing firmly with elbows against the body, should suffice. Here, maintaining image composition while releasing the shutter is sometimes a problem. It should be borne in mind that as film-to-subject distance decreases, the effect of any camera motion is heightened and will become noticeable as blur in the copy. For light sources fixed horizontally, a more formal copy stand, in which the camera is aimed downward over the center of the view box, should be obtained or improvised. Figure 9-10 shows an inexpensive copy stand with a separate view box placed on its base; the photofloods are used for copying by reflected light. Figure 9-11 is a more elaborate device with integrated view box, electronic shutter control, and greater flexibility in positioning the camera.

Whether copied vertically or horizontally, the radiograph or camera may be moved to allow the copying of a selected area of the film, with two caveats. First, the film plane of the camera must be parallel to the

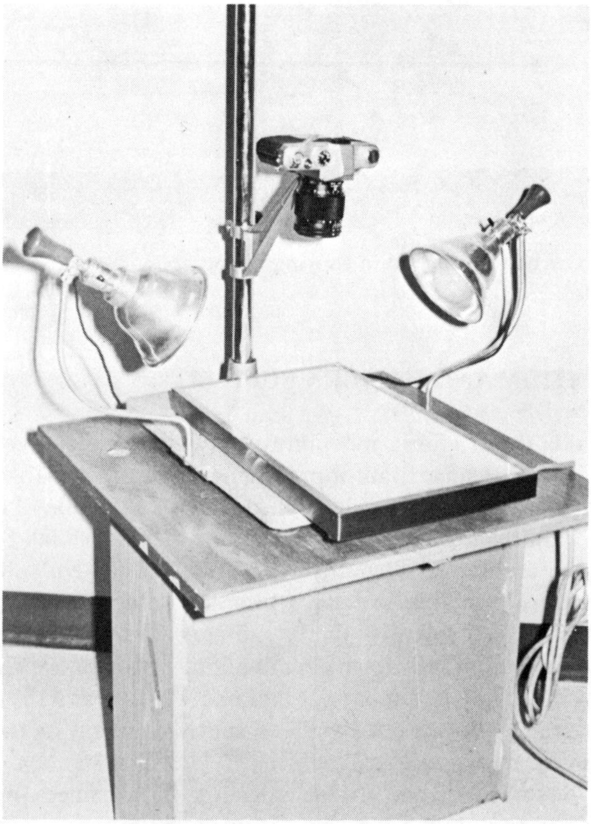

Figure 9-10 Copy stand with separately mounted radiograph illuminator.

radiograph being copied. As a dental analogy, the "central ray" through the camera's lens should be normal or perpendicular to both film and radiograph planes. Second, the light source should be visibly uniform over the copy field.

For copy work, the areas of the radiograph immediately *outside* the camera's field of view should be masked with opaque black construction paper or fully exposed sheets of film. Similarly, areas of light spillover from the view box *into* the metered area of the field of view will lead to underestimation of correct exposure, and inclusion of opaque masks in the same area will lead to overexposure. Therefore, it is important that the portion of the field of view on which the exposure is determined, as specified by the manufacturer, contains only the radiograph being copied. Radiographs that do not lie flat may be overlaid with a sheet of clean plate glass after focusing. To avoid reflections and to aid focusing, room lights should be extinguished. As visual dark adaptation is best for reading diagnostic films, so, too, is focusing for copy purposes made easier.

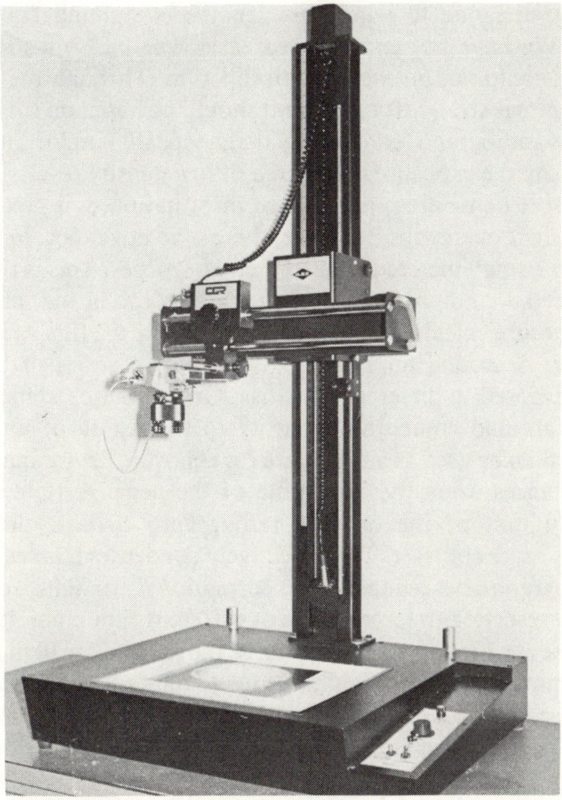

Figure 9-11 Copy stand with integral illuminator and electronic timer for lengthy B exposures.

NEGATIVE FILMS AND EXPOSURE

Although there are a number of films suitable for producing slides or negative intermediates from radiographs,[14,15] only a few have gained currency, and undoubtedly none has precisely the same tonal range as the original radiograph. For obtaining negatives with fine grain suitable for moderately enlarged photographic prints without loss of image quality, Kodak Panatomic-X is rated at ASA 32 and developed with Kodak Microdol-X 1:3 for 11 minutes at 24 °C in standard tanks agitated for 5 seconds every 30 seconds. While this has proven suitable in our hands, other film/developer/time combinations are employed. In general, the negative should contain detail (density differences) in all areas in which the original contained detail. If the negatives consistently have too much contrast, a starting point for experimentation would be a lengthened exposure and shortened development time or pre-exposure of the film, as described below. Panatomic-X is available in standard 35 mm magazines of 20 or 36 exposures as well as in long bulk rolls, which have the advantage of allowing one to wind film lengths containing fewer than 20 exposures. We have not encountered cases where diagnostically useful radiographs could not be copied with this film. Through-the-lens metering of exposure is straightforward and should be based on the most dense area of the radiograph containing diagnostically important information.[1,16] Basing the exposure on an area of low density results in underexposure of more dense areas and loss of information; it is better to err on the side of *slight* overexposure. Here, there is an advantage in the use of a camera with a small metered area for copy purposes. This is the ability to position a detail-containing area of the radiograph in the small metered field for exposure calculation, and then to relocate the film as appropriate for copying. A second approach is to employ a series of blank films uniformly exposed to different densities. One of these "standard" films of appropriate and comparable density to the region of interest being copied may then be used as a surrogate for exposure determination. There may be instances when the grey scale of the negative (intermediate) is shorter than that of the original radiograph; that is, the copy has significantly more contrast. This effectively condenses nuances of density in the radiograph and reduces the informational content. To overcome this without resorting to large stocks of different film types, it is possible to pre-expose the film used for copying to the same white light that will be used to illuminate the radiograph, *but* for 1/100 to 1/200 of the exposure time to be used for the final copy.[16,17,18] This pre-exposed frame is then rewound and the copy made as a double exposure. Intentional double exposures are difficult to make with the SLR because the camera's focal plane shutter spring is tensioned in the film advance operation. There is frequently a problem in obtaining reregistration of the pre-exposed frame.

Negative intermediates of 35 mm film will always be enlarged, and it is at this stage that additional control over the copy image can be exercised by cropping the image to exclude unwanted areas from the final print. It is also possible to make black-and-white prints from color negatives.[19] The contrast of the print can be increased by using enlarging paper grades such as 3 or 4 and an F or glossy surface, or may be reduced by using paper grade 1. Paper grade 2 is most frequently used as it minimally reduces or heightens contrast, but obviously requires a uniform and well-exposed subject. Such photographic contrast shifts are roughly analogous to grey-scale lengthening or shortening via kilovoltage changes. Increasing overall density in the copy by means of lengthening the exposure time functions much as varying the mAs controls on the x-ray machine. By dodging, in which light transmitted through low density areas of the negative is held back from the enlarging paper by rapidly moving the hands or other opaque objects to intercept the light rays, detail in dense areas of the radiograph may be heightened. Burning-in is the opposite of the dodging procedure and augments the exposure of low density areas of the radiograph by selectively overexposing the corresponding high density areas of the negative through suitable masks or cones formed by the cupped palms. One must be cautious not to "introduce" pathology through injudicious use of these techniques. These procedures are confined to the darkroom inasmuch as the fractional second exposures yielding the negative intermediate do not permit such manipulations.

Figures 9-12, 9-13, and 9-14 are different treatments of the same sialogram. Figure 9-12 is a straightforward copy of the film with the exposure based on the average density of the entire film (large, center-weighted meter area). The glandular tissue is indistinct because exposure was biased by the large, low density area corresponding to bone. Figure 9-13 is the same negative intermediate printed with the bony areas burned in to reveal their detail. Figure 9-14 is a spot meter exposure based on the glandular tissue. The sialogram was positioned with the salivary gland tissue in the spot meter field, the correct exposure for this structure set, the film repositioned, and the exposure made. The appearance of the filling of the tissue is heightened at the expense of other, less critical structures. The exposure technique used in Figure 9-14 is applicable to copies yielding negative intermediates from which prints will be produced as well as the production of direct positives.

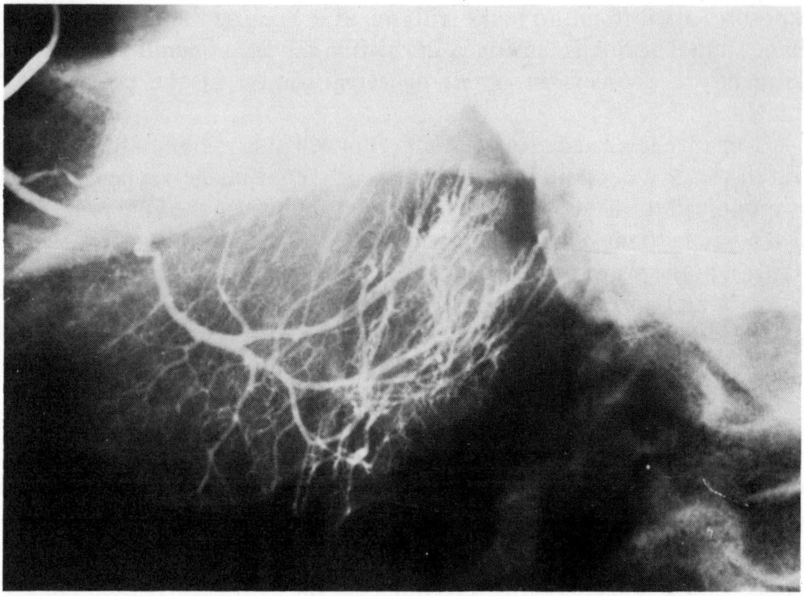

Figure 9-12 Photograph of sialogram copied with 60 mm macro lens on Kodak Panatomic-X film. Exposure was based on average density of radiograph and the negative intermediate was printed on enlarging paper grade 2. Note glandular tissue and lack of detail in bony structure.

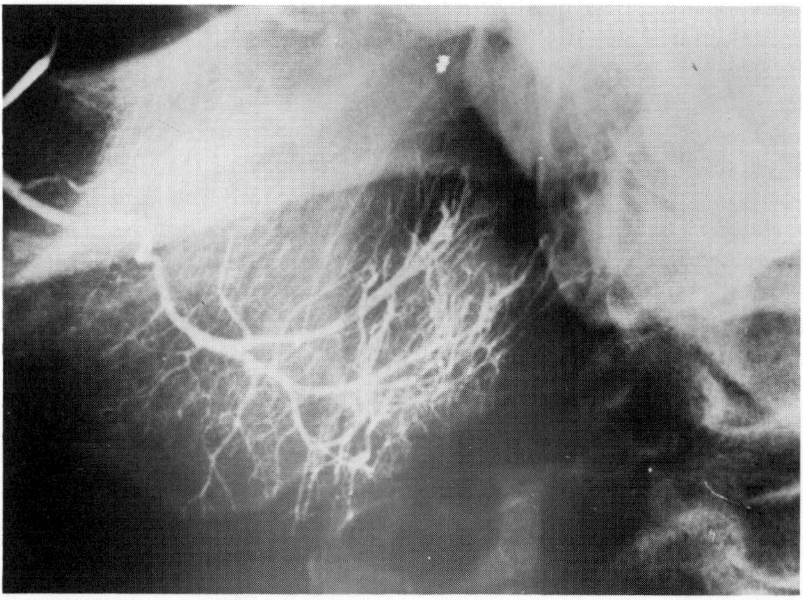

Figure 9-13 Print of same negative as Figure 9-12 with detail in bony area burned-in by selective overexposure during enlargement.

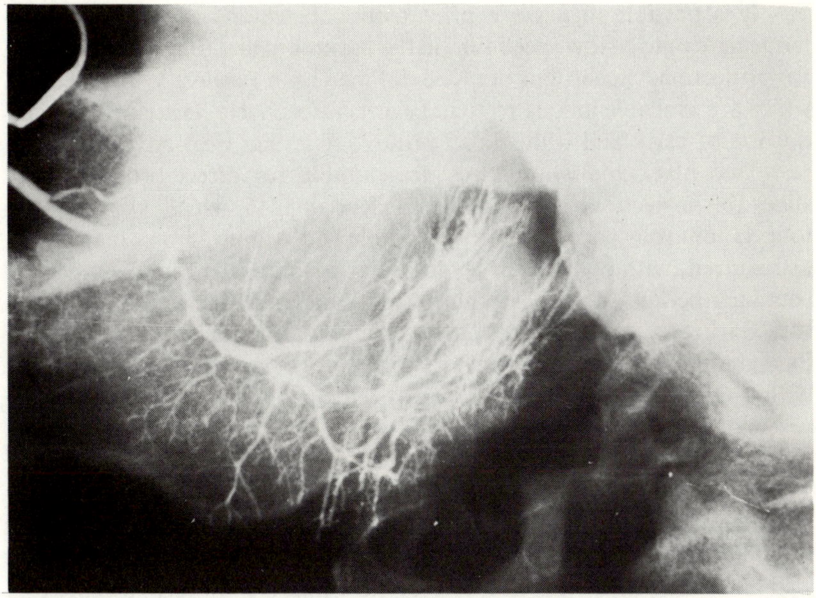

Figure 9-14 Same sialogram as Figure 9-12 but with exposure based on glandular tissue through the use of a spot exposure meter.

DIRECT POSITIVE FILMS AND EXPOSURES

For copies of a direct positive type, which yield slides for projection, color slide film may be the most readily available, especially if the camera serves a dual function in clinic and/or home. While no 35 mm film, black-and-white or color, will have precisely the same tonal scale as a radiograph, daylight color slide film introduces the problem of color balance associated with the light source. Thus, film balanced for daylight or electronic flash (5500 °K) will yield yellow-green slides of x-rays when exposed by fluorescent or tungsten illumination (3200 °K to 3400 °K). It is possible, knowing the temperature of the light source and the light balance of the film, to bring both into reasonable harmony with supplementary filters such as those of the Kodak 81 series, which reduce light temperature, or those of the 82 series, which raise it. Larger magnitude changes are affected with 85 series and CC (color compensating) filters used in concert with 81 or 82 series or with the Tiffen FL-D.[15,20] As more filters are added, the exposure time increases and so indicates the use of a fast color slide film.[21] Therefore, it becomes important to standardize film and light source (bulb age and manufacturer), or inordinate amounts of time and material may be spent in trial and error filter substitutions. In any event, the images will have a bluish tint that may be subjectively bothersome, and the film may require pre-exposure to mute contrast.

It is possible to make a print from a black-and-white negative intermediate onto a slow speed film in the darkroom and to mount the image for projection.[6] Such films are Kodak Fine Grain Positive 5302 and 7302, which are available in long rolls and sheets respectively. However, the production of black-and-white direct positive slides has clear advantages.

Two black-and-white films are suitable for direct production of slides for projection.[16,22,23] The first is Kodak 5246, which is available in long 35 mm rolls and is therefore suitable for loading 35 mm magazines, as required, with convenient lengths. For loading, the film should be at room temperature for several hours and handled with clean dry hands in total darkness. Its ASA speeds of 64 for tungsten illumination and 80 for daylight mean conveniently short exposures, perhaps even hand-held with a suitably bright view box. However, processing this direct positive reversal film entails eight steps and more than one hour with special chemistry or the services of a commercial photo laboratory.

With Kodak SO-185 film, however, rapid processing (RP) equipment and chemistry is used to produce direct positive slides of copied radiographs. For all its convenience and its availability in 36-exposure as well as in long rolls, this film is very slow and has no meaningful ASA value that can be used in setting the camera's exposure meter. It absolutely requires rigid camera support during exposures, which commonly are over 15 seconds in length. Processing with RP chemistry in a Kodak X-Omat or equivalent machine is simply done and requires no resetting of machine time or temperature. If care has been taken not to rewind the film fully into its magazine, the leader end may be cut straight across, butted against a piece of clean scrap x-ray film, and secured top and bottom with heat-stable tape—Scotch Electrical Tape No. 3—to withstand the drying temperatures that soften most tape adhesives. The lights are switched off, and the leader started into the processor pulling the film, emulsion side up, out of the magazine. The film is cut off flush with the magazine opening when resistance is felt. Alternatively, the film may be developed in a tank with standard x-ray processing chemicals, once loaded onto a suitable reel. In either case, the dry finished slides are cut apart and mounted in suitable snap-together binders.

As implied above, the slow speed of SO-185 requires a fair amount of experimentation to find the optimum exposure time with the particular light source employed. These determinations are customarily made with the lens fully open. Frequently, for every radiograph a series of several different exposures is made, and the one appearing to be the most reasonable compromise is selected for use. (This selection should be made based on the light reflected from a screen by the projected image rather than by the more expedient method of viewing the film strip with transmitted light.)

We have employed a technique with SO-185 that assigns an arbitrary

ASA speed to the film. This technique has four advantages. 1) It permits elimination of the test series of exposures for every radiograph being copied. 2) Exposure correction is possible for radiographs of different densities. 3) The exposure of the film can be based on a selected area of either high or low density that contains detail of interest associated with normal or pathologic conditions. 4) There are savings in material. To determine the duration of exposure time, which will become a constant in this procedure, an average radiograph is selected, and the viewed image is composed and focused with suitable precautions to exclude from the metered area both light spill from the view box and opaque masks. A shutter speed and ASA film speed are selected arbitrarily and set such that the camera's built-in exposure meter indicates correct exposure with the lens stopped down 1 to 1.5 stops from fully open. (These two settings are flexible and serve only to establish two constants for further work. Depending on the intensity of the light source, for example, these values can be 1/125 second with ASA 64.) The two values at which the exposure meter was nulled with the "average" radiograph subject are recorded. Then the shutter speed is changed to Bulb and a trial series of exposures from 10 to 60 seconds by 10 second increments is made. The slides are processed and mounted, and the best projected image is selected. The time for this exposure should be recorded inasmuch as it will be used for all subsequent radiograph copying with that view box and initially selected ASA and shutter speeds. The only variable is the lens opening or f-stop, and this is used to compensate for radiographs of different average density as well as for basing exposure of an entire film on a selected area of atypical density. For copying all subsequent films, the initial shutter and ASA speeds (1/125 second, ASA 64) are set and the f-stop is used to null the exposure meter and thereby to correct for differences between radiograph densities. The shutter speed control is reset to Bulb, and the film exposed at the newly set f-stop for the time determined by the initial exposure series. This procedure is summarized in Table 9-2.

For making same-size, 1:1, copies of small intraoral films (for projection) or of larger extraoral films, Kodak RP-D X-Omat film has the added convenience of rapid or conventional x-ray processing.[14,16,23] A range of sizes from 8 × 10 inch to 14 × 17 inch is available, and the film may be handled under Kodak 6B safelight conditions. Several periapical films may be copied at once on a single sheet of RP-D film and, after processing, cut apart into 35 × 37 mm sizes for mounting. This film is most accurately exposed and radiograph density differences most faithfully maintained by ultraviolet light. The use of other types of light, such as the tungsten or fluorescent illumination of a typical photographic contact printer, yields copies with more contrast than the original. For these reasons, a printer with appropriate light source, timer, and means of ensuring close contact between original(s) and copy film is recommended.

Table 9-2
Determining Exposure with Kodak SO-185 Copy Film

STEPS

1. Select average radiograph, compose, focus, and mask to exclude extraneous light as required.
2. Close lens aperture 1 to 1.5 f-stops from fully open, eg, to f4 or f4.5 with an f2.8 lens.
3. Arbitrarily select and set an ASA film speed and shutter speed to obtain correct exposure as indicated by camera's light meter.
4. Record this film speed and shutter speed, eg, ASA 64, 1/125 second.
5. Reset shutter to Bulb and make trial series of exposures from 10 to 60 seconds in 10 second increments.
6. Process, mount, project, and select most suitable image.
7. Record this slide's exposure time, eg, 20 seconds.
8. For subsequent copies of other films, reset shutter to values recorded in step 4 (verify ASA setting) and adjust f-stop to give correct exposure.
9. Return shutter to Bulb and expose for time recorded in step 7.

SUMMARY

1. Constants: ASA speed, initial shutter speed, final exposure time.
2. Variable: f-stop.

NOTE

These procedures are applicable to cameras with a spot meter instead of or in addition to an averaging meter by noting the spot meter setting at steps 3 and 8. A hand-held exposure meter, separate from the camera, may also be used, provided its angle of acceptance is sufficiently narrow that when held at or near the film plane it "sees" only radiograph.

However, it is possible to expose RP-D X-Omat film by room light or by the light of a fluorescent view box and to process it manually if several variables can be controlled. Complete, close, and uniform contact must be assured between the original(s) and the copy film to obtain the sharpest image. To facilitate this, in a darkroom, the demounted intraoral films are placed over the copy film in a spring-loaded printing frame, which resembles an x-ray film cassette with a glass front, or at least are placed under the weight of a piece of heavy plate glass. The room lights or view box may be switched on for an exposure time determined by prior experimentation. For reproducibility, the distance from the light source and its intensity should be constant and have been adjusted to require no less than a 5-second exposure. If the fluorescent tubes tend to flicker before lighting, it may be best to store the loaded printing frame in a drawer or beneath an opaque cover until the exposure source has stabilized.

REFERENCES

1. Brownell, C.G. Making copies of radiographs. *Med Radiogr Photogr.* 27:114–120, 1951.

2. Tribe, H.E. Photographic copying for the dentist. *Dent Clin North Am.* Nov:773–783, 1968.

3. Corney, G.M., and Splettstosser, H.R. Intensifying underexposed radiographs. *Med Radiogr Photogr.* 27:128–129, 1951.

4. Kattan, K.R., Caplan, M.L., and Felson, B. A method for improving roentgenographic illustrations for publication—blurred undersubtraction (BUS). *Med Radiogr Photogr.* 49:21–22, 1973.

5. Maurer, R.E., Yule, J.A.C., and Cornwell, W.S. A masking technique for making radiographic paper duplicates. *Med Radiogr Photogr.* 27:121–125, 1951.

6. Seidler, B. Duplicating and dodging in copying radiographs. *Dent Radiogr Photogr.* 43:12–18, 1969.

7. Winestock, D.P., and White, E.T. Mask for use in cropping radiographs. *Med Radiogr Photogr.* 53:16–18, 1977.

8. Hetherington, W.I., and Freehe, C.L. Single lens reflex cameras and associated equipment for use in dental photography. *Dent Clin North Am.* Nov:699–729, 1968.

9. Manuel, W.B. Extraoral small-object photography. *Dent Clin North Am.* Nov:757–762, 1968.

10. Gibson, H.L. Practical optics and basic lightings in dental photography. *Dent Clin North Am.* Nov:675–693, 1968.

11. Purves, F., and Mannheim, L. In *The Focal Encyclopedia of Photography.* London: Focal Press, 1965, Vol. 1, pp. 251–255, 352–356.

12. Close-up photography. In *The Encyclopedia of Practical Photography.* Vol. 3. Edited by Eastman Kodak. New York: Amphoto, 1978.

13. Copying. In *The Encyclopedia of Practical Photography.* Vol. 4. Edited by Eastman Kodak. New York: Amphoto, 1978.

14. Gibson, H.L. Direct duplicates of dental radiographs. *Dent Radiogr Photogr.* 38:60–63, 1965.

15. Hurtgen, T.P. Understanding photographic parameters—guides to film selection. In *Biomedical Photography.* A Kodak Seminar in Print. Rochester, N.Y.: Eastman Kodak, 1976.

16. *Copying Radiographs.* Rochester, N.Y.: Eastman Kodak, 1975.

17. Gibson, H.L. Copying radiographs with miniature Kodachrome film. *Med Radiogr Photogr.* 27:125–127, 1951.

18. Gibson, H.L. Copying dental radiographs with Kodachrome film. *Dent Radiogr Photogr.* 25:57–60, 1952.

19. Gibson, H.L. Black and white prints from color negatives—a discussion of Kodak Panalure paper. *Dent Radiogr Photogr.* 31:71–72, 1958.

20. Sherrill, C.A. Professional techniques in dental photography. In *Biomedical Photography.* A Kodak Seminar in Print. Rochester, N.Y.: Eastman Kodak, 1976.

21. Hurtgen, T.L. Kodak color films for dental photography. *Dent Radiogr Photogr.* 50:48–53, 1977.

22. Gibson, H.L. Making direct positive slides with Kodak Panatomic-X film, 35 mm. *Dent Radiogr Photogr.* 31:71, 1958.

23. *Kodak RP/D X-Omat Radiograph Duplicating Film Technique Guide.* Rochester, N.Y.: Eastman Kodak, 1975.

SECTION II

DIAGNOSIS

10 Principles of Interpretation

There is a common misconception about the role of radiology in dental diagnosis and treatment planning. Because two-thirds to three-quarters of all tooth structures lie within bone and cannot be examined clinically, many dentists assume that an x-ray examination is a mandatory or routine procedure for all patients. Such a position cannot be supported for several important reasons. First, the best available information defining the effects of x-irradiation on human tissues indicates that there are small but important hazards.[1] Second, x-ray examinations constitute a significant cost in the overall perspective of our health care system and, therefore, the elimination of unnecessary examinations is a productive step toward cost containment.[2] Finally, if one examines the rationale behind the routine use of x-ray examinations, one experiences great difficulty in justifying the continued use of the practice. The examination of any part of the body must be based on the anticipation of positive findings arising from clues obtained during a careful history and physical examination.

X-RAY DIAGNOSIS

Criteria

In recent studies, Phillips[3] and Bell and Loop[4] demonstrated that it is possible to develop criteria or indications for a specific type of x-ray examination so that the yield of useful findings is high without significant chance of diagnostic error resulting from omission of an exam or an inappropriate examination. The development and application of these high yield criteria to skull examinations in trauma patients lead to a 60% reduction in the number of examinations with no apparent effect on the success of therapy.

The criteria that can be most productively used in dentistry come from the history and physical examination of each patient. A history of pain, diminished sensation, trauma, systemic disease, certain habits, or the chronic use of medication may be indications for an x-ray examination. Developmental anomalies including delayed or premature eruption of teeth or family histories of missing or supernumerary teeth may require investigation. Independent of a history obtained from any individual, it must also be recognized that impactions of some teeth occur with predictably high frequency, as do developmental cysts, supernumerary teeth, and congenitally missing teeth. These abnormalities occur during development and should be assessed by x-ray of appropriate anatomic sites at predetermined intervals during development. It is often possible to derive several types of information from a single examination. For example, the use of a number 2 film for a bitewing examination in a seven- or eight-year-old child will often produce evidence of a congenitally missing premolar at a time when space problems can be most flexibly managed. Obviously, the likelihood of finding a developmental cyst or a supernumerary tooth in an adult is extremely unlikely if that individual has had dental care during his or her developmental years.

Physical findings constitute the most obvious indication for radiographic examination. Unexplained swelling, trauma, missing teeth, deep caries, or displaced teeth clearly require further evaluation unless adequate information is obtainable from the patient's history. Physical abnormalities at other sites of the body or evidence of systemic disease may also raise the clinician's index of suspicion to a point where radiographic examination becomes advisable. At each point, however, judgement is important. The probability of alveolar bone destruction in an uncontrolled diabetic is quite high while the probability of detecting metastatic lesions in the jaws is relatively low and should be assessed in terms of the site and type of the primary lesion.

Once the history and clinical examination have been completed, the need for x-rays and other supplemental studies can be determined. The entire data base must then be considered for its completeness and adequacy. If the data are sufficient, a differential diagnosis can be developed, and the findings can be sequenced according to appropriate priorities. If the data are insufficient, the need for additional tests will become apparent.

Treatment Components

Treatment can be divided into three components. The first phase of treatment deals with acute problems and preparation of the patient for definitive therapy. Local and systemic diseases must be arrested and stabilized. Relief of pain is a primary consideration. Radiographic examination may be required at this time. The second phase of treatment is concerned primarily with corrective therapy. At this stage, restorations and prosthetic devices may be constructed. The need for radiographs during corrective treatment is unusual. Restorative margins and the placement of prosthetic devices can usually be established by clinical examination. In those instances in which radiographic examination is essential, extreme care must be paid to the technical aspects since small errors in film placement, tube angulation, processing, or the choice of exposure factors can distort the image and create a deceptive picture (Figure 10-1).

The final phase of treatment planning is the formalization of plans for follow-up or recall. Again, it is important to exercise judgement in determining the frequency and extent of follow-up examinations. Individuals with a history of a high caries attack rate or rapidly progressing periodontal disease may require frequent bitewing examinations. Other individuals who have undergone endodontic treatment or have had extensive restorative work may require evaluation of the periapical areas of involved teeth. With increasing periods of post-treatment stability, the length of time between recall examinations (x-rays) can be progressively extended.

Choice of Examination

The information content of each x-ray film depends upon a great many factors and can be varied by the imaging process. Therefore, it is extremely important to choose the type of examination to be performed on any patient on the basis of a specific need of that patient. First, it is essential to define the diagnostic information that is required. It is then necessary to consider the biologic and economic costs that are involved. Based on these considerations it is possible to decide whether or not to proceed and, if so, how.

Some technical factors should be kept in mind. For example, the detail of a conventional nonscreen film is several times greater than that obtainable with screen film. In general, the amount of detail decreases as the speed of the imaging system increases. Tomographic examinations,

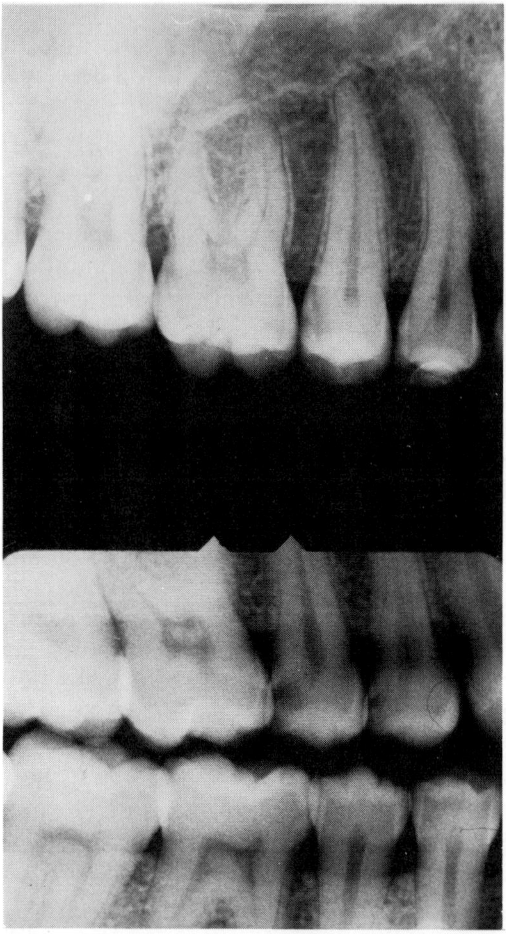

A

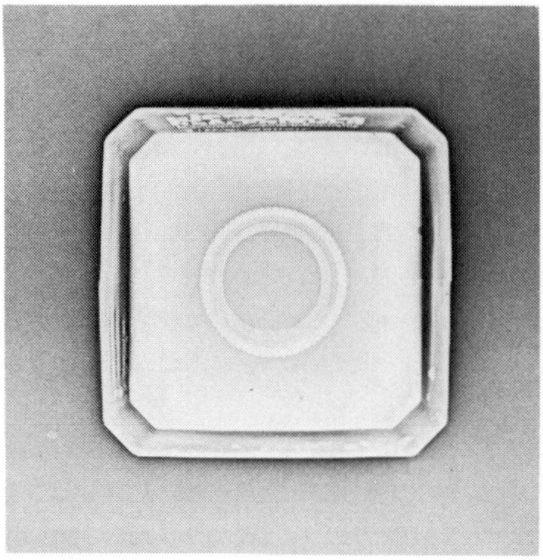

B

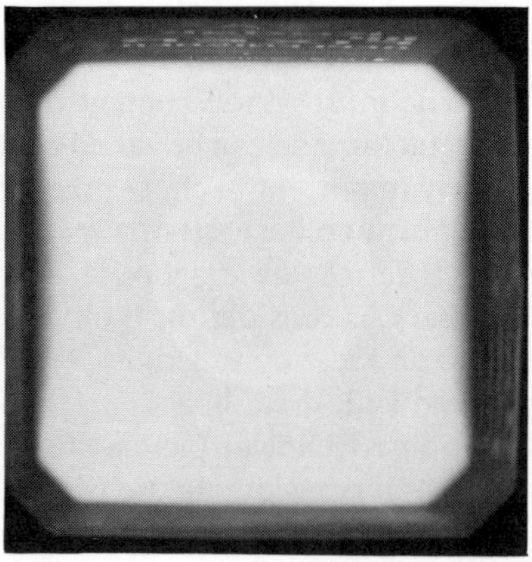

C

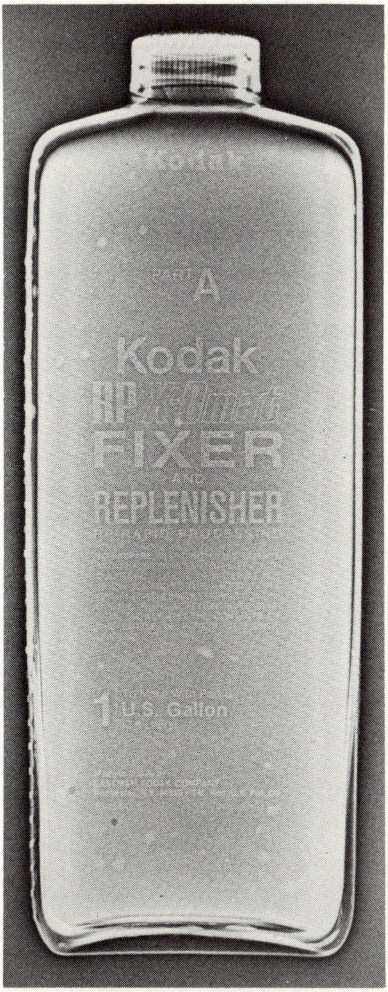

D

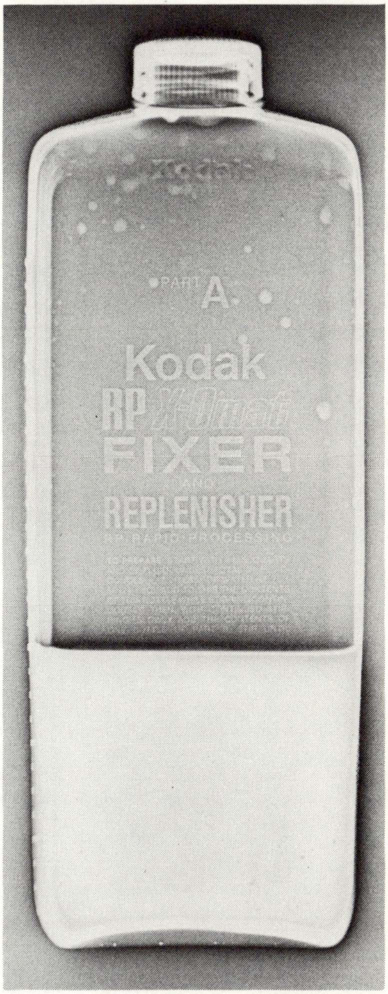

E

Figure 10-1 Distortions in radiographic films. **A.** A small change in vertical angulation makes a dramatic difference in the appearance of the carious lesions in the premolar teeth. **B.** Radiographs are two-dimensional representations of three-dimensional objects. Orientation of an object to the x-ray source in the film will greatly affect the ease with which the object can be recognized. In this radiograph of a bottle, the x-ray beam passed through its long axis toward a film which lay below. **C.** By changing the relative distance between the x-ray source, the object, and the film, the magnification of an image can be altered. In this radiograph, the bottle was moved away from the film and toward the x-ray source to produce magnification. **D.** Gravity also plays a role in the evaluation of dynamic structures. It is impossible to tell whether a vessel is empty or partially filled with fluid if it is radiographed in a horizontal position. **E.** By turning the bottle right side up and directing the x-ray beam perpendicular to its long axis, it is possible to determine its contents. Similar situations exist in the evaluation of sinuses, parts of the genitourinary system, and the gastrointestinal tract.

including panoramic examinations, are information-limited when compared to conventional films. Not only do these procedures use screen films but the movement required during the exposure is intended to degrade the images of structures outside of the plane of interest. Unfortunately, some degradation of the useful image plane also occurs.

RADIOGRAPHIC IMAGES

The interpretation of radiographic images must take into account several important factors. First, anatomic variation within individuals and between individuals is extensive. Second, calcified tissues, including teeth and bones, are dynamic structures that can change their size, shape, and density from time to time (Figure 10-2). Third, three-dimensional biologic structures are reduced to two-dimensional images by the radiographic process. Fourth, radiography is not precise. Even with rigorous controls, its ability to demonstrate small changes is limited.[5]

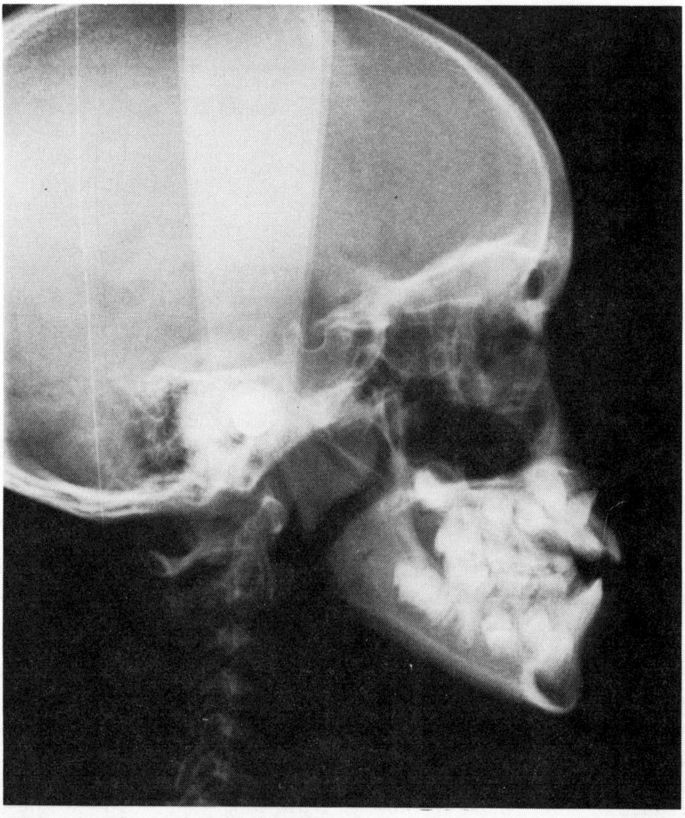

A

Figure 10-2 **A.** The cephalometric film shows a central incisor which appears to be maloccluded.

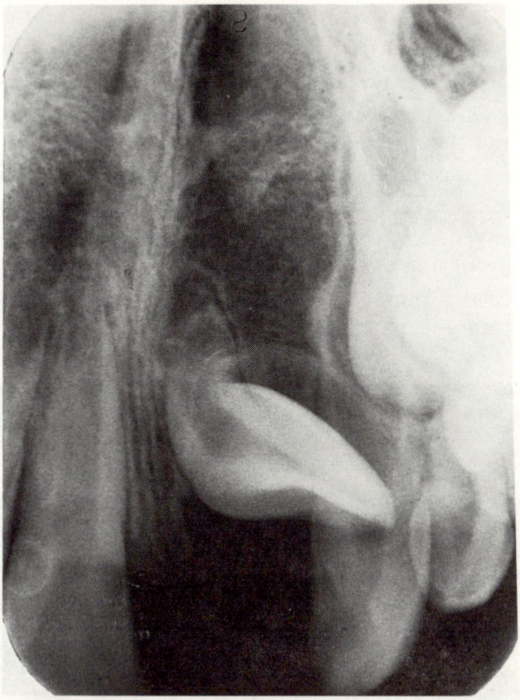

B

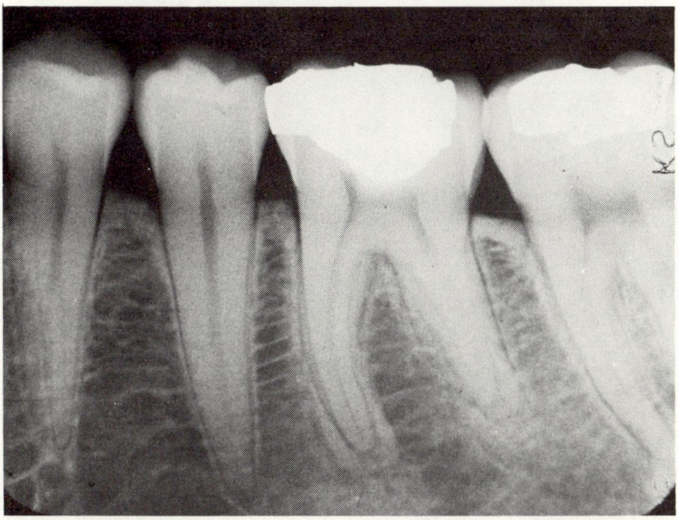

C

Figure 10-2 **B.** Closer inspection reveals that the crown of the central incisor lies at right angles to the developing root. This phenomenon, referred to as dilaceration, is believed to be the result of trauma. **C.** A physiologic response to stress is the thickening of surrounding bone. The lamina dura around the mesial root of the first molar demonstrates this response.

Under ordinary circumstances, radiographic technique is poorly controlled and significant errors can result from confusion between image artifact and biologic change. Fifth, the progress of a pathologic process is influenced by a variety of factors, including the aggressiveness of particular lesions and the resistance of the host. The image produced in one individual with a specific disease can vary dramatically from the image produced by the same disease process in another individual. Finally, the eyes of the observer are designed to deal with three-dimensional objects through the use of binocular vision. In many instances, physiologic characteristics of the human visual system can lead to erroneous conclusions (Figures 10-3 and 10-4).[6]

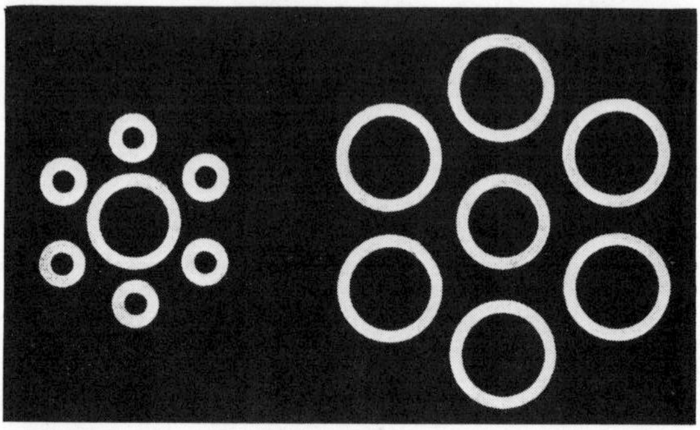

Figure 10-3 Misinterpretation of size. The circles lying in the center of each cluster are the same size, but the bone to the right appears smaller because of its size relative to structures at the periphery.

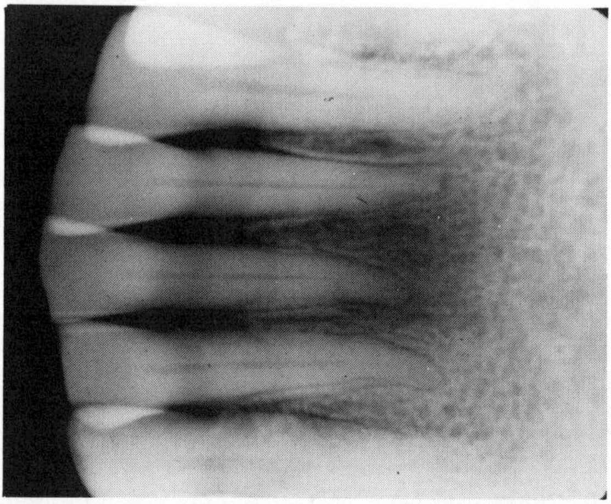

Figure 10-4 Misinterpretation of density. In areas where teeth overlap, dark lines appear to separate single and double thickness of enamel. These dark lines result from a physiologic phenomenon called lateral extinction. The dark lines are a visual artifact and do not exist in the image.

It should be apparent that the characterization of pathology by precise and specific radiographic criteria is virtually impossible. Contrary to popular belief and teaching practices, radiographic interpretation by pattern recognition can lead to serious mistakes. Except in unusual circumstances, it is impossible to arrive at a definitive diagnosis as the result of image analysis (Figure 10-5). Radiographic data can be used most effectively in the development of a differential diagnosis. They can also provide important supporting evidence to validate a clinical diagnosis. In some instances, such as a fracture that is clinically apparent, the radiograph will help to identify the number and position of fragments. This may be essential to the correct management of the patient. The x-ray image *alone* should not be used as the basis for developing a definitive diagnosis or establishing the most appropriate mode of therapy.

A

B

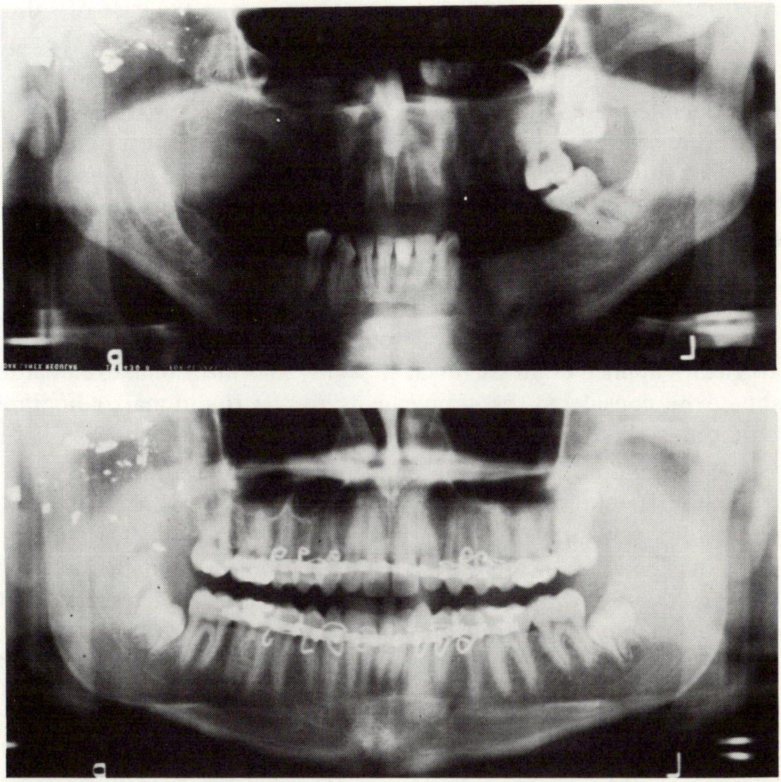

Figure 10-5 Flecks of opaque material are seen around the right temporomandibular joint regions of these two individuals. **A.** The opaque material lies within the base of the skull (retained contrast media from a myelogram), but has been projected to the side. **B.** The opaque material represents metal fragments resulting from a gunshot injury. A distinction between the two cannot be made on the panoramic film.

Before any attempt to analyze radiographic images, many factors should be considered. As previously mentioned, three-dimensional structures are reduced to two dimensions. The human visual system is not well suited to this transition. It is desirable, when practical, to view objects on two or more films and, in appropriate circumstances, it is helpful to have views that are at right angles to one another.

Radiographs that give the most direct and unobstructed views of the anatomic parts under study are obviously the most desirable. When body parts are paired, it is usually useful to obtain views of both sides for comparison. Although symmetry is not exact, gross discrepancies between two sides of the body often indicate the presence of an abnormality.

When body parts are movable or perform some specific function, different views should be obtained to show the range of movement or function. In the case of joints, for example, it is desirable to see anatomic relationships during flexion and extension; and in the case of salivary glands it is helpful to observe the rate of filling and emptying of the gland.

When a particular problem requires continued surveillance, the most reproducible views should be selected for serial comparisons. Special precautions may be necessary to obtain serial comparisons. In orthodontics, cephalometers are commonly used to place the head in a reproducible position. The application of a wax or compound bite to an intraoral film holder can achieve the same objective.

When ordinary views do not provide adequate information, it is reasonable to use either under- or overpenetrated film, stereoscopic views, oblique projections, and tomograms. The use of fluoroscopy, artifically applied contrast, nuclear scans, and ultrasonic examinations should be considered, as supplements to the traditional radiographic procedures.

Radiographic images represent density differences in film that result from the differential attenuation of x-rays by objects of different quantity or with different attenuation characteristics (Figure 10-6). The amount of difference between the densities seen on a film is a complex function of the quality of the x-ray beam, the absorption characteristics of the materials within the object being examined, the contrast properties of the film or recorder, and the type of processing employed. Small density differences that may be measurable by machine often may escape visual detection.[7] It is, therefore, essential to recognize radiographic features that are directly attributable to density differences within the subject as compared to those that may result from artifacts within the radiographic or visual systems.

The initial step in radiographic interpretation must be the careful analysis of the image with a clear and accurate description of its specific characteristics. These include such factors as size, both absolute and

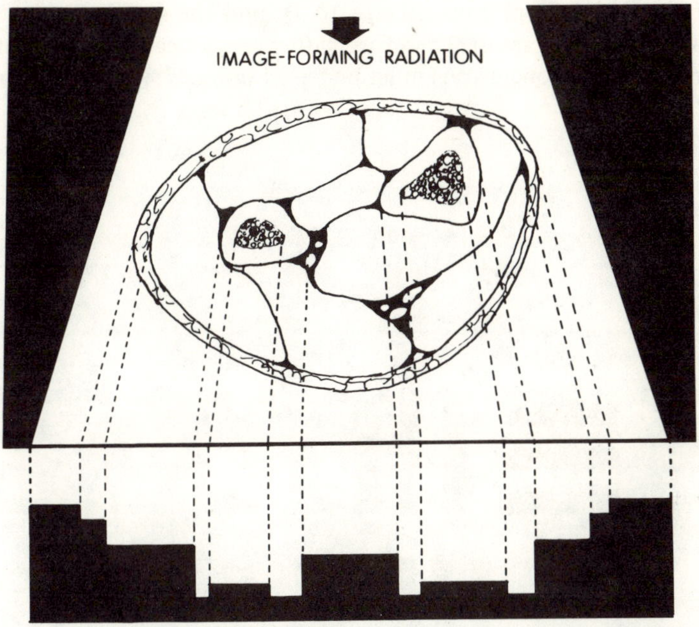

Figure 10-6 The image on the film represents a summation of the total absorption or transmission of the x-ray beam through a complex object. Many characteristics of the object may be obscured as a result of overlap or the varying densities of different components.

relative, architecture, density, orientation, and margination. These observations should be placed in the perspective of available clinical data. In general, there are five to seven distinct densities which can be recognized in dental radiographs. These include air, fat, soft tissues and blood, trabecular bone, cortical bone, dentin and cementum, and enamel. As already noted, the ability to distinguish among these materials depends not only upon their absolute density but also on the relative quantity of material present. The detectability of material of any density is also influenced by its position, by the projection geometry used in producing the film, and by the overall sharpness of the image. In some instances, particular types of image processing can be used to enhance particular image features.[6]

The extraction of information from a radiograph also depends heavily upon a number of other factors that can be optimized by the observer. These include the intensity and the spectrum of the light that is transmitted through the radiograph, the presence or absence of extraneous light from the periphery of the film, and the eyesight and/or physical alertness of the observer. Intraoral radiographs in particular are capable of extremely high resolution (Figure 10-7), and the structures that are imaged are extremely small. Therefore, either magnification or projection is desirable. Since conclusions must be based on facts, it is important to make clear distinctions between fact and artifact.[8]

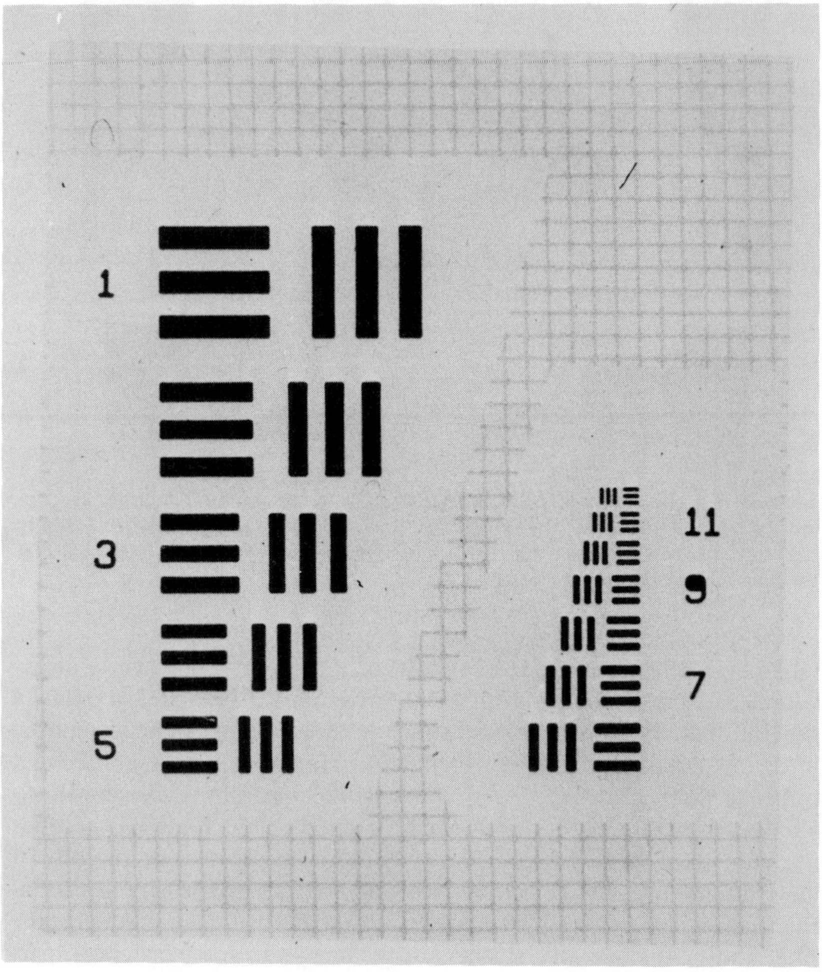

Figure 10-7 **A.** This bar pattern is one test target used to measure the resolving power of film.

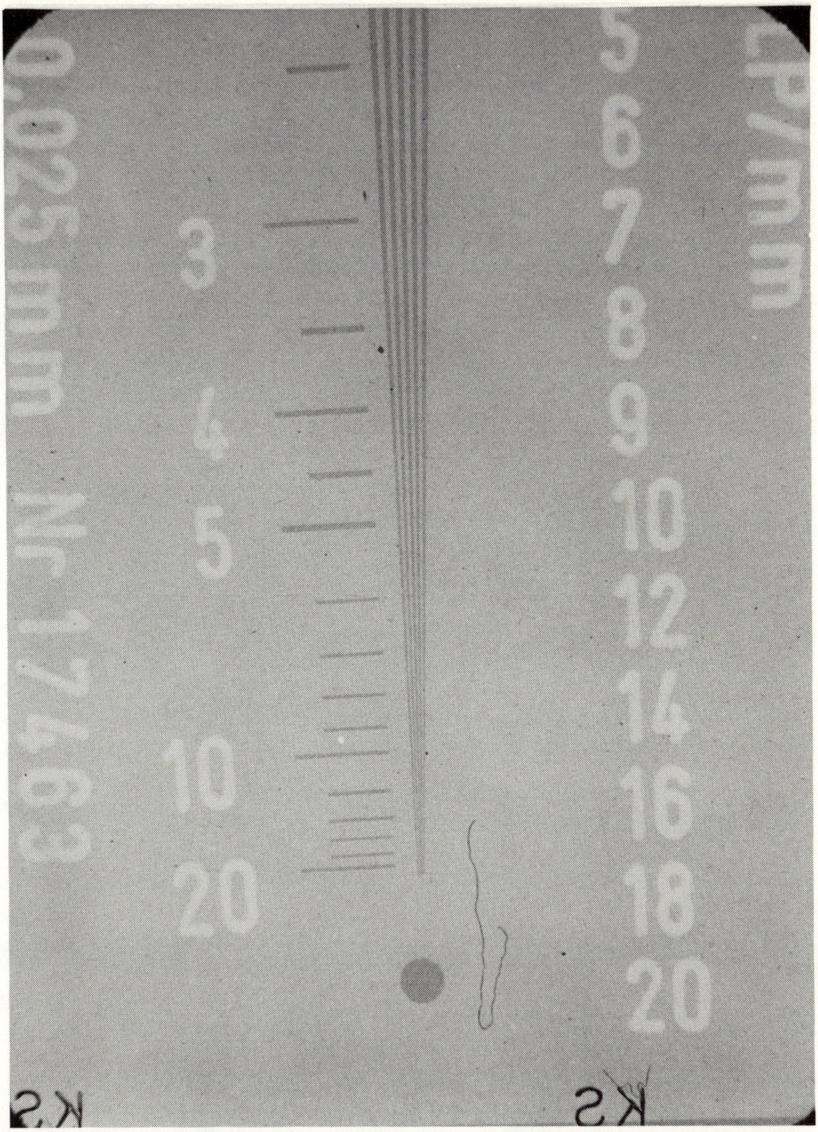

Figure 10-7 B. Converging lines represent an alternative test pattern. This image was produced on intraoral film and shows a resolving capacity of 20 line pairs per millimeter.

Analysis of the x-ray image should take into account the fact that calcified tissues are dynamic. Their dimensional properties, including shape, length, breadth, and contour, are changeable (Figure 10-8). Owing

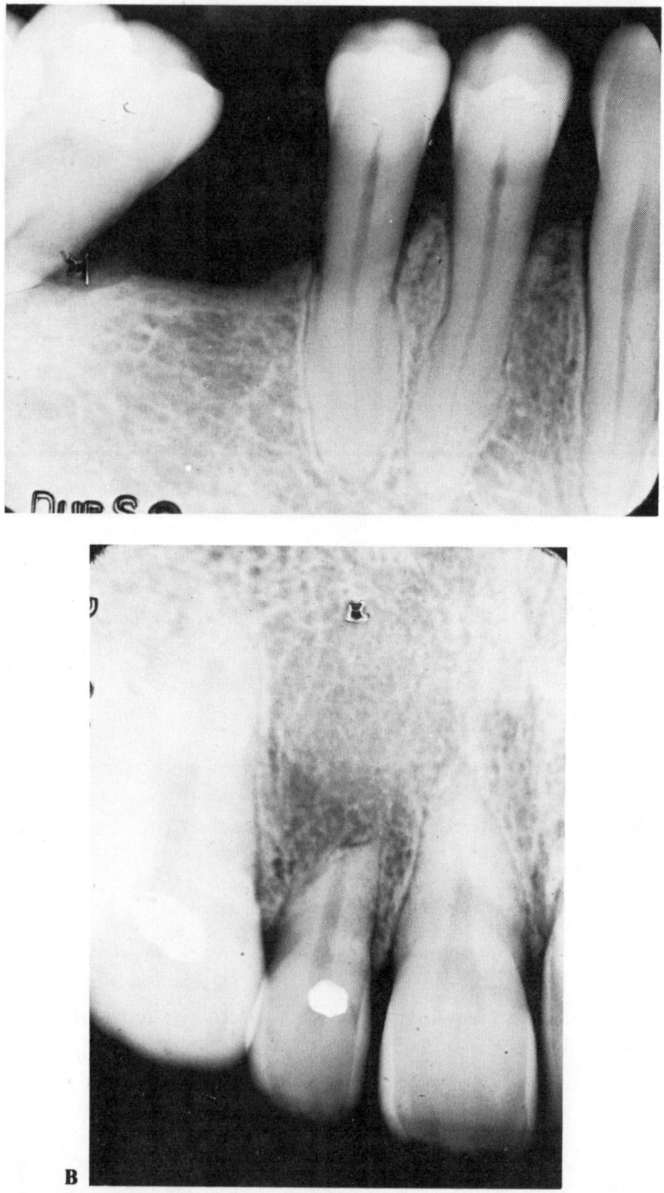

A

B

Figure 10-8 **A.** The roots of developed teeth can become enlarged as in hypercementosis, demonstrating the dynamic nature of calcified dental structures. **B.** Root structure can also be removed or remodeled after it has developed in response to an appropriate stimulus. This is exemplified by the phenomenon of external resorption.

to geometric considerations, size must be considered in absolute as well as relative terms. Magnification and/or distortion can be introduced artifically and should not be mistaken for actual changes in biologic structure. Calcified tissues respond to mechanical and functional stresses and have the ability to repair certain types of injuries. Evidence of these processes is usually demonstrated by changes in density with the specific characteristics of the density change depending upon the process involved (Figure 10-9). The physical properties of calcified tissues change during development so that immature structures, which are relatively pliable, will respond differently to a particular stimulus than will fully developed tissues, which are relatively hard and inelastic. The responsiveness of tissues at different stages of development are therefore reflected in different types of radiographic images.

A

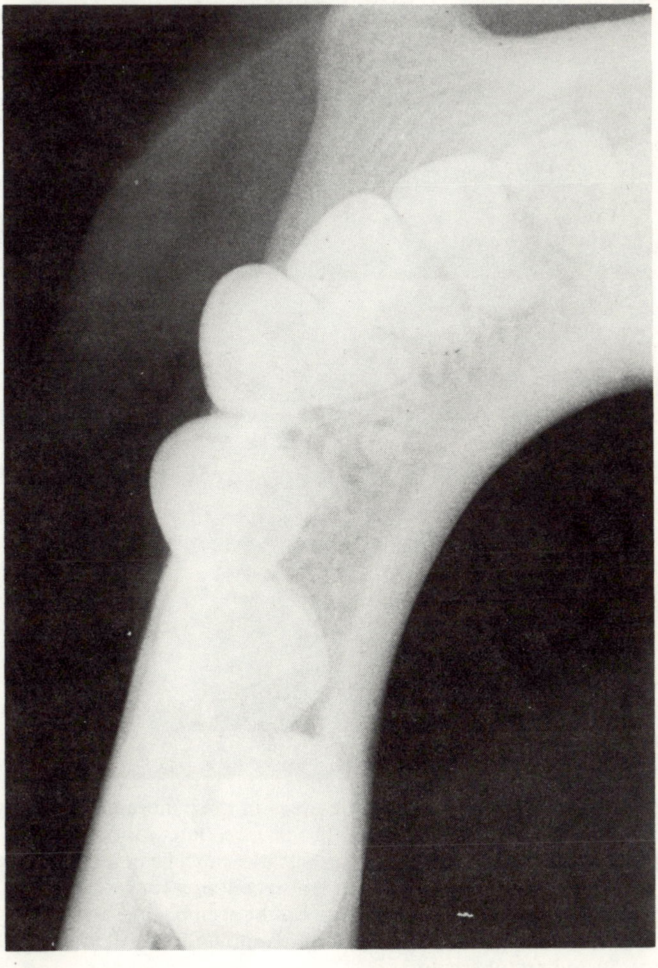

Figure 10-9 A. Benign bony growths often retain the same architectural characteristics as the structures from which they are derived.

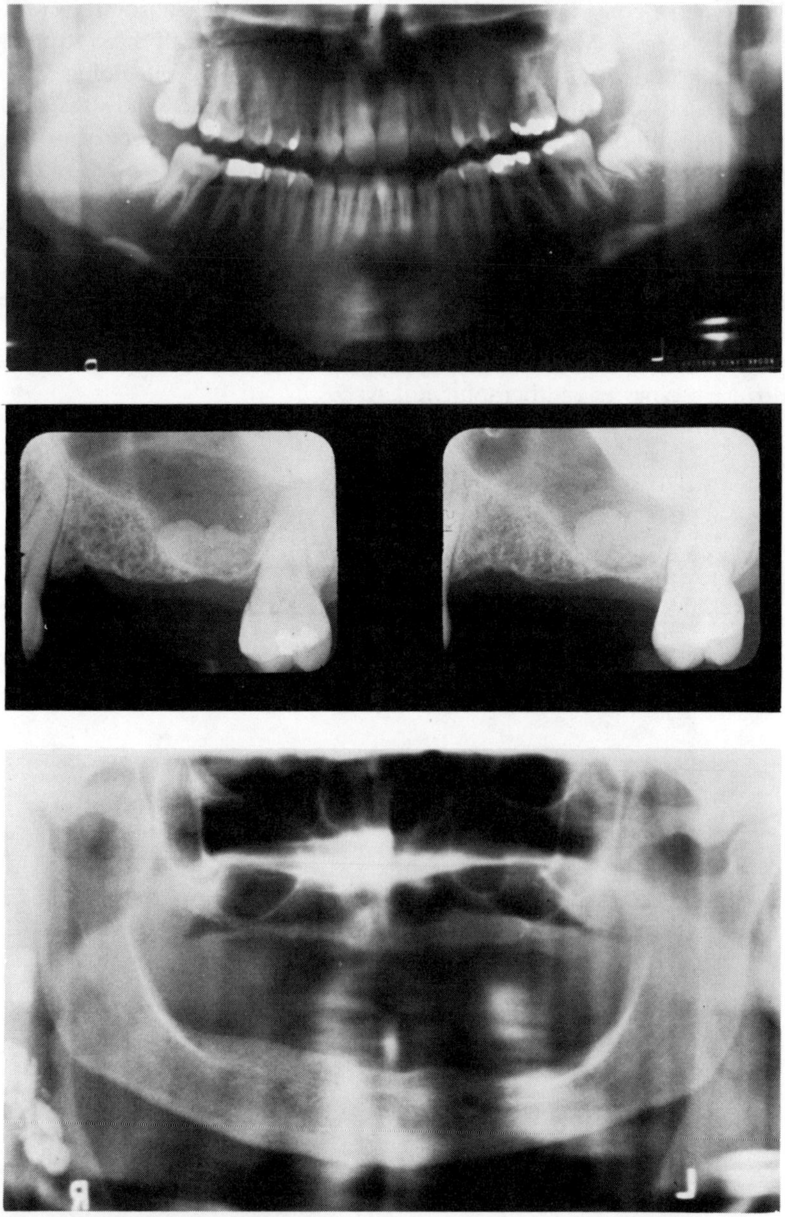

B

C

D

Figure 10-9 **B.** The abnormality can be seen in the panoramic view, but the architectural details are less distinct. **C.** Chronic infection or inflammation can lead to calcification within soft tissues. In this instance, a stone or antrolith is observed in the floor of the maxillary sinus. **D.** It is also common for calcifications to occur in lymph nodes or in salivary glands, as can be seen behind and below the right mandibular angle. Calcification of cervical lymph nodes is often the result of old infections, including tuberculosis.

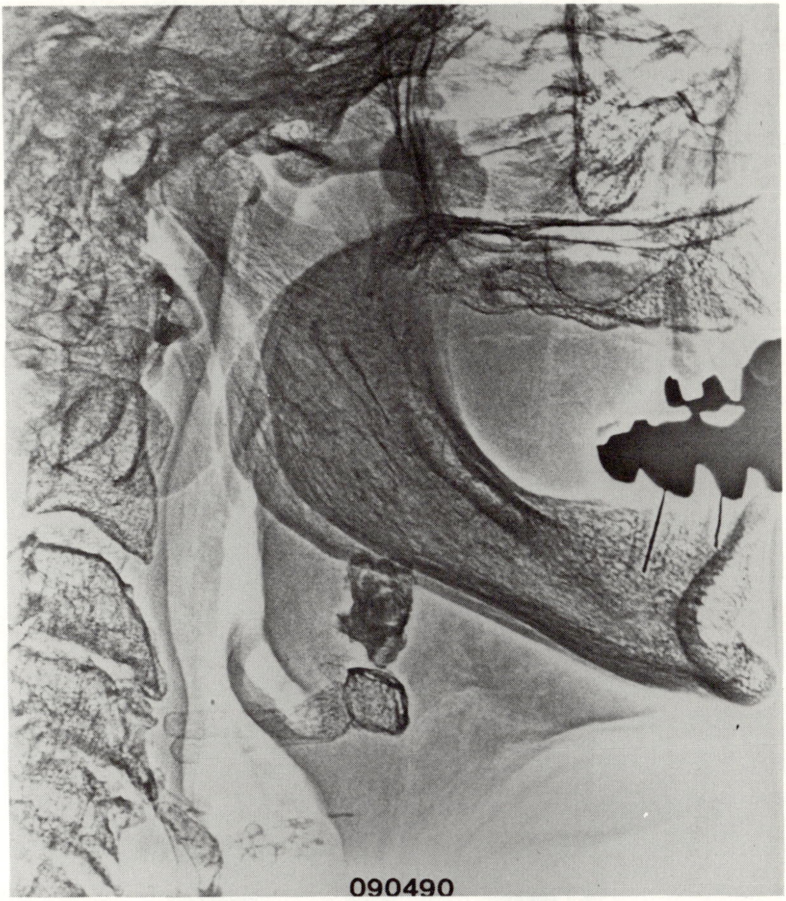

E

Figure 10-9 **E.** This calcification has a shape reminiscent of tooth structure and may represent an odontogenic tumor.

Even with immature tissues, certain types of variability are predictable. For example, von Wowern[9,10] found that trabecular bone is more dense in the incisor regions of the mandible than in the premolar or molar regions, although the overall bone mass is similar at these different sites. She also demonstrated that variations in trabecular pattern appear to be independent of the state of the dentition and that bone mass is fairly uniform on the lingual surfaces of the mandible but varies considerably along buccal surfaces from one region to another.

In addition to demonstrating the dynamic nature of calcified tissues, Figure 10-10 illustrates that these tissues can participate either actively or passively in a variety of physiologic functions. In this case, the proliferation of bone marrow elements in an individual with sickle cell anemia has caused a dramatic alteration in the appearance and organization of trabecular structure in the skull. Calcified tissues are covered with and held together by soft tissue. Changes in the soft tissues can alter the appearance of either bone or tooth. For example, inflammation of gingival tissues can lead to demineralization of alveolar bone, and the presence of calculus on interproximal surfaces may obscure the presence of carious lesions.

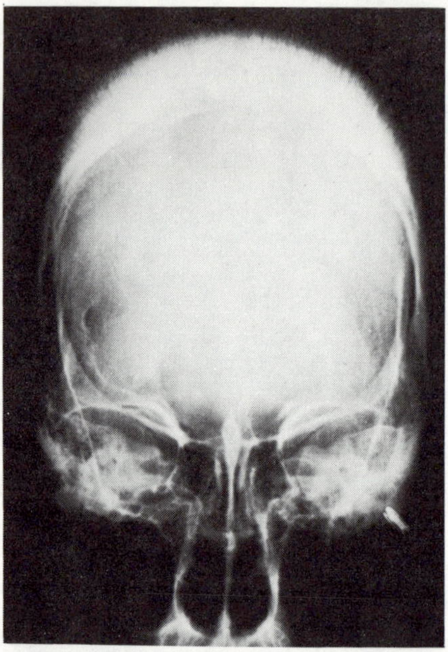

A

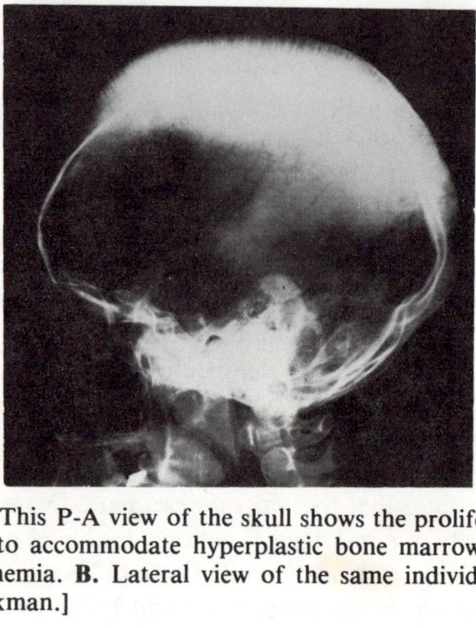

B

Figure 10-10 **A.** This P-A view of the skull shows the proliferation of bone in the cranial vault to accommodate hyperplastic bone marrow in an individual with sickle cell anemia. **B.** Lateral view of the same individual. [Courtesy of Dr. Thomas Spackman.]

Time discrepancies may exist between the appearance of symptoms in a patient and the appearance of changes in a radiograph. The physiologic and pathologic processes that alter the density of calcified tissues progress slowly. Because of the relatively low contrast of most films, only substantial changes in density are perceptible on a radiograph. Depending upon the precision with which a radiograph is made, a 30% to 60% change in mineral content may be required to produce a radiographically detectable lesion.[5] Therefore, an acute abscess or infection may not be demonstrable on a radiograph at the time symptoms first appear; conversely, recovery from a fracture or an infection may be inapparent for days or weeks after there is unequivocal evidence of clinical improvement. The lack of correlation between clinical and radiographic findings is explainable on a reasonable physical basis. The fact that an absolute correlation is missing should never be taken as evidence that the clinical diagnosis is incorrect. Rather, the possibility that the observation is untimely or inadequate should always be borne in mind.

In summary, the observer must be familiar with the normal range likely to be encountered. The normal appearance of calcified structures on radiographs changes with age and differs in males and in females. The appearance of bone in premenopausal and postmenopausal adult women is different. The quality of bone changes as its functional state varies. Alveolar bone without teeth becomes atrophic.

Although radiographs are obtained to examine a selected anatomic site, the entire radiograph should be carefully evaluated. It is not uncommon for one's eye to be distracted by obvious pathology, and as a result miss other equally important but less conspicuous changes. Once an abnormality is detected, it should be precisely located. The nature of an abnormality often depends upon its association with the particular anatomic structures. Careful location may require multiple views. Figure 10-11 is an example of how the two-dimensional nature of the radiograph can be deceptive. It is also important to establish the relationship of an abnormality to anatomic surfaces so that one may distinguish between lesions that are erosive in nature and those that undermine from within. In a salivary gland, a filling defect may be caused by the presence of a stone, fibrosis around the duct, extrinsic pressure resulting from peripheral swelling, or local reaction to an irritant. The determination of the type of defect is often associated with its position and its association with natural boundaries.

The nature of an abnormality should also be carefully characterized. The density should be determined both in absolute terms and in relation to surrounding structures. A determination should be made as to whether the density of the abnormality is homogeneous or regular and whether it is hollow or solid. The size of the abnormality should be carefully considered because it bears on the timing of its development and the

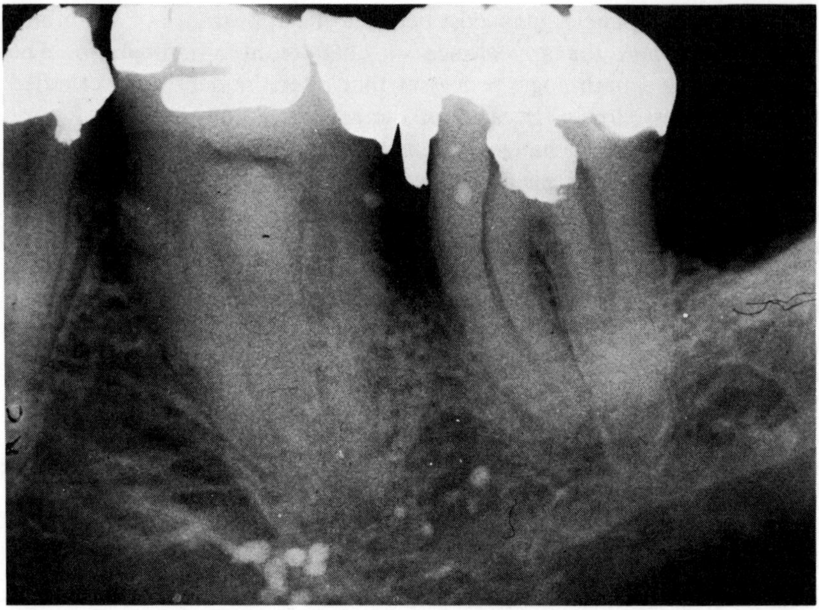

Figure 10-11 The opaque material observed in this periapical film might be mistaken for an amalgam tattoo. The dense particles, however, lie in adjacent soft tissue and result from the injection of an oil-based contrast agent.

likelihood of its affecting adjacent structures. The shape is also of great importance and may provide important insight into the nature of the lesion by helping to distinguish between passive and aggressive pathogenic processes.

Many different approaches to radiographic interpretation are currently used or have been used successfully by different practitioners in the past. There is no magic formula. One must start with a sound understanding of normal anatomy and physiology. To this base, an understanding of the pathogenesis of disease is added. The manner in which these two parameters are altered by the radiographic process must be thoroughly understood. The particular approach to interpretation used by any individual should be determined primarily as a matter of personal preference and convenience.

GAMUTS IN RADIOLOGY

Reeder and Felson[11] compiled comprehensive lists of roentgen diagnoses, which they referred to as *gamuts* (gamut being the whole range). The gamuts are lists of causes of roentgenographic pictures and are grouped anatomically for convenience. The gamuts dealing with the skull and brain; facial bones, jaws, sinuses, and neck; spine; and bone, joints, and soft tissues are of particular interest in dental radiology.

Although an attempt has been made to provide comprehensive lists, there are occasional omissions. When possible, gamuts based upon radiographic signs are divided into common and uncommon pathologic conditions or listed as syndromes. When the causes of the particular problem such as the delayed eruption of teeth are numerous, an attempt is made to categorize the causes according to traditional criteria. In some instances, subroutines follow the main gamuts. Examples of gamuts relevant to dental diagnosis follow.*

SALIVARY DUCT STRICTURE ON SIALOGRAPHY

1. Carcinoma
2. Inflammation (scarring)
3. Radiation therapy
4. Stone
5. Trauma, including surgical

SALIVARY GLAND ENLARGEMENT

Common

1. Mumps
2. Stone
3. Suppurative sialitis
4. Tumor

Uncommon

1. Alcoholism
2. Hormonal disturbance
3. Idiopathic
4. Kwashiorkor
5. Mikulicz's disease
6. Mucoviscidosis
7. Nutritional deficiency, cirrhosis
8. Sarcoidosis
9. Sjögren's syndrome (associated with rheumatoid arthritis, lupus, or scleroderma)
10. Stricture of duct

---

*M.M. Reeder and B. Felson. *Gamuts in Radiology*. Cincinnati: Audiovisual Radiology of Cincinnati, Inc., 1975. Reproduced with permission.

DELAYED ERUPTION OR NONERUPTION OF TEETH

I. Congenital Syndromes
  1. Acrocephalosyndactyly (Apert's syndrome)
  2. Chondroectodermal dysplasia (Ellis-van Creveld's syndrome)
  3. Cleidocranial dysplasia
  4. Down's syndrome
  5. Goltz's syndrome
  6. (Hypophosphatemic rickets)
  7. Incontinentia pigmenti
  8. Oculomandibulofacial syndrome (Hallermann-Streiff)
  9. Osteopetrosis
  10. Progeria
  11. Pseudohypoparathyroidism
  12. Pyknodysostosis

II. Endocrinopathies
  1. Hypoparathyroidism
  2. Hypopituitarism
  3. Hypothyroidism

III. Familial Tendency

IV. Idiopathic

V. Local Factors
  1. Developmental
    a. Cleft lip and/or palate
    b. Disorientation of tooth germ
    c. Ectopic eruption
    d. Lack of space
    e. Prolonged retention of deciduous teeth
    f. Submersion and ankylosis
    g. Supernumerary teeth
  2. Hereditary (eg, amelogenesis imperfecta)
  3. Iatrogenic
    a. Improperly contoured restoration
    b. Lack of space
    c. Over-retained roots of deciduous teeth
  4. Inflammatory (eg, Garré's chronic sclerosing osteomyelitis)
  5. Mechanical (eg, fibrosis of alveolar mucosa, dilaceration, impaction)
  6. Neoplastic

b. Odontogenic tumor
    (1) Adenoameloblastoma
    (2) Ameloblastic fibroma
    (3) Ameloblastic odontoma
    (4) Neuroectodermal tumor of infancy (melanotic progonoma)
    (5) Odontogenic fibroma
    (6) Odontoma
c. Nonodontogenic tumor
    (1) Central giant cell (reparative) granuloma
    (2) Ossifying fibroma, fibrous dysplasia, cherubism

7. Traumatic

LOSS OF LAMINA DURA OF THE TEETH

Common

1. Local inflammatory disease (eg, gingivitis, periodontitis, caries, periapical granuloma, apical cyst)
2. Senile osteoporosis

Uncommon

1. Burkitt's lymphoma
2. Cushing's syndrome
3. Fibrous dysplasia
4. Histiocytosis X
5. Hyperparathyroidism
6. Hyperphosphatasia
7. Leukemia
8. Metastasis
9. Multiple myeloma
10. Neoplasm, primary (eg, benign cementoblastoma)
11. Osteomalacia
12. Paget's disease
13. Removal of opposing tooth
14. Scleroderma
15. Traumatic cyst

CYST-LIKE LESION OF THE JAW

Common

1. Ameloblastoma
2. Brown tumor of hyperparathyroidism
3. Dentigerous (follicular) cyst
4. Fibrous dysplasia, cherubism

5. Odontogenic cyst (eg, keratocyst, primordial cyst, Gorlin cyst)
6. Radicular cyst, periapical granuloma
7. Traumatic (hemorrhagic) cyst

Uncommon

1. Adenomatoid odontogenic tumor (adenoameloblastoma)
2. Ameloblastic fibroma
3. Aneurysmal bone cyst
4. Bone cyst
5. Cementoma
6. Central giant cell (reparative) granuloma
7. Fissural developmental cyst (eg, globulomaxillary, median palatal, median mandibular, median alveolar, incisive canal)
8. Giant cell tumor
9. Histiocytosis X (especially eosinophilic granuloma)
10. Hydatid cyst
11. Malignant neoplasm, primary or metastatic
12. Odontogenic fibroma or myxoma
13. Ossifying fibroma, cementifying fibroma
14. Pindborg tumor

LOCATION OF CYST-LIKE LESION OF THE JAW

I. At apex of root

1. Apical scar
2. Cementoma (early)
3. Periapical (dental) granuloma or abscess
4. Radicular cyst

II. Midline of maxilla

1. Cyst of papilla palatina
2. Incisive canal cyst (nasopalatine duct cyst)
3. Median alveolar cyst
4. Median palatal cyst

III. Lateral to midline of maxilla

1. Globulomaxillary cyst
2. Nasolabial cyst (soft tissue)
3. Surgical ciliated cyst of maxillary sinus

IV. Around impacted or unerupted tooth

1. Adenoameloblastoma
2. Ameloblastoma
3. Dental follicle

4. Dentigerous (follicular) cyst
5. Melanotic progonoma
6. Odontogenic fibroma or myxoma
7. Odontogenic keratocyst
8. Odontoma, compound
9. Pindborg tumor

UNILOCULAR RADIOLUCENT LESION OF THE JAW

Well-Defined Borders

1. Adenoameloblastoma
2. Ameloblastoma
3. Bone cyst
4. Cementoma (immature)
5. Central cementifying fibroma (immature)
6. Dentigerous (follicular) cyst
7. Fissural cyst (eg, nasopalatine, globulomaxillary, median palatal, median alveolar, median mandibular)
8. Neurofibroma, neurilemmoma
9. Odontogenic cyst (eg, keratocyst, primordial cyst)
10. Radicular cyst, periapical granuloma

Ill-Defined Borders

1. Cementoma (immature)
2. Giant cell tumor
3. Histiocytosis X
4. Metastasis
5. Myeloma
6. Odontogenic cyst (eg, Gorlin cyst)
7. Osteoporotic bone marrow defect

EXPANSILE MULTILOCULAR RADIOLUCENT LESION OF THE JAW

Expansile with Discrete Margins

1. Ameloblastoma
2. Aneurysmal bone cyst
3. Brown tumor of hyperparathyroidism*
4. Calcifying epithelial odontogenic tumor (Pindborg tumor)
5. Central giant cell (reparative) granuloma*
6. Central hemangioma, arteriovenous malformation

*Common.

7. Dentigerous (follicular) cyst*
8. Eosinophilic granuloma (histiocytosis X)
9. Fibrous dysplasia, cherubism, ossifying fibroma*
10. Myeloma, plasmacytoma
11. Odontogenic cyst (eg, keratocyst, primordial cyst)*
12. Odontogenic myxoma or fibroma

Expansile with Ill-Defined Margins

1. Bone sarcoma (eg, chondrosarcoma)
2. Calcifying epithelial odontogenic cyst (Gorlin cyst)
3. Fibrous dysplasia*
4. Giant cell tumor
5. Metastasis
6. Myeloma*

MIXED RADIOLUCENT AND RADIOPAQUE LESION OF THE JAW

Common

1. Fibrous dysplasia, cherubism, ossifying fibroma
2. Odontoma, compound or complex
3. Paget's disease

Uncommon

1. Adenoameloblastoma
2. Ameloblastic fibro-odontoma
3. Ameloblastic odontoma
4. Calcifying epithelial odontogenic tumor (Pindborg tumor)
5. Cementoma
6. Chondrosarcoma
7. Gorlin cyst
8. Metastasis (eg, from breast or prostate)
9. Osteoblastoma
10. Osteosarcoma

RADIOPAQUE LESION OF THE JAW

Common

1. Condensing osteitis, focal sclerosing osteitis†
2. Fibrous dysplasia, ossifying fibroma
3. Odontoma, compound or complex†

---

*Common

†Localized.

4. Paget's disease
5. Torus palatinus or mandibularis†
6. [Unerupted tooth; retained root]†

Uncommon

1. Cementoma (late stage)†
2. Chondrosarcoma†
3. Infantile cortical hyperostosis (Caffey disease)
4. Osteoblastic metastasis†
5. Osteoma (eg, Gardner's syndrome)†
6. Osteopetrosis
7. Osteosarcoma†
8. Sclerosing osteomyelitis (eg, Garré osteomyelitis; chronic diffuse sclerosing osteomyelitis)
9. [Superimposed sialolith, phlebolith, foreign body]†

DEFORMITY, ASYMMETRY, OR OPACIFICATION OF THE NASAL CAVITY

Common

1. Congenital deformity of nasal septum
2. Fracture of nasal plates or septum
3. Mucosal swelling (inflammatory, allergic, traumatic)
4. Pseudopolyp
5. Rhinolith, foreign body
6. Turbinate abnormality (eg, enlargement, congenital absence)

Uncommon

1. Benign tumor (eg, fibroma, neurofibroma, ossifying fibroma, osteoma)
2. Carcinoma of nose or antrum
3. Choanal atresia or stenosis
4. Dermoid cyst
5. Encephalomeningocele
6. Hypoplasia of nasal bones in various congenital syndromes
7. Rhinoscleroma with granulomatous mass
8. Wegener's granuloma

Taybi[12] has also included a gamut index in his text, *Radiology of Syndromes,* which provides an alphabetical list of syndromes and their synonyms and cites the most important clinical and radiologic manifestations of these syndromes. Selected radiographs and abundant references are also provided.

---

†Localized.

A slightly different approach to radiographic diagnosis has been described by Eversole and Rovin.[13,14] These clinicians also categorized lesions according to their radiographic characteristics. In their system of classification lesions are described on the basis of density and location so that radiographic characteristics can be associated with pathologic changes in or affecting specific structures. An attempt is made to correlate the radiographic features of particular lesions with the underlying pathologic process. These investigators also emphasized that although many lesions occurring in the jaws produce characteristic images on film, there is considerable overlap of radiographic features from one type of lesion to the next. They point out that microscopic examination is often required to confirm the radiographic impression, particularly when the image characteristics are ambiguous. The following are examples of their system of classification.*

CLASSIFICATION OF RADIOGRAPHIC ABERRATIONS ENCOUNTERED IN LESIONS OF THE JAWS

I. Radiolucencies
  A. Unilocular
    1. Well-defined borders
      a. Sclerotic border absent (punched-out effect)
      b. Sclerotic border present
    2. Ill-defined borders
  B. Multiocular
    1. Well-defined borders
    2. Ill-defined borders (moth-eaten pattern)

II. Radiopacities
  A. Well-demarcated
  B. Diffuse

III. Mixed radiopaque/radiolucent
  A. Unilocular radiolucencies with central opacities
  B. Multiocular radiolucencies with central opacities (cotton wool)
  C. Diffuse radiopaque-lucent (ground glass)

IV. Periosteal reactions
  A. Cortical redundancy (onion skin)
  B. Osteophyte reaction
  C. Cortical osteolysis
    1. Well-defined border

*Source: L.R. Eversole and S. Rovin. Differential radiographic diagnosis of lesions of the jawbones. *Radiology* 105:277–284, 1972. Reproduced with permission.

2. Ill-defined border

V. Peridental reactions
  A. Periapical
    1. Radiolucent
    2. Radiopaque
    3. Mixed lucent/opaque
  B. Periodontal
    1. Loss of lamina dura
    2. Widened periodontal ligament space
      a. Localized
      b. Diffuse
  C. Radicular involvement
    1. Root divergence
    2. Root resorption
  D. Coronal involvement
    1. Radiolucent
    2. Mixed lucent/opaque

LESIONS PRODUCING UNILOCULAR RADIOLUCENCIES IN THE JAWS

Well-defined borders

1. Fissural cysts
2. Odontogenic cysts
3. Cementoma
4. Benign neural neoplasms
5. Static bone cyst
6. Adenoameloblastoma
7. Immature central cementifying fibroma

Ill-defined borders

1. Fissural cysts
2. Odontogenic cysts
3. Cementoma
4. Osteoporotic bone-marrow defect
5. Multiple myeloma
6. Metastatic disease
7. Eosinophilic granuloma
8. Hand-Schüller-Christian disease

LESIONS PRODUCING MULTILOCULAR RADIOLUCENCIES IN THE JAWS

Expansile with discrete margins
1. Central giant cell granuloma
2. Ameloblastoma
3. Calcifying epithelial odontogenic tumor
4. Myxoma
5. Central hemangioma or arteriovenous shunt
6. Aneurysmal bone cyst
7. Familial fibrous dysplasia
8. Odontogenic keratocyst
9. Fibrous dysplasia

Expansile with indiscrete margins
1. Osteomyelitis
2. Central sarcomas
3. Fibrous dysplasia
5. Calcifying epithelial odontogenic cyst

Nonexpansile with discrete margins
1. Traumatic bone cyst

LESIONS PRODUCING RADIOPACITIES

Solitary well-defined
1. Cementoma
2. Focal sclerosing osteitis
3. Osteosclerosis
4. Superimposed sialoliths, phleboliths, and foreign bodies
5. Maxillary antrolith

Multiple discrete or diffuse opacities
1. Diffuse sclerosing osteomyelitis
2. Paget's disease of bone
3. Osteomas (Gardner's syndrome)
4. Superimposed sialoliths, phleboliths, and foreign bodies
5. Osteoblastic osteosarcoma

LESIONS PRODUCING TARGET LUCENCIES WITH CENTRAL OPACITIES

1. Ameloblastic adenomatoid tumor

2. Calcifying epithelial odontogenic cyst
3. Ameloblastic fibro-odontoma and dentinoma
4. Ameloblastic odontoma
5. Odontoma
6. Central cemento-ossifying fibroma
7. Cementoma (periapical cemental dysplasia)
8. Benign cementoblastoma
9. Osteoid osteoma

LESIONS PRODUCING A MIXED RADIOLUCENT/ RADIOPAQUE APPEARANCE

Ill-defined lucencies with diffuse central opacities

1. Paget's disease
2. Fibrous dysplasia
3. Calcifying epithelial odontogenic tumor
4. Benign osteoblastoma
5. Osteoblastic metastasis
6. Osteogenic sarcoma
7. Chondrosarcoma

Ground-glass pattern

1. Fibrous dysplasia
2. Hyperparathyroidism

LESIONS PRODUCING CORTICAL ABERRATIONS

Cortical redundancy

1. Garré's osteomyelitis
2. Ewing's sarcoma
3. Infantile cortical hyperostosis

Cortical osteophytic reaction

1. Benign aggressive odontogenic and central mesenchymal tumors and reactive processes
2. Juxtacortical osteosarcoma
3. Peripheral ossifying fibroma of gingiva

Cortical expansion

1. Benign aggressive odontogenic and central mesenchymal tumors and reactive processes
2. Malignant neoplasms
3. Odontogenic cysts
4. Fibrous dysplasia
5. Paget's disease of bone

Cortical erosion

1. Underlying bone lesion
   a. Osteomyelitis
   b. Malignant epithelial or mesenchymal tumors
   c. Histiocytosis X
   d. Multiple myeloma
2. Overlying soft tissue lesion
   a. Invasive squamous-cell carcinoma
   b. Salivary adenocarcinoma
   c. Sarcoma
   d. Peripheral giant cell granuloma
   e. Soft-tissue odontogenic or fissural cysts

TRADITIONAL RADIOGRAPHIC INTERPRETATION

A more traditional approach to radiographic interpretation involves the association of a radiographic image with broad classifications of disease, including trauma, infection or inflammation, congenital abnormalities or abnormalities of growth and development, metabolic diseases, neoplasia, and others. Specific entities that fall in any one of these categories are likely to be recognized by general characteristics of the group.

Trauma

In general, radiographs are not an essential part of the primary diagnosis of trauma.[4,15] Under most circumstances there will be clinical evidence of soft tissue injury or the fracture of calcified tissues. Radiographs are of greatest value in defining the exact location and the nature of the injury. They may also be important for ruling out indirect and contrecoup injuries.

Trauma to soft tissue is usually characterized by the presence of foreign bodies and/or increased density that results from swelling. Radiographic evidence of trauma in hard tissues is most often seen as fracture lines that are sharp and irregular and extend through bony cortices or margins.

It should be remembered that fractures can occur without displacement of adjacent bony segments. In such cases, fracture lines may be difficult to visualize on conventional radiographs. Often, after a period of approximately ten days to two weeks, the nondisplaced fracture becomes visible because the injured periosteum reacts by producing layers of new bone or callus.

Examination of radiographs obtained for the evaluation of traumatic injuries should be thorough. In many instances, evidence of trauma is indirect. Fluid in the maxillary sinus may be the only radiographic clue of a fractured maxilla. Similarly, air trapped within soft tissues may provide evidence of more extensive injury than can be appreciated by clinical examination.

Trauma may have an iatrogenic origin. In many instances, the radiographic findings can be used to establish the nature of an injury and the extent to which additional studies might be of value.

Metabolic, Nutritional, and Endocrinologic Diseases

Diseases of metabolic, nutritional, or endocrinologic origin can produce varied radiographic images. These diseases, however, can often be distinguished from other types of problems because they tend to occur with a diffuse and symmetrical pattern (Figure 10-12). With few exceptions, one would not anticipate seeing focal changes in bone or in teeth as

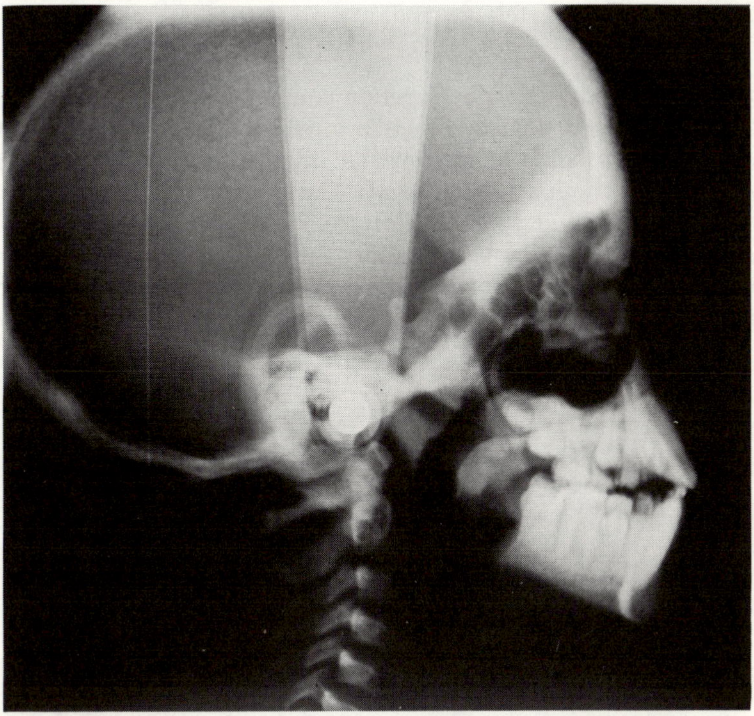

Figure 10-12 This individual suffering from a kidney disorder cannot maintain normal calcium balance. **A.** As a result, architecture of the skull is dramatically changed.

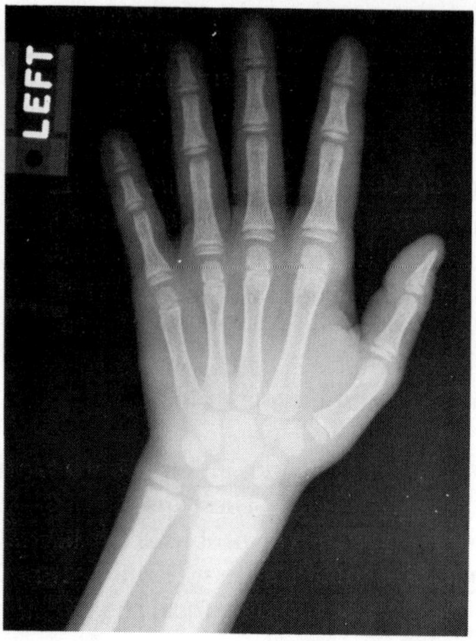

Figure 10-12 **B.** The extremities also show evidence of osteoporosis and other calcification defects.

a result of altered endocrine function or nutritional deficiency (Figure 10-13). The loss of bone density that often occurs as a result of hyperparathyroidism should be recognizable in most parts of the body, particularly in the cranium (Figure 10-14). The hypothesis that changes in the lamina dura around the roots of teeth are a specific indicator of parathyroid dysfunction has been extremely popular, but such changes are not pathognomonic for this disease and may not be as dramatic as more general alterations in bone density and architecture.[16]

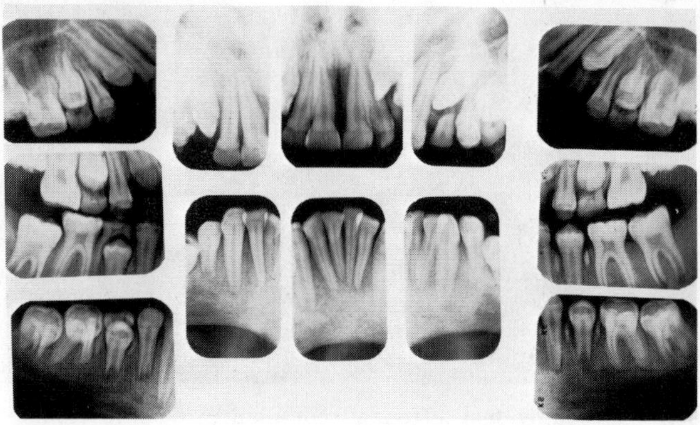

Figure 10-13 Calcium imbalance also results in altered morphology of the teeth and in late development in eruption of the teeth, as can be seen in this 14-year-old.

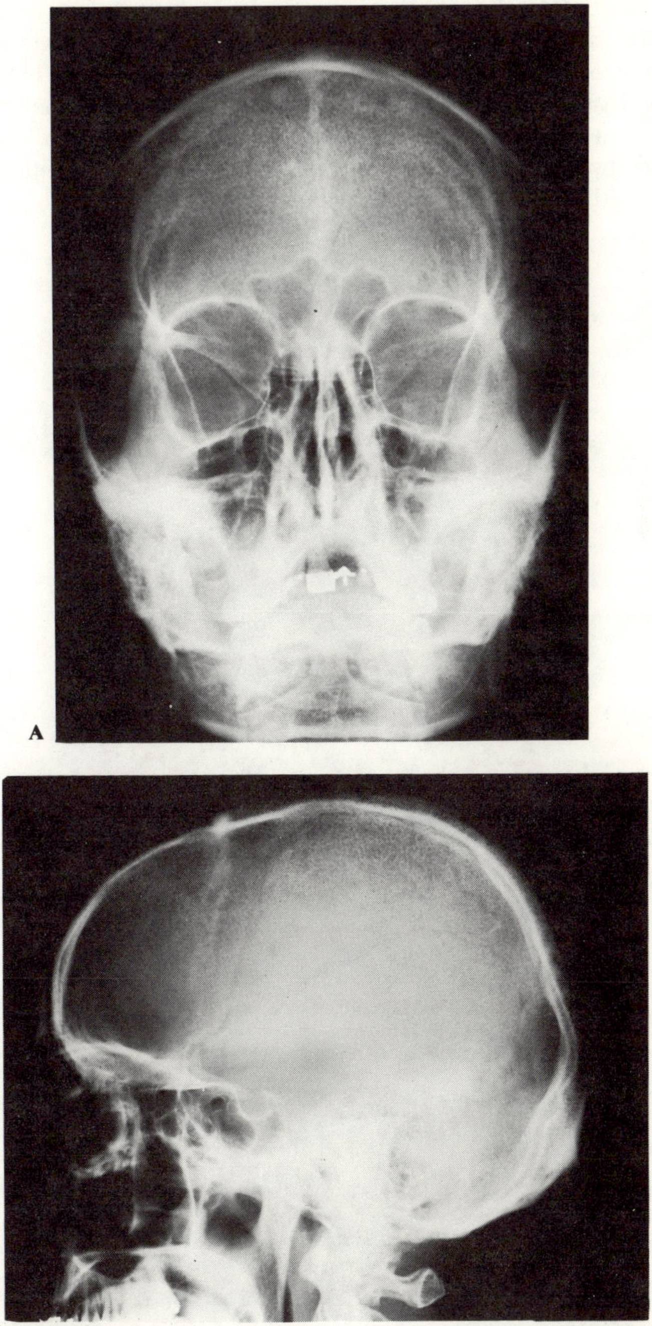

A

B

Figure 10-14 **A.** Stippled appearance which often occurs in the cranial vault as a result of hyperparathyroid disease. **B.** The effect is somewhat less pronounced in lateral view.

In addition to altering the normal radiographic appearance of bones and teeth, metabolic, nutritional, or endocrinologic disorders may be recognized indirectly. Figure 10-15 shows a fractured mandible in a patient suffering from hypothyroidism. The initial reduction of the fracture failed to produce a bony union. After the patient was placed on thyroid replacement therapy, bone formation occurred. Fractures may occur with minimal stress in nutritionally impaired individuals (Figure 10-16).

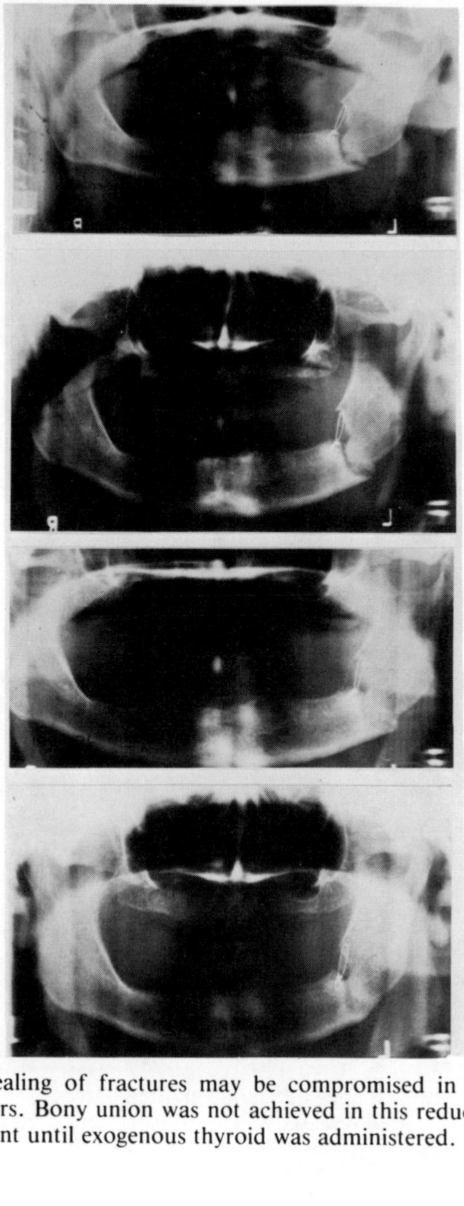

Figure 10-15 Healing of fractures may be compromised in individuals with endocrine disorders. Bony union was not achieved in this reduced fracture of a hypothyroid patient until exogenous thyroid was administered.

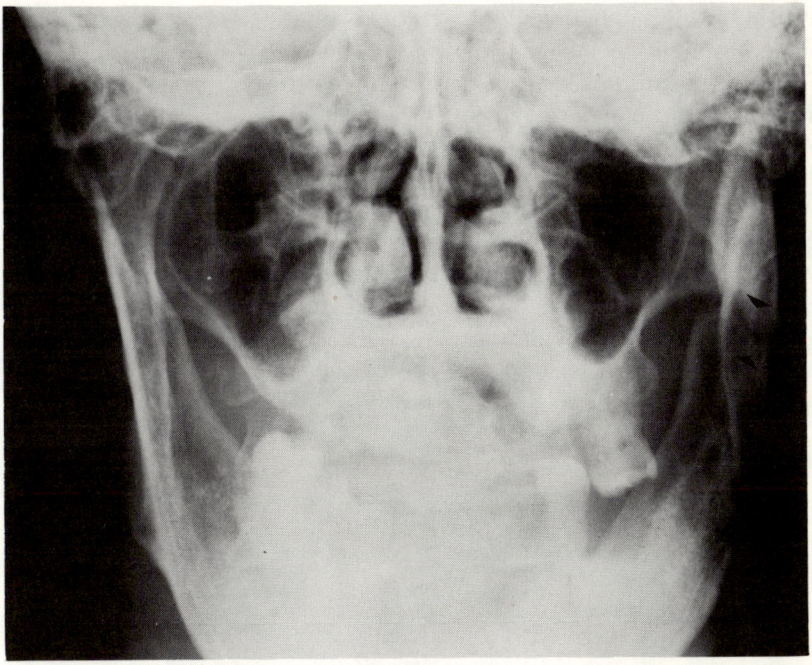

Figure 10-16 This older woman sustained a fracture through the coronoid process and condylar neck without a history of significant trauma. Fractures may occur without significant trauma in older individuals, particularly when their mobility and nutrition are compromised.

Congenital Anomalies and Abnormalities of Growth and Development

Defects that fall into this category are often recognized by alterations in the size, shape, or number of structures. Congenital defects may be limited to specific parts of the body or may involve multiple organ systems. In either event, missing teeth, supernumerary teeth, or deformed teeth may occur as a clinical manifestation of aberrant growth.

In normal individuals there is a close parallel between growth measured in chronologic units and growth measured by both skeletal maturation and dental development. Many of the pathologic conditions that cause altered rates of osseous development can be recognized by changes in the developing dentition. For example, accelerated skeletal and dental development tend to occur with hyperthyroidism, androgenic syndromes, tumors of the ovary, testes, pineal gland, and hypothalamus, and with obesity or polyostotic fibrous dysplasia. Delayed skeletal and dental development is often associated with hypothyroidism, Addison's disease, hypopituitarism, malnutrition, chronic illness, Hurler's syndrome, mongolism, and hypogonadism or gonadal agenesis.[17] Evaluation of the developing dentition is particularly useful in neonatal years when there is insufficient skeletal development for a meaningful assessment.

Local trauma associated with birth or congenital or acquired disease can have a variety of effects. For example, growth of the mandible is primarily a function of growth centers in the condylar heads. Injury to these growth centers may lead to either hypertrophy or hypoplasia. Malocclusion of teeth in individuals can often be attributed to a condylar or subcondylar fracture or to disease that alters this growth plate. Although condylar growth normally ceases during adult life, a potential for growth is retained and hypertrophic changes can occur later in life (Figure 10-17).

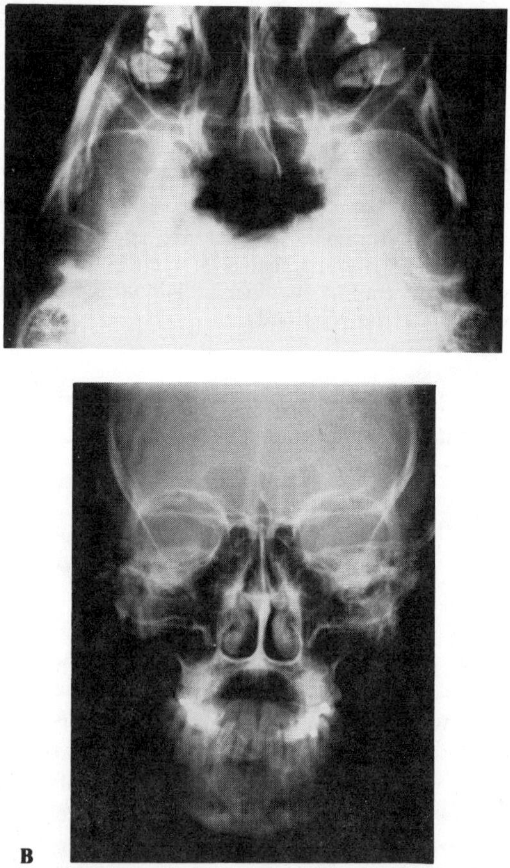

A

B

Figure 10-17 **A.** In this base view, a prominent difference can be seen in the mediolateral dimensions of the two mandibular condyles. **B.** Condylar hypertrophy may produce deviation of the midline.

Deficiencies in organ systems that affect calcium absorption, metabolism, or excretion also influence the development of the skeleton and the teeth. Figure 10-18 shows a child suffering from renal failure. Quantitative and qualitative alterations in the development of teeth and bone are evident.

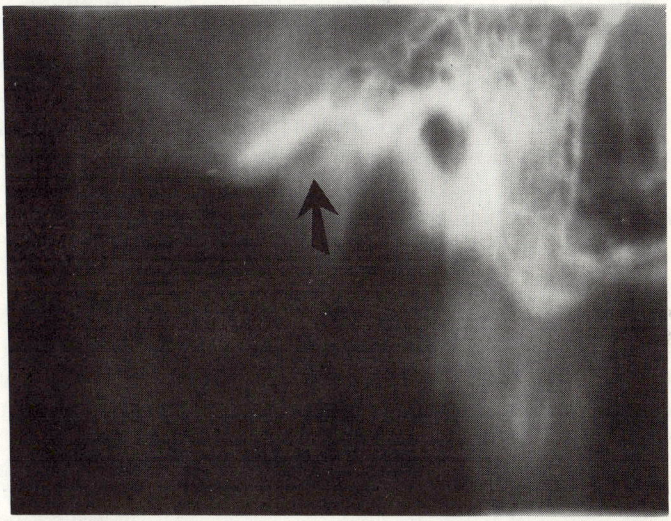

Figure 10-18 Child suffering from renal failure. A large crescent-shaped defect is noted on the superior-anterior surface of this mandibular condyle. The joint space is also narrowed.

Iatrogenic Lesions

Some radiologic signs have distinctive features that permit a diagnosis by recognition of a specific pattern of change. More commonly, radiographic abnormalities are obscure and their interpretation requires careful correlation with many different types of information about the patient.

For example, sex and age play an important role in the radiographic appearance of bones. Not only are certain diseases found to have a particular age and sex distribution but many physiologic changes occur in response to varied levels of hormonal activity that occur during development and maturation. Similarly, race and ethnic background play a role in radiographic interpretation. There are many diseases that have a genetic association or are related to the dietary practices that can be attributed to specific cultures.

Geography is also important since unusual infections, which can be mistaken for other pathologies, may be recognized when there is a history of recent travel or residence in a particular area where such infections are endemic. The occupation of the patient is a significant factor. Many skeletal changes occur as a result of exposure to toxic chemicals, including organic solvents and a variety of plastic derivatives. In dentistry, materials that irritate the maxillary sinuses are of particular concern since inflammatory or allergic reactions of this site can often mimic simple toothache or infection.

Unusual forms of trauma must be taken into account. For example, the patient shown in Figure 10-8 presented with extensive destruction of one condylar head. This aggressive lesion might easily have been mistaken for a neoplasm if a careful history had not indicated possible trauma associated with the use of general anesthetic and surgical extraction of the third molars. Figure 10-19 shows evidence of a healing subcondylar fracture in the same patient. Injuries to different parts of the jaws may occur inadvertently as a response to the application of force during therapy. The temporomandibular joints are common sites for injury secondary to endodontic and oral surgical procedures in which mouth props and other similar devices are used. Aggressive orthodontic movement of teeth may result in root resorption, which can mimic pulpal or periodontal disease once the orthodontic appliances have been removed.

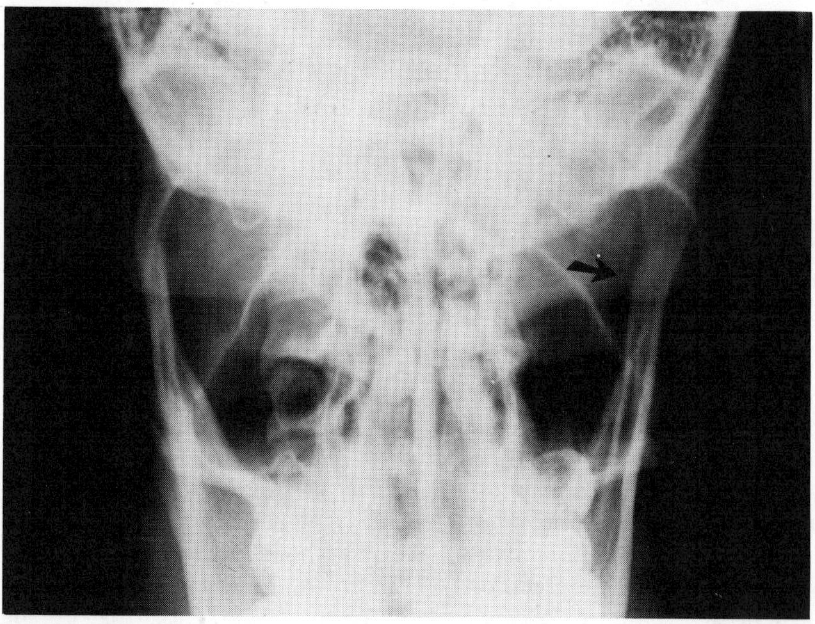

Figure 10-19 An irregularity in the subcondylar region is the result of remodeling following bony union after a fracture which occurred during a third molar extraction.

Chronic trauma resulting from unusual habit patterns can also be mistaken for dental or skeletal disease. The erosion or abrasion of tooth surfaces that result from poorly fitting prosthetic clasps or the inappropriate use of toothpicks and oral hygiene devices are common examples. Excessive gum chewing can produce muscle spasm and radiographic changes of the temporomandibular joints. The use of musical instruments can contribute to the development of both dental and salivary gland disorders.

Among the more serious but more subtle problems that may be encountered in the evaluation of radiographs are a series of iatrogenic disorders of metabolism that result from different therapies. These problems can often be divided into two main categories, diet and drugs. Nutritional deficiencies may occur as a result of inadequate dietary intake of essential substances because patients are inadequately counseled with regard to balanced nutrition. Radiographically, the most significant elements include calcium and vitamin D. Primary rickets and rickets secondary to renal disorders still exist in our population (see Figure 10-12). The lack of adequate calcium or vitamin D or the presence of calcium intolerance may lead to osteomalacia. In some instances the treatment of such disorders can also lead to bony abnormalities. Patients who suffer from gastrointestinal problems may undergo surgical procedures that may ultimately induce their own metabolic disturbances. Gastrectomy, for example, may ultimately lead to osteomalacia because of altered patterns of calcium absorption.

The use of various drugs may be the most significant cause of radiographically evident abnormalities in the bone. Some anticonvulsant drugs alter the metabolism of vitamin D and lead to calcium depletion. This effect is sometimes exaggerated by the combined use of anticonvulsants and barbiturates.

The use of steroids can lead to a reduction in osteoid formation with generalized osteoporosis (Figure 10-20). Steroids initially suppress normal inflammatory reactions and may produce an erroneous picture of radiographic health during the early stages of their administration. Prolonged use, however, can lead to the deterioration of bony surfaces, particularly when they are stressed, as is the case with the articular surfaces of the joints. Destruction changes mimicking primary articular disease may result.

Osteoporosis also occurs with long-term therapy of thromboembolic disease involving heparin. The exact mechanism by which osteoporosis is produced remains unclear.

Other drugs, including heavy metals, excess vitamins, and anti-inflammatory agents, may produce a variety of disorders that can be mistaken on radiographs for primary bone disease. The subject of iatrogenic lesions of the skeleton has been reviewed by Murray.[18]

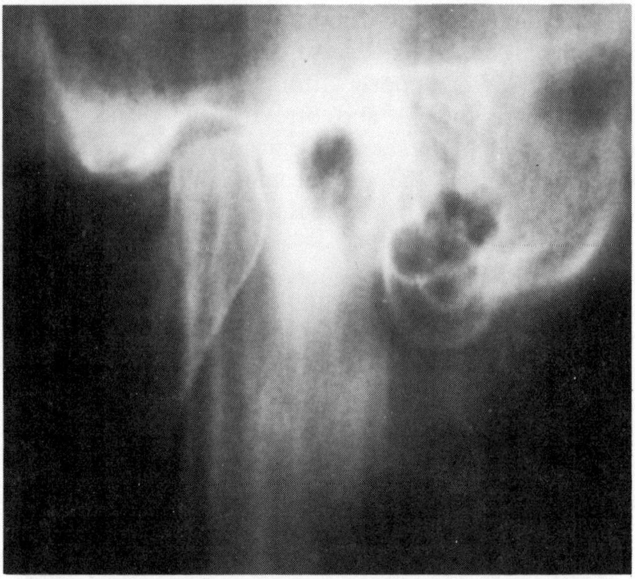

A

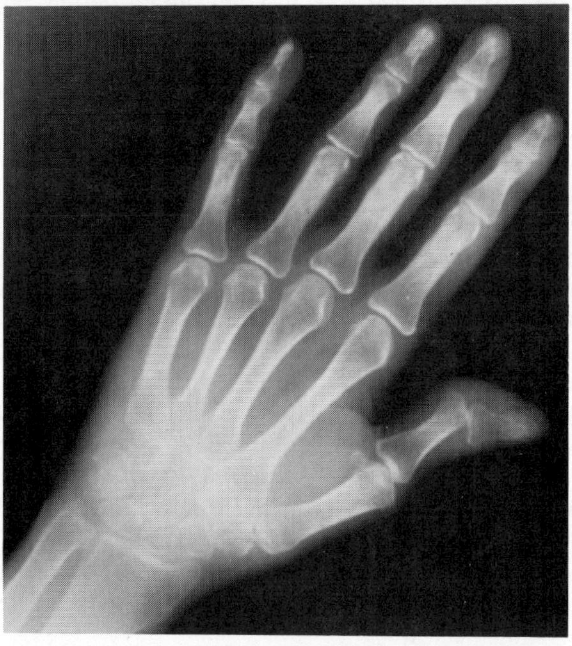

B

Figure 10-20 The prolonged administration of many drugs can alter the radiographic appearance of bone. This individual has been on long-term steroid therapy for lupus erythematosus. **A.** Osteoporosis of the temporomandibular joints. **B.** Osteoporosis of the extremities. The deformity of the thumb is the result of the primary disease and not of the medication.

Neoplastic Diseases

Tumors of bone can be classified as benign or malignant. Benign neoplasms are often asymptomatic and may be recognized on radiographs taken for other reasons. In contrast, most primary malignant tumors cause significant symptoms in the region of bony involvement. Metastatic bone tumors may or may not be symptomatic, and the radiographic search for such lesions is often unrewarding. Most head and neck neoplasms originate in soft tissue and are not visible on conventional radiographs until they invade bone. Soft tissue tumors can be demonstrated by special techniques (Figure 10-21). There is little

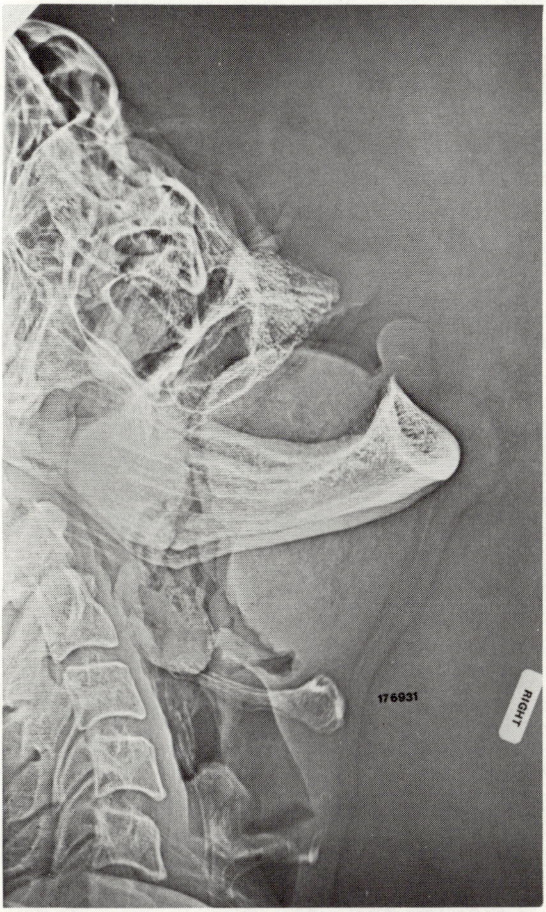

Figure 10-21 This older black male complained of facial pain and difficulty in swallowing. A xeroradiograph taken to demonstrate soft tissues revealed a mass within the pharynx. Histologic examination indicated that the mass was composed of a leukemic infiltrate.

evidence, for example, that panoramic or other surveys of the face and jaws contribute significantly to the detection of metastatic disease in symptom-free patients who are known to have primary neoplasms at other sites.[19] The accurate distinction between benign and malignant disease requires careful correlation of the radiographic evidence with the patient's clinical signs and symptoms, history, age, sex, ethnic background, and occupation. The size, location, and morphology of the lesion are of obvious importance. Radiographic study of suspected neoplastic lesions is of particular importance in determining the most useful site for biopsy and in formulating a therapeutic plan.

Malignant tumors that originate in soft tissue but invade bone may be difficult to distinguish from osteomyelitis or other inflammatory conditions that may affect peripheral bone. Primary or metastatic lesions in the jaws may be difficult to recognize and to distinguish from other types of lesions. Figure 10-22 demonstrates a lymphomatous lesion occurring at the apices of mandibular anterior teeth. A diagnosis was made from tissue obtained during retrograde filling of the root canals. It should be noted that the teeth were not carious and had not been traumatized. Apical lesions associated with sound teeth must be viewed with suspicion.

Figure 10-23 shows an extremely unusual retinal analogue tumor occurring in an infant. Excess tissue is evident in the maxilla, and the developing teeth have been displaced. The trabecular pattern is grossly atypical, presenting with a sunburst configuration often associated with osteogenic sarcomas.

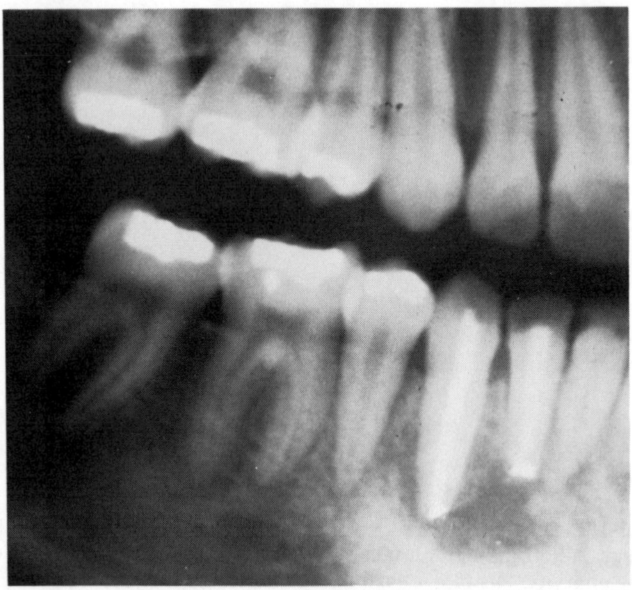

Figure 10-22 **A.** Section of a panoramic film showing bone destruction resulting from disseminated lymphoma. The lack of sharpness made it difficult to distinguish this lesion from other more common radiolucent processes.

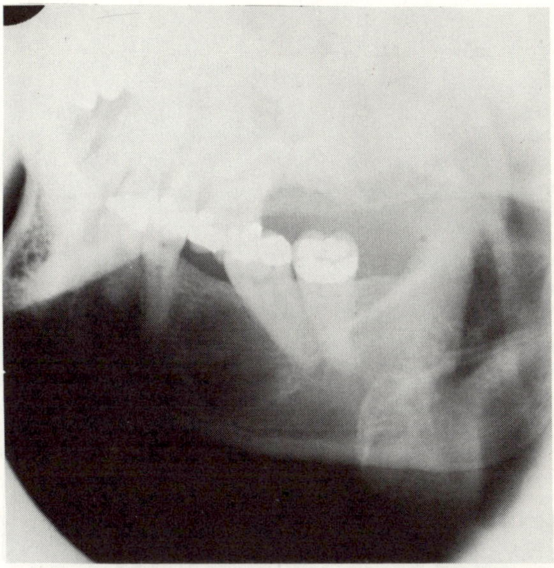

Figure 10-22 **B.** For comparison, a poorly defined lucent lesion is noted between the premolar and molar teeth. Root displacement has occurred as a result of the expanding lesion of multiple myeloma although radiographically it appears as if the molar is tilted mesially into the edentulous space.

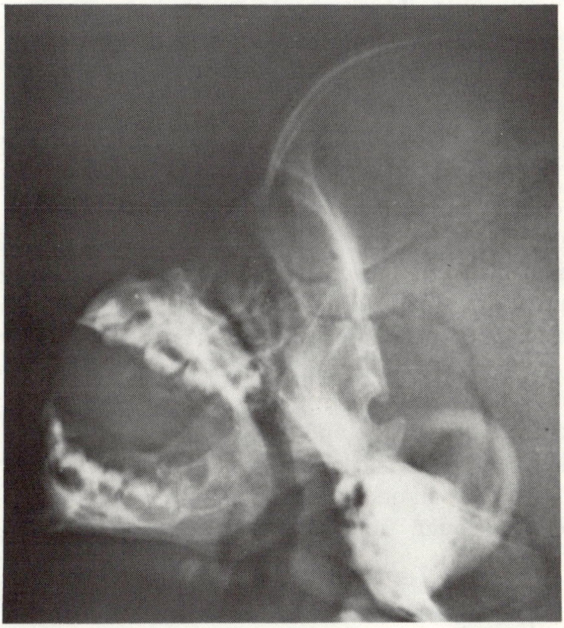

Figure 10-23 **A.** Lateral view of the facial bone in a newborn shows a soft tissue mass in the oral cavity.

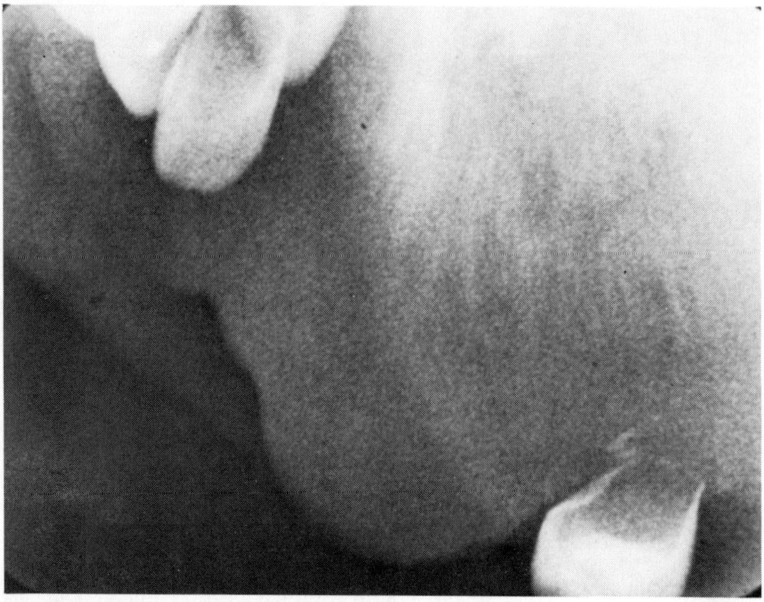

Figure 10-23 B. Intraoral radiograph shows displacement of teeth, a large soft tissue mass, and atypical bony trabeculation.

Benign Tumors

Several benign tumors are found in the jaws, facial skeleton, skull, and hands. Enchondromas are well-demarcated, benign, lytic lesions that most frequently occur in the fingers (Figure 10-24). They are most likely to be detected by orthodontists who use hand and wrist films for purposes of determining skeletal aging. Enchondromas may cause expansion of cortical bone but rarely cause its destruction, although fractures secondary to trauma are not uncommon. Osteomas are benign tumors of cortical bone that occur in the outer table of the skull (Figure 10-25), in the mandible, and in the paranasal sinuses with some frequency. Osteomas frequently have a broad base and may be associated with Gardner syndrome, which includes dermal lesions and intestinal polyposis. The largest category of benign tumors occurring in the jaws are those that are characterized as benign fibro-osseous lesions of odontogenic origin. Benign fibro-osseous lesions have been reviewed in detail by Waldron and Giansante.[20,21] Common lesions include exostoses (see Figure 10-9) and tori (Figure 10-26).

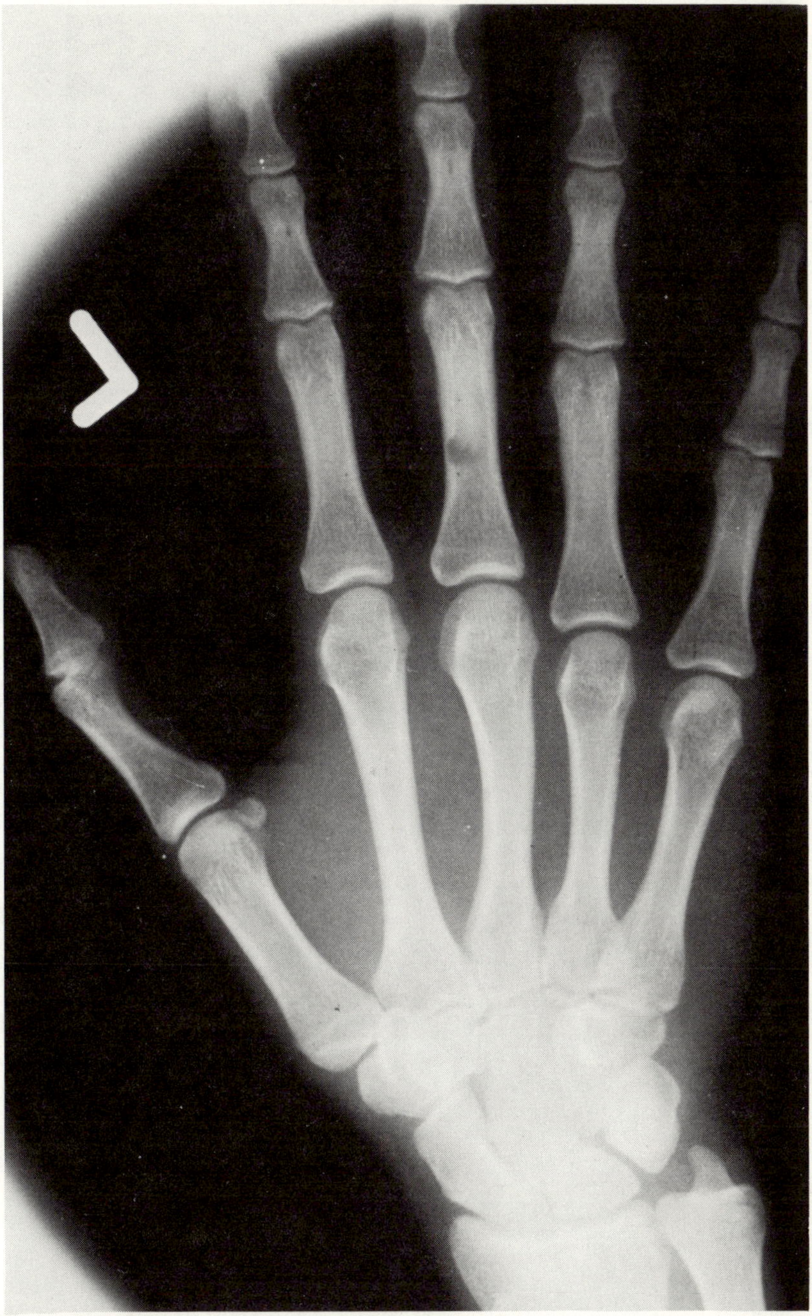

Figure 10-24 The small lytic lesion evident in this radiograph was discovered accidentally during an orthodontic evaluation. The radiographs were taken for the purpose of ascertaining skeletal aging in a patient who was symptom free.

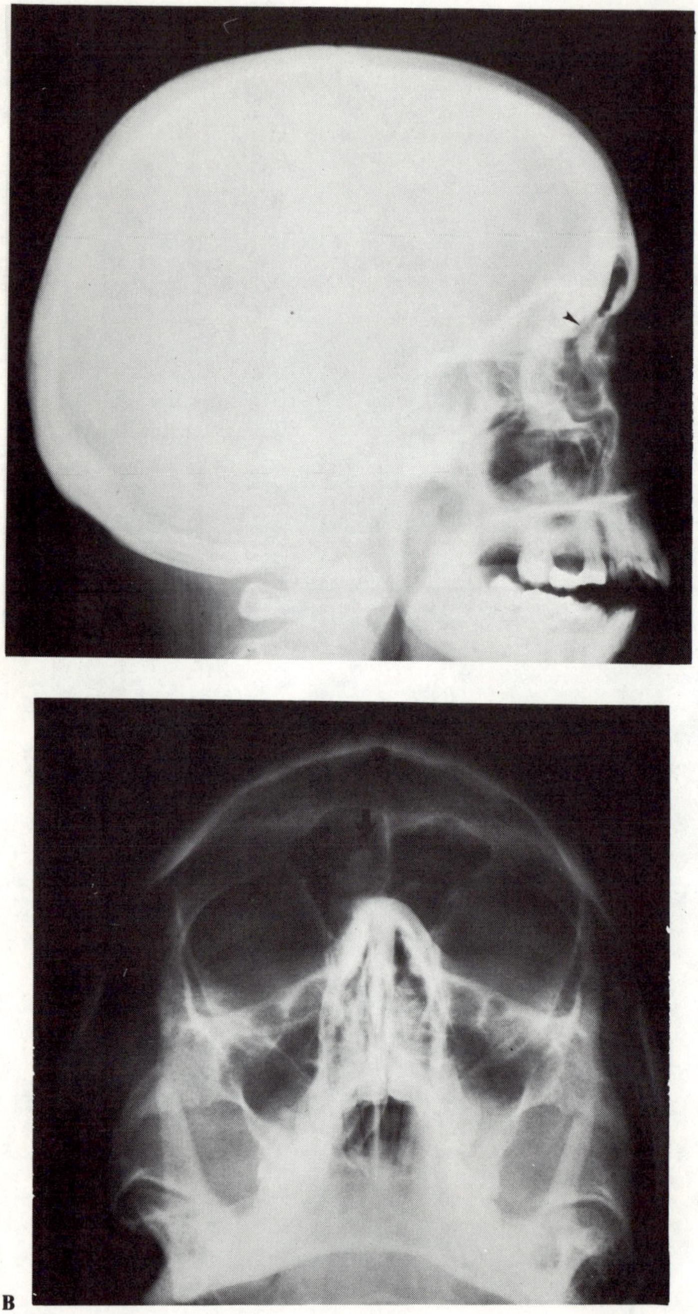

A

B

Figure 10-25 **A.** In a lateral cephalometric film, an area of increased density is noted above the bridge of the nose. **B.** A Waters' view shows the osteoma most distinctly, overlying the frontal sinuses.

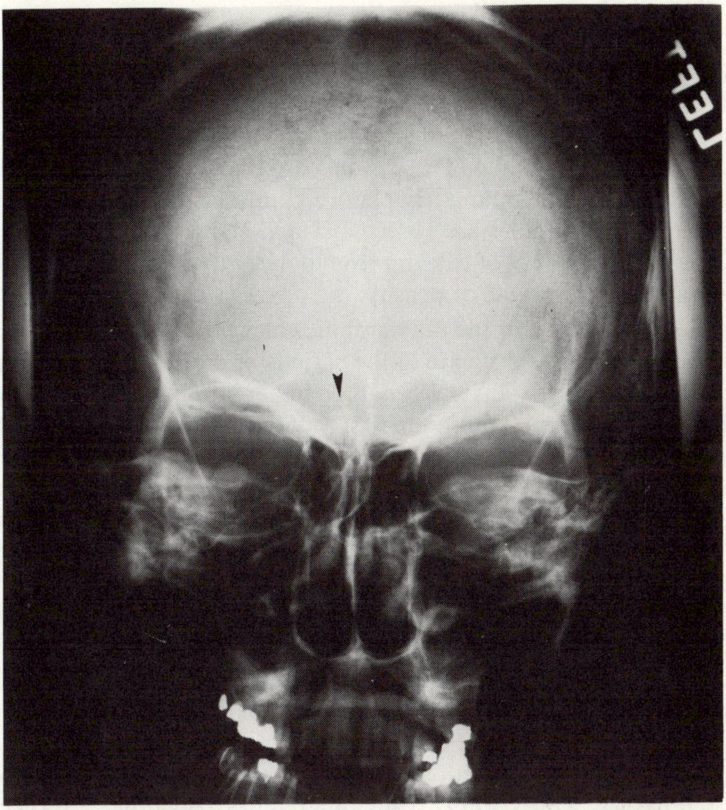

C

Figure 10-25 **C.** A P-A view of the skull shows the osteoma, although it is less distinct than when surrounded by an air-containing cavity.

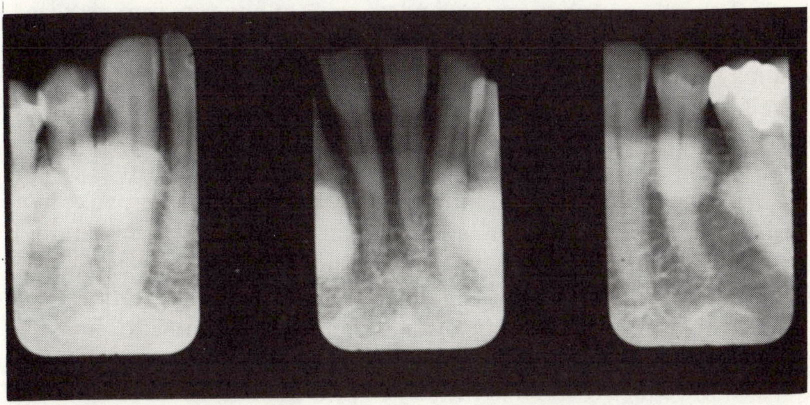

Figure 10-26 Tori are sometimes considered benign fibro-osseous lesions or benign tumors. They appear as areas of increased density, usually in the premolar regions of the mandible. They are most often bilateral.

Infection and Inflammation

Inflammatory disease in bone is usually the result of infection. Regardless of the primary cause, inflammatory processes are usually characterized by increases in the local blood supply and regional changes (usually reductions) in pH. These events are reactions to injury that can result from physical trauma, but more commonly follow invasion by pathogenic microorganisms. Hyperemia and reductions in pH tend to result in the withdrawal of calcium from bone and/or teeth, which is seen radiographically as a loss of density.

The exact nature of the radiographic change is determined by many factors, including the virulence of the organism, the anatomic site, portal of entry, and host resistance. When infection or inflammation is the result of changes in the dental pulp, the first radiographic evidence is usually a widening of the periodontal ligament space. This appears to be the result of fluid accumulation secondary to periapical hyperemia, which causes hydraulic extrusion of a tooth and accounts for sensitivity to percussion.

If the hyperemia persists, calcium depletion follows. Since the solubility of calcium in bone is greater than in tooth structure, widening of the periodontal ligament space is followed by loss of lamina dura. If the process is allowed to continue, the area of decreased density increases in size, producing an apical radiolucency that is commonly referred to as a periapical rarefying osteitis. When the inflammatory process is relatively benign, a reaction may become evident in the surrounding area. Radiographically, this reaction is seen as an increase in the density of calcified tissues, which results from an attempt to lay down a protective area of new bone. This is referred to as a reactive or condensing osteitis.

When the area of involvement is sufficiently large, segments of bone may become isolated from their blood supply. These bony segments retain their calcium whereas surrounding areas of bone are demineralized. The isolated, calcified, but dead areas of bone are referred to as sequestra and may remain within the infected or inflamed tissue. New or reactive bone produced at the margins of the area is called involucrum and the presence of the involucrum, sequestration, and irregular density are signs of diffuse involvement referred to as osteomyelitis (Figure 10-27).

Although infections and inflammatory processes may provoke bone formation at the margins of a lesion, they are primarily lytic in nature. It therefore becomes necessary to distinguish infections from cysts, early benign fibro-osseous lesions, vascular tumors or malformations, and other neoplastic processes. In most instances, the distinction must be made on the basis of histologic rather than radiographic evidence. Figure 10-28 shows a lucent lesion at the angle of the mandible that has many of the radiographic characteristics of a simple residual or primordial cyst. Its boundaries are smooth and appear to have a dense regular margin.

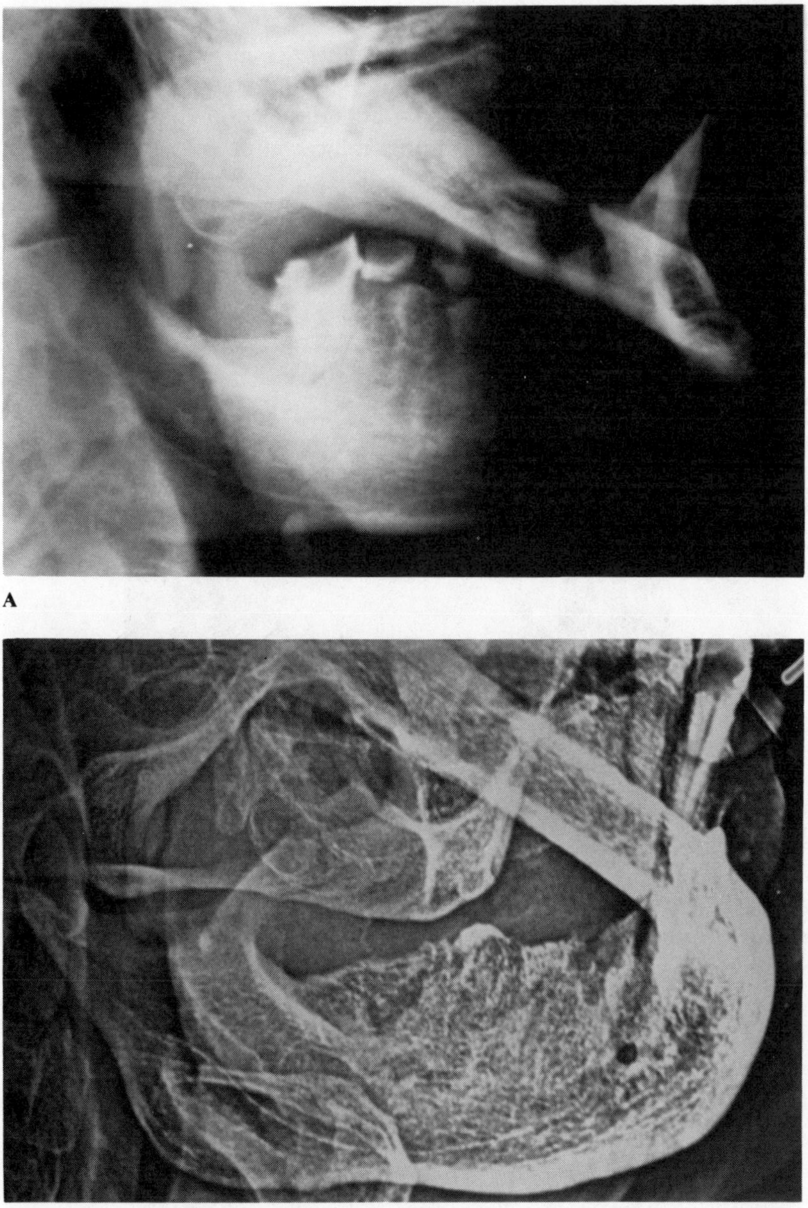

A

B

Figure 10-27 **A.** This preoperative lateral oblique film shows multiple retained root tips. **B.** In the postoperative xeroradiograph, areas of irregular trabeculation are visible near the crest of the ridge. A small sclerotic sequestrum is also seen at the crest of the ridge.

Histologically, however, this lesion proved to be a keratocyst, which requires more aggressive clinical management. Figure 10-29 illustrates a second keratocyst. This time the lesion is in the anterior portion of the mandible. There is a distinct impression that this lesion may be of dental or periodontal origin and its radiographic characteristics differ from Figure 10-28 in several respects, including a less clearly defined margin and evidence of resorption of the root of an approximating tooth. Figure 10-30 illustrates a lucent lesion around the crown of an impacted third molar that is similar in nature to the lesion in Figure 10-28. Histologically,

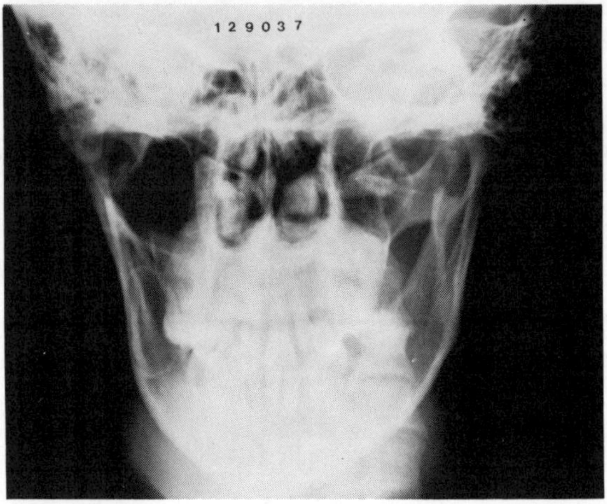

A

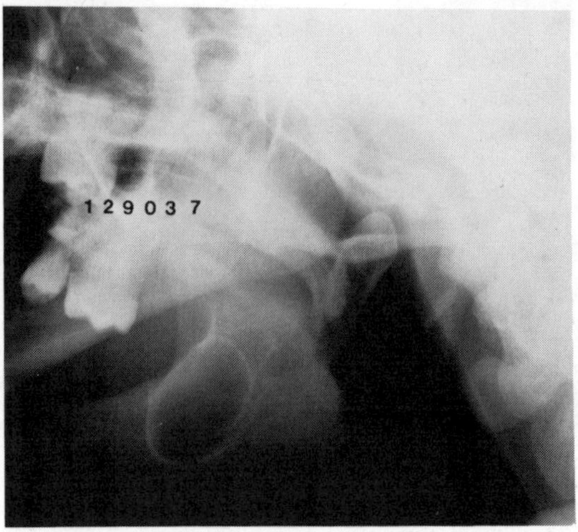

B

Figure 10-28 **A.** The lucent area in the mandibular ramus appears to have a dense cortical margin. The dense margin may, however, be an optical illusion resulting from erosion of the lesion through cortical plates, causing sharp density differences. **B.** In a lateral view the same lesion appears to be a simple residual cyst.

this proved to be a simple dentigerous cyst. The lucent area around the premolar teeth in Figure 10-31 is reminiscent of the keratocyst involving the mandibular anterior teeth illustrated in Figure 10-29, but this lesion represents a histiocytic lymphoma. Again, the lack of evident dental disease associated with teeth bordering the lesion should increase the level of suspicion.

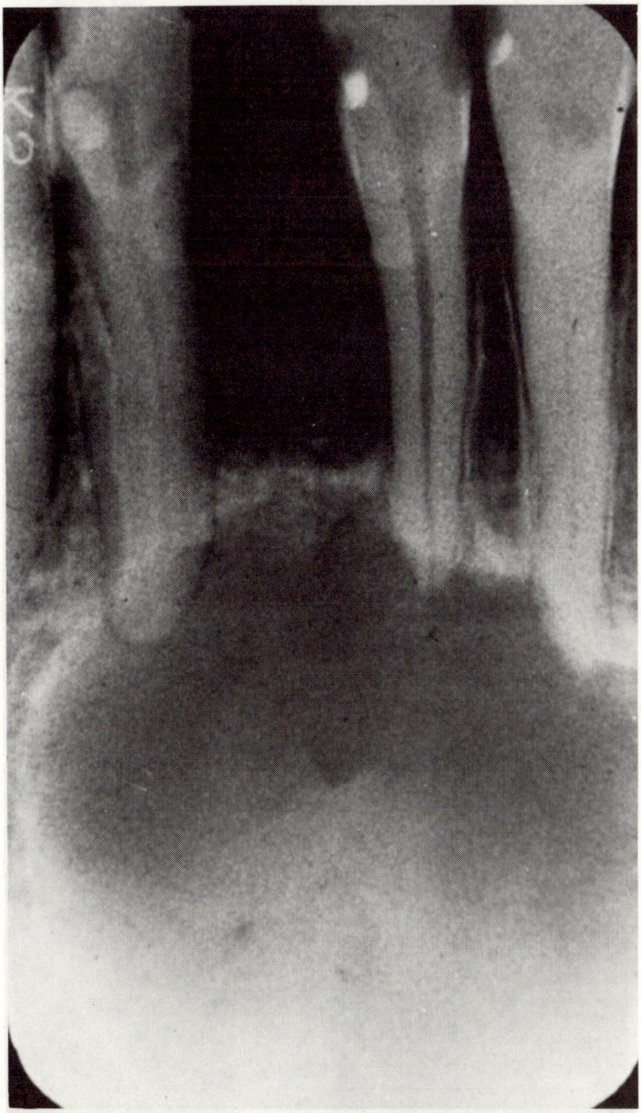

Figure 10-29 **A.** This keratocyst occurring in the anterior part of the mandible has margins which appear somewhat indistinct on this periapical view.

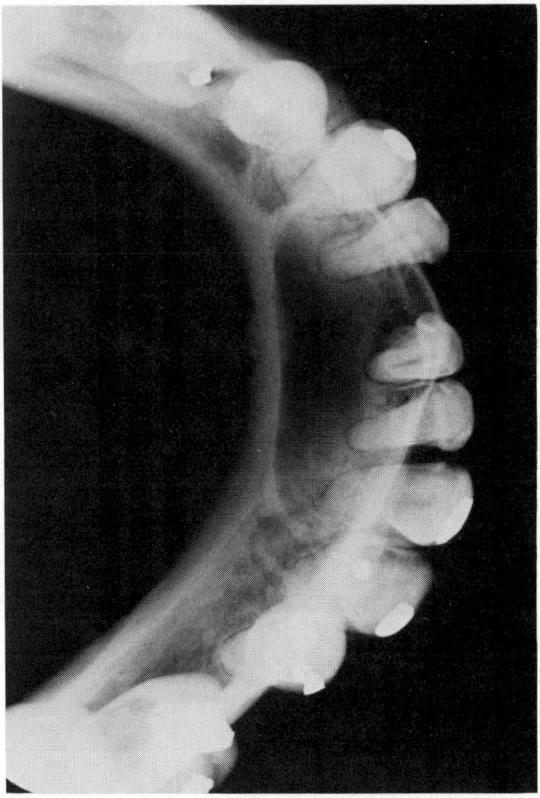

Figure 10-29 **B.** An occlusal view in which the lesion is seen encroaching upon the inferior cortex appears to have better definition. A lucent area around one incisor suggests the possibility of periodontal involvement.

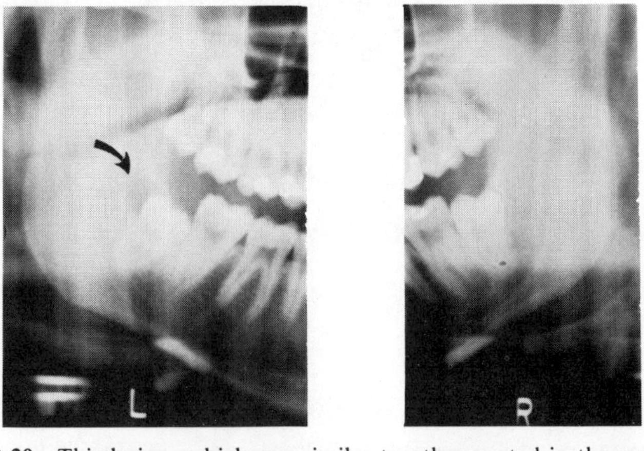

Figure 10-30 This lesion, which was similar to others noted in the mandibular rami, was histologically proven to be a simple dentigerous cyst.

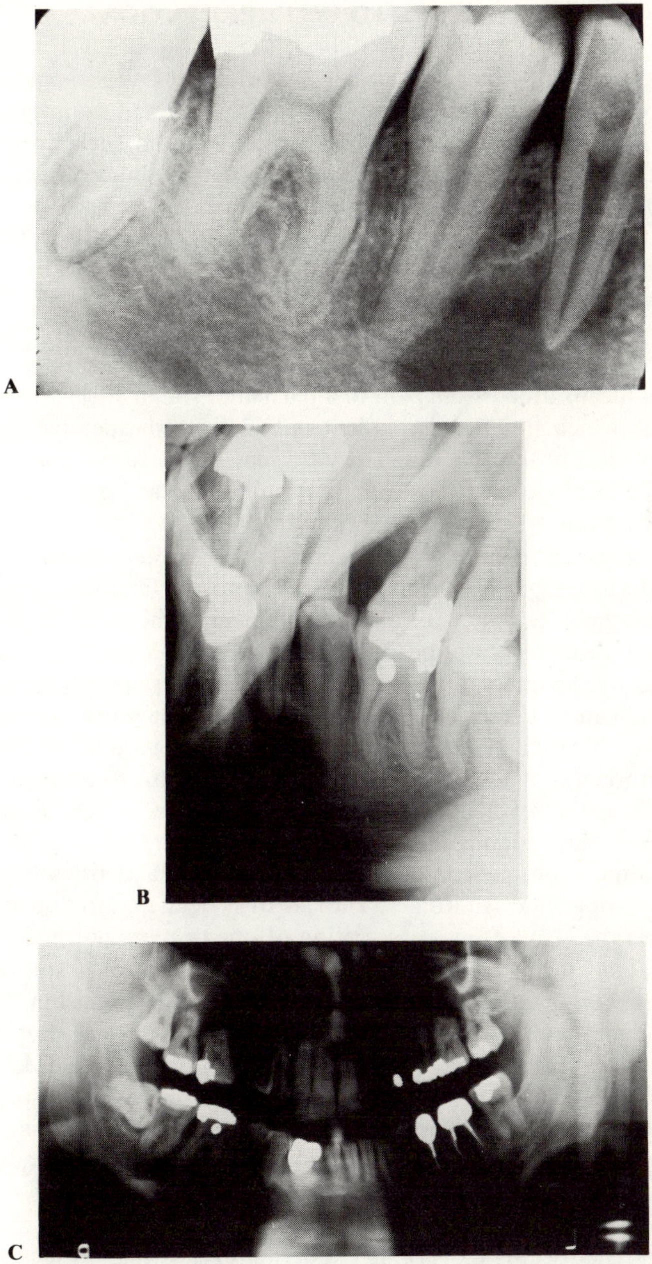

Figure 10-31 **A.** This poorly defined lucent lesion seen on a periapical view appears to involve the two premolar teeth. **B.** A change in geometry obtained with a lateral oblique view appears to localize the lesion to the first premolar and associate it with the mandibular canal. **C.** The lesion is also recognizable on a panoramic view.

ALTERNATE APPROACHES TO INTERPRETATION

As described by Potchen, Koehler, and Davis,[22] it is also possible to approach radiologic diagnosis from the point of view of symptoms and systems. For example, one may focus on a symptom such as pain to establish the basis for deciding whether or not a patient should be examined radiographically and what type of examination should be performed. Individuals with pain that has characteristics of muscular stress or that can be attributed to psychological causes should be followed clinically before a decision is made to proceed with radiographic evaluation.

When sufficient time has passed to increase the likelihood of positive findings on x-ray examination, the choice of examination should be based on careful localization of the pain to a particular site or sites. Survey examinations, which are often convenient and relatively inexpensive, usually have a low yield of information. The yield may be increased dramatically by selecting local views of those anatomic sites that can be related to the specific symptoms of an individual (Figure 10-32).

Disorders of particular organ systems have characteristics that can be useful in the development of a differential diagnosis. Nutritional deficiencies, for example, can alter skeletal development as measured by height, weight, and skeletal maturation. Just as the chronologic age of a patient is established by the interval between birth and the present, a bone age or skeletal age can be determined by comparisons of the size and shape of centers of ossification in one individual with the same parameters in other average, normal individuals within a similar population. Techniques for assessing skeletal development have been described by Greulich and Pyle.[23] Bone maturation is slowed by many factors, including prolonged illness, malnutrition, endocrine deficiencies, emotional deprivation, and a variety of congenital syndromes. The rate of skeletal maturation usually increases as the result of excess secretion of one or more hormones.

Characteristically, disorders of nutrition or hormonal status will affect many or most skeletal structures, thereby distinguishing these diseases from more clearly localized conditions. In some instances, however, the specific nature of the nutritional or hormonal disorder may be traceable to a specific anatomic defect. For example, malabsorption syndromes that interfere with normal nutrition can often be recognized by the radiographic presentation of the intestines; and endemic goiter, which is caused by insufficient dietary iodine, may be recognized by special radiographic or scintiscan characteristics of the thyroid.

Similarly, diseases of various endocrine organs may also produce local evidence of pathology as well as more generalized radiographic changes. Pituitary tumors may cause demineralization, erosion, or expansion of the sella turcica, while thyroid goiters may produce abnormal patterns of calcification within the neck.

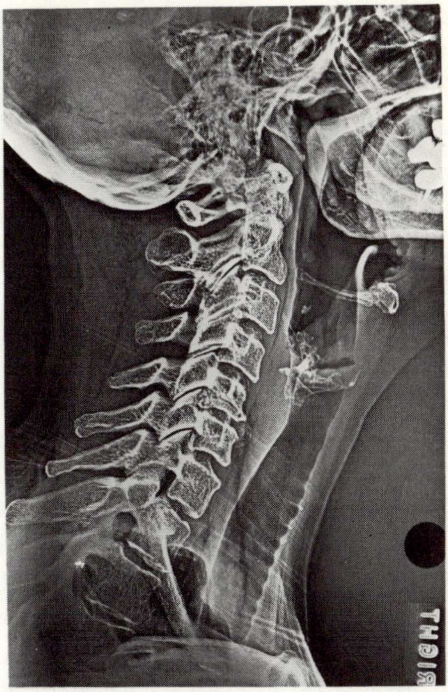

Figure 10-32 This middle-aged woman experienced a period of discomfort and lymphadenopathy after the endodontic treatment of the mandibular molar. Her symptoms included discomfort on swallowing. A xeroradiograph showed evidence of a mass in the posterior wall of the pharynx and an osteophyte bridging the gap between two vertebral bodies.

Disorders of blood forming organs can alter the trabecular pattern of bone at any site, but will have the most pronounced effect at those sites where the production of blood elements is most active. Anemias resulting from a variety of causes may produce radiographic changes in the skull and mandible.[24-27]

Trapnell[8] approaches the interpretation of radiographs of the skull, face, and teeth from a combined densitometric, anatomic, and physiologic point of view. Radiographic changes are first divided into those that cause increased density. Trapnell points out that increased density can result from changes on top of the skull or within the scalp, including opaque dressings and cosmetic preparations that may overly the scalp or foreign bodies, calcified hematomas, sebaceous cysts, and parasites that may lie within the scalp. Within the skull itself, Trapnell divides areas of increased density into normal variants, which include hyperostosis frontalis interna and similar entities, as well as abnormal conditions, which include meningioma, fibrous dysplasia, osteomyelitis, and neoplastic diseases (Figure 10-33). These entities tend to produce focal areas of increased density whereas Paget's disease, hemoglobinopathies, osteopetrosis, and hypervitaminosis-D produce more generalized increases in cranial density (Figure 10-34).

Many calcifications also occur within the brain itself. These must be recognized and localized by the evaluation of multiple right angle views. It is extremely important, particularly for orthodontists and oral surgeons who rely most heavily on skull films, to distinguish between those

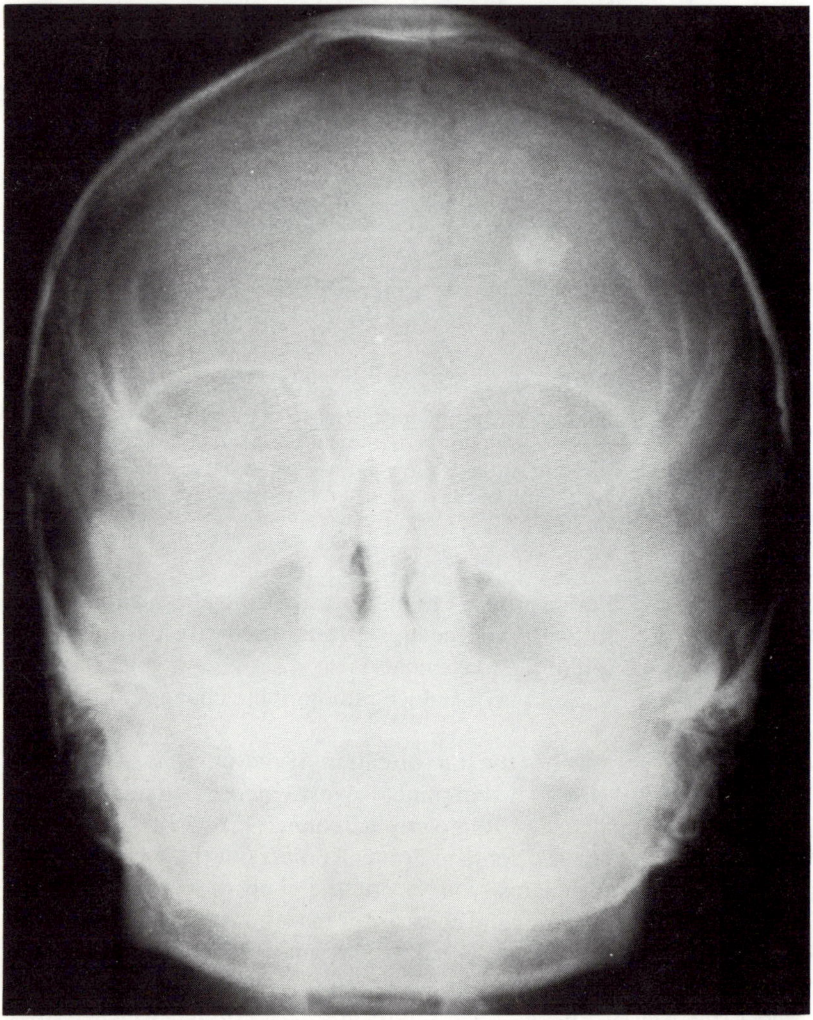

Figure 10-33 **A.** A density is noted on this P-A view but its position in an anteroposterior direction cannot be established.

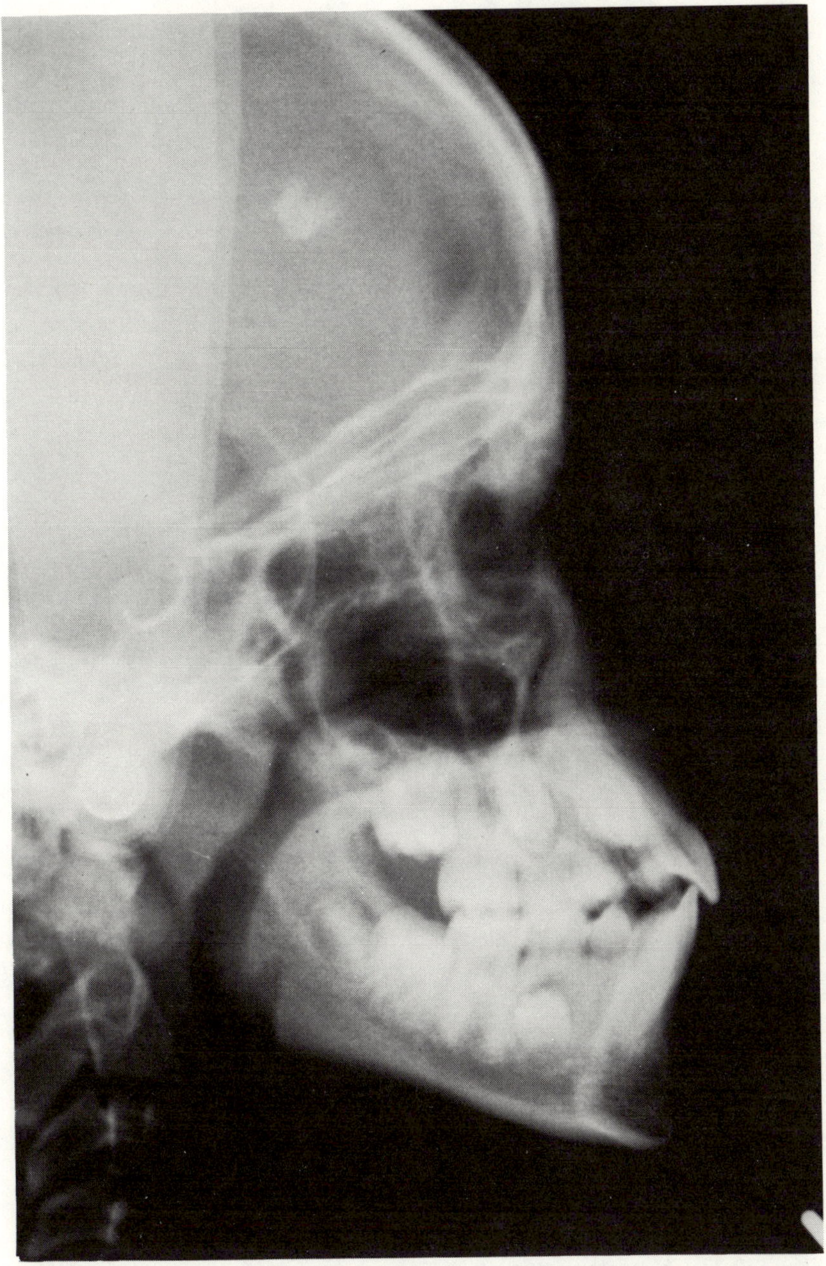

Figure 10-33 B. The lateral view localizes the density to the anterior cranial fossa. The lesion was diagnosed as tuberous sclerosis.

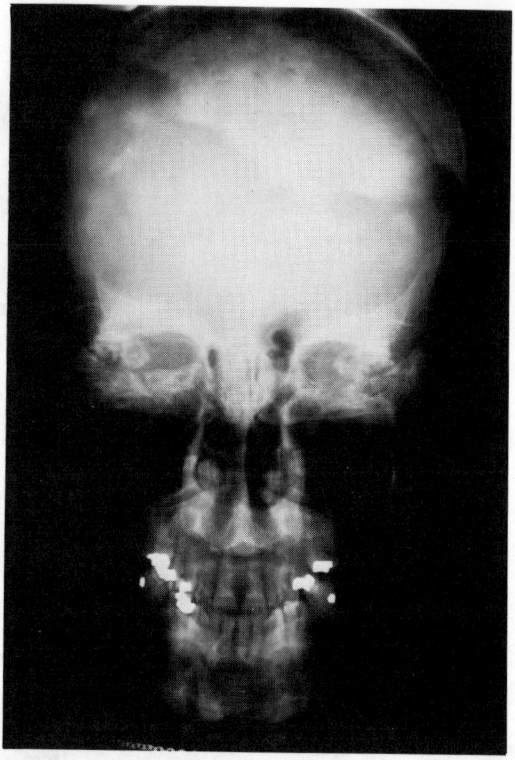

A

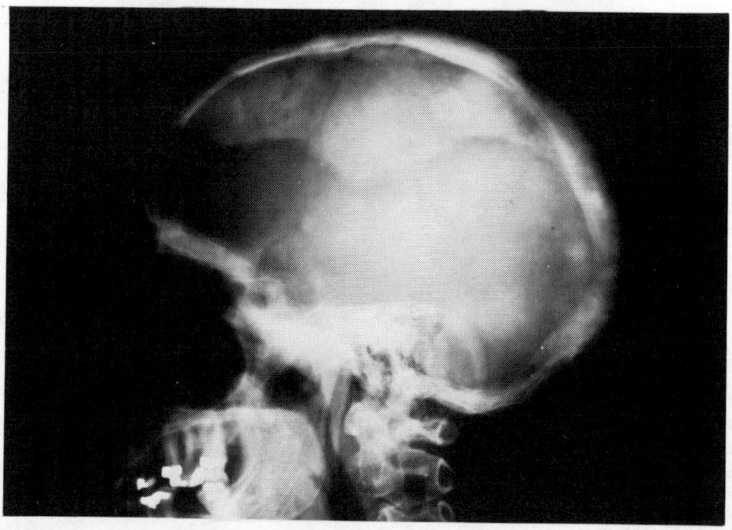

B

Figure 10-34 **A.** A circumspect area of increased density is noted at the top of the cranial vault. **B.** The sharp difference in density as well as patchy opacification of the cranial vault is noted in the lateral view.

calcifications that are normal and those that are pathologic. Ozonoff and Burrows[28] have summarized the so-called physiologic and pathologic types of intracranial calcifications. Physiologic intracranial calcifications include:

1. The pineal gland. Calcification is evident in approximately 60% of adults. Calcification is commonly visible in lateral projections and occasionally in frontal views. A calcified pineal lies in the midline when it is visible in a frontal projection and serves as a useful index of midline shift. Habenular neuroglial nodules on the surface of the habenular commissure are visible on lateral projections in approximately 30% of adults. The calcification lies several millimeters anterior to and above the pineal and is characterized by a C-shaped structure.

2. Basal ganglia and dentate nucleus. These calcifications are rarely visible on radiographs, but may be seen on frontal views where they assume a V-shaped configuration.

3. Choroid plexus. Calcification of the choroid plexus is most common in individuals after the age of 40. The particular configuration of this calcification may vary from amorphous to nodular and the size of the calcified area is extremely variable.

4. Falx. Midline calcification of the falx cerebri occurs in fewer than 10% of adults. Falx calcification may appear as a linear streak or may present with a lamellar pattern.

5. Pituitary. On rare occasions nonpathologic calcifications occur within the pituitary gland. Since pituitary tumors with calcifications can also occur, they must be considered as alternative diagnoses. Pathologic calcifications can occur in a large number of situations and as a consequence of many syndromes and diseases. Dental practitioners are not likely to find it profitable to study the wide variety of pathologic calcifications that may occur. When roentgen examination of the skull reveals calcifications that cannot be included in the category of normal or physiologic, the patient should be referred to a practitioner with greater expertise.

Trapnell has summarized signs of an intracranial mass that are likely to be evident in plain radiographs. In the case of increased intracranial pressure that may produce headache or other neurologic signs, radiographic findings include widened sutures, a beaten copper appearance to the skull vault, and demineralization or fuzziness of the lamina dura around the pituitary fossa. Displacement of the pituitary may provide evidence of a space-occupying lesion. Tumors are radiographically demonstrated by the presence of bone sclerosis, enlargement of foramina, alteration in the normal pattern of vascular channels, asymmetries, or atypical patterns of calcification.

REFERENCES

1. Committee on Commerce, Science, and Transportation. United States Senate. *Report on Radiation Health and Safety.* Washington, DC: US Government Printing Office, December, 1978.

2. Phillips, L. *Comparative Evaluation of the Effect of a High Yield Criteria Test upon Skull Radiography Utilization in Emergency Rooms.* Contract Report #223-76-6019 FDA, BRH, Washington, DC: US Government Printing Office, 1977.

3. Phillips, L. *A Study of the Effect of High Yield Criteria for Emergency Room Skull Radiography.* DHEW Publ. No. (FDA) 78-8069. Washington, DC: US Government Printing Office, 1978.

4. Bell, R.S., and Loop, J.W. The utility and futility of skull examination for trauma. *N Engl J Med.* 284:236–239, 1971.

5. Lachman, E. Osteoporosis: the potentialities and limitations of its roentgenographic diagnosis. *Am J Roentgenol.* 74:712, 1955.

6. Webber, R.L. Intensity-coded pseudostereoscopic image enhancement of radiographic displays. *Invest Radiol.* 8:170–177, 1973.

7. Hellewell, A.B., and Beljan, J.R. A new *in vivo* method of quantitating the rate of magnitude of mineralization of an experimental osseous defect. *Invest Radiol.* 12:467–473, 1977.

8. Trapnell, D.H. *Principles of X-Ray Diagnosis.* London: Butterworth, 1967.

9. von Wowern, N. Variation in bone mass within the cortices of the mandible. *Scand J Dent Res.* 85:444–455, 1977.

10. von Wowern, N. Variations in structure within trabecular bone of the mandible. *Scand J Dent Res.* 85:613–622, 1977.

11. Reeder, M.M., and Felson, B. *Gamuts in Radiology.* Cincinnati: Audiovisual Radiology of Cincinnati, Inc., 1975.

12. Taybi, H. *Radiology of Syndromes.* Chicago: Year Book Medical Publishers, 1975.

13. Eversole, L.R., and Rovin, S. Differential radiographic diagnosis of lesions of the jawbones. *Radiology* 105:277–284, 1972.

14. Eversole, L.R., and Rovin, S. Differential radiographic diagnosis of lesions of the jawbones. *Dent Radiogr Photogr.* 46:71–81, 1973.

15. Boulis, Z.F., Dick, R., and Barnes, N.R. Head injuries in children—aetiology, symptoms, physical findings and x-ray wastage. *Br J Radiol.* 51:851–854, 1978.

16. Berry, H.M. The lore and the lure of the lamina dura. *Radiology* 109:525–528, 1973.

17. Marshall, D. Radiographic correlation of hand, wrist, and tooth development. *Dent Radiogr Photogr.* 42:51–59, 1976.

18. Murray, R.O. Iatrogenic lesions of the skeleton. *Am J Roentgenol.* 126:5–22, 1976.

19. White, S.C., and Weissmann, D.D. Relative discernment of lesions by intraoral and panoramic radiography. *J Am Dent Assoc.* 95:1117–1121, 1977.

20. Waldron, C.A., and Giansante, J.S. Benign fibro-osseous lesions of the jaws: A clinical-radiological-histological review of sixty-five cases. *Oral Surg.* 35:190–201, 1973.

21. Waldron, C.A., and Giansante, J.S. Benign fibro-osseous lesions of the jaws. *Oral Surg.* 35:340–350, 1973.

22. Potchen, J.E., Koehler, P.R., and Davis, D.O. *Principles of Diagnostic Radiology.* New York: McGraw-Hill, 1971.

23. Greulich, W.W., and Pyle, S.I. *Radiographic Atlas of Skeletal Development of the Hand and Wrist.* 2nd Ed. Stanford: Stanford University Press, 1959.

24. Baker, D.H. Roentgen manifestations of Cooley's anemia. *Ann NY Acad Sci.* 119:641, 1964.

25. Caffey, J. Cooley's anemia: A review of the roentgenographic findings in the skeleton. *Am J Roentgenol.* 78:381, 1957.

26. Moseley, J.E. *Bone Changes in Hematologic Disorders.* New York: Grune and Stratton, 1963.

27. Moseley, J.E. Patterns of bone change in leukemia and myelosclerosis. *J Mt Sinai Hosp.* 18:1, 1961.

28. Ozonoff, M.B., and Burrows, E.H. Intracranial Calcification. Edited by T.H. Newton, and D.G. Potts. In *Radiology of the Skull and Brain.* St. Louis: C.V. Mosby, 1971.

11 Temporomandibular Joints

Diseases of the temporomandibular joints as presumed causes of facial pain and headache have received growing attention from dental practitioners during the last decade. Several schools of thought have developed based on principles of occlusion, orthopedics, surgery, and psychology. Specialists in prosthodontics, orthodontics, oral surgery, otorhinolaryngology, psychiatry, and neurology treat patients who are presumed to have the same general pathology; and, interestingly enough, remarkably similar results are reported by individuals using dramatically different approaches to therapy. An understanding of temporomandibular joint anatomy in health and disease is an essential component of the diagnosis and management of patients.

ANATOMY

The glenoid fossa, which lies at the base of the middle cranial fossa, is formed by the articular eminence anteriorly and the tympanic plate posteriorly. Behind the tympanic plate lies the external auditory canal and the middle ear. The head of the mandibular condyle forms the second bony component of the joint. The surfaces of the glenoid fossa and the condylar head are covered with a white fibrocartilage that is different from the hyaline cartilage that covers the bony surfaces of other joints. An oval fibrocartilage disc lies between the glenoid fossa and the mandibular condyle. This disc or meniscus is attached at its periphery to a capsule that encloses the joint. The capsule also attaches to the condyle and to the glenoid fossa, dividing the joint into an upper and a lower compartment. The disc derives its blood supply from the posterior attachment, which is also important to retrusive movements of the mandible. Under most conditions, the disc is held in a relatively fixed position in relation to the condylar head while the attachments of the disc and capsule to the glenoid fossa are loose and flexible.

The capsule enclosing the temporomandibular joint is lined by a synovial membrane that extends to the edges of the fibrocartilage. The synovial membrane is backed by connective tissue and produces fluid. The joint is supported or reinforced by accessory ligaments. The temporomandibular ligament arises from the lateral surface of the zygomatic arch and runs downward to its attachment on the lateral surface of the neck of the condyle. This ligament strengthens the joint and prevents excessive forward and backward lateral movements. The sphenomandibular ligament runs from the angular spine of the sphenoid bone to the lingula of the mandibular foramen. The stylomandibular ligament extends from the top of the styloid process to the angle of the mandible.

The temporomandibular joint and its associated musculature are innervated by branches from the mandibular division of the trigeminal nerve and by branches of the facial nerve. The mandibular division of the trigeminal nerve lies in close association with the accessory meningeal artery and the middle meningeal vessels. The meningeal branch of the mandibular nerve re-enters the skull through the foramen spinosum. The area immediately around the joint is supplied by the auriculotemporal nerve.

The joint receives its blood supply from a branch of the deep auricular artery and from branches of the superficial, middle meningeal, anterior tympanic, and ascending pharyngeal arteries. Lymphatic drainage is via the deep parotid nodes. The anatomy and histology of the temporomandibular joint is reviewed by Orban,[1] Sicher,[2] and Woodburne.[3]

The complex nature of the innervation and blood supply of the joint may account for the broad spectrum of symptoms that have been associated with temporomandibular disease or dysfunction. A list of the presenting symptoms in a retrospective study of 90 patients is shown in Table 11-1.

Joints serve several functions.[4] Their primary purpose is to connect different body parts. In some instances they also serve to transmit forces

Table 11-1
Presenting Symptoms of Temporomandibular Disease or Dysfunction

Symptoms	No. patients
Fullness, tinnitus, vertigo	17
Recurrent temporal pain	15
Variety of symptoms with no apparent organic basis	12
Fullness, subjective hearing loss	9
Inability to open or close mouth	8
Pain in zygomatic arch, fullness in cheek	7
Nerve V trigger zones	6
Toothache	5
Ear, deep head pains	4
Earache, weakness in facial muscles	2
Ear and mastoid pain	2
Pain in preauricular area, gonial angle, swelling	2
Resorption of condyles	1

From L.R. House et al. Clinical evaluation of TMJ arthroplasties with insertion of articular eminence prosthesis on ninety patients (an eight year study). *Laryngoscope* Vol. LXXXVII, No. 7, pp. 1182–1187, July, 1977. Reproduced with permission.

and to permit free movement. The temporomandibular joint is a synovial joint that is enclosed within a connecting ring or capsule. The lining of the capsule is a synovial membrane that is continuous with the periosteum but ends where fibrocartilage covers the continuous bony surfaces of the joint.

The joint is separated into upper and lower compartments by an intervening fibrocartilaginous articular disc. The shape of the articular disc is determined largely by functional requirements of the joint. The range of motion of the joint is determined by the laxity or tightness of the capsule and by supporting ligaments. In the adult, cartilaginous parts of the joint are essentially avascular, aneural, and relatively acellular. The cartilage is resilient and is not seen on radiographs.

Articular cartilage is nourished by synovial fluid and material which reaches it from the underlying bone. Some cartilage at the periphery of the joint is nourished by vascular bundles that abut the area.

Degenerative changes are often characterized by ulceration of the cartilaginous surface. Erosion is more common in central areas while excrescence is more typical at the periphery. Once cartilage is damaged, repair is unusual.

Most sensory function lies within the capsule and ligaments, which are composed of collagenous fibers. The sensitivity of these tissues protects the joints and provides a mechanism for functional feedback to control movement. Excessive stretching of the capsule or ligaments is usually responsible for producing protective muscle contraction. As described by Hilton's law, "The same trunk of nerves whose branches supply the groups of muscles moving a joint also furnishes a distribution of nerves to the skin over the insertion of those muscles, and the interior of the joint receives its nerves from the same source."

The major concentration of sensory articular nerve endings is located in the capsule, ligaments, and adjacent fat pads. No nerve endings are found in synovial membrane, although some nerve endings have been observed in vessels supplying the synovium.

Although the two primary functions of joints are to provide a mechanism for movement and a means of transmitting forces, the architecture of the temporomandibular joint appears to be poorly suited to the latter. The roof of the glenoid fossa is extremely thin. Under ordinary circumstances, the teeth, rather than components of the joint, establish the terminal position of the condyle in its fossa. The joint space is normally symmetrical and approximately 2 mm wide. Collapse of the occlusion, loss of teeth, muscle spasm, and a variety of intra-articular diseases can change the dimensions of the joint space.

At the margins of the joint where the synovial membrane joins the fibrocartilage, there are small bony surfaces that lack a protective layer. These regions are particularly vulnerable to inflammatory processes. The points of attachment of the capsule are also vulnerable and may show changes resulting from excessive mandibular excursions.

In most joints the articular cartilage is the surface that bears both static and dynamic forces during compression, tension, or shearing. Interwoven collagen fibers and long-chained mucopolysaccharides make up the cartilage of most joints, but the cartilaginous surfaces of the temporomandibular joints are more fibrous in nature. Therefore, temporomandibular joint cartilage is likely to be somewhat less elastic. Its capacity to deform under stress should be significantly less than that of hyaline cartilage and, therefore, the propensity for wear or damage may be increased. This is particularly important because of the poor capacity of articular cartilage to repair damage. It is also of interest to note laboratory studies suggest that cartilage from an osteoarthritic joint is less resistant to damage than is cartilage from the normal joint. Once a degenerative process is initiated, it may tend to be self-perpetuating.

The durability of articular cartilage is also dependent upon the nature of the material with which it is lubricated. Synovial fluid does not reduce friction by coating the surface; instead, it reacts with the articular surfaces to reduce friction.

Under ordinary circumstances, no single area of articular cartilage carries a continuous load. This is particularly true in the temporomandibular joint, where the teeth determine the point of terminal closure and because a space is normally maintained between the teeth during function. As force is applied and relaxed, synovial fluid coats the articular surfaces.

It is clear that the examination of the temporomandibular joints must be accomplished in a way that permits the demonstration of the joint space, joint alignment, mobility, and the articular surfaces. One should also bear in mind that the joints are three-dimensional structures that are reduced to two dimensions in any radiographic procedure.

RADIOGRAPHIC EXAMINATION

Several techniques have been used for the examination of the temporomandibular joints. Thin sectioned tomography is, however, the only reasonable way of demonstrating the articular surfaces and joint relationships without the superimposition of confusing shadows from adjacent structures. Oblique views demonstrate the lateral margins of the joint (Figure 11-1). In a typical adult, the condyle lies in an area between 10 and 30 mm in from the skin surface.

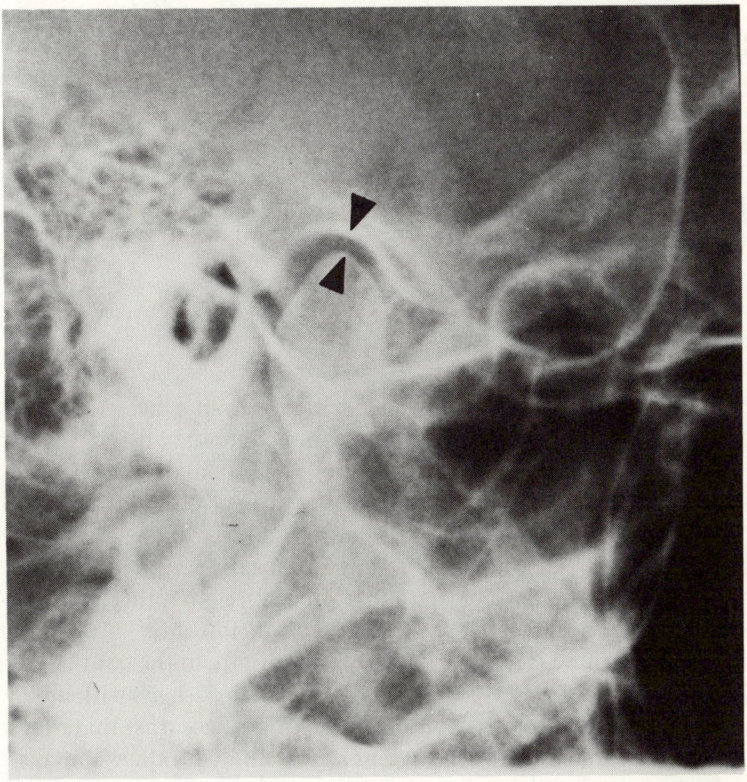

Figure 11-1 The arrows point to the lateral margin of the glenoid fossa and the lateral pole of the condyle. The head of the condyle lies below and is superimposed onto other structures. The separation between condyle and fossa does not represent the joint space in this view.

As a result of the anatomic variability of different individuals, it is usually necessary to make several tomographic sections at different levels to establish the exact position of the joint. Typically, these "scout" films are made at 15, 20, 25, and 30 mm from the skin surface. In some individuals these preliminary films provide all the necessary diagnostic information. In other circumstances it is necessary to obtain additional films at other levels as well as radiographs of the condyles in different functional positions. In those patients who are undergoing therapy with an occlusal appliance (which alters jaw position), it may be desirable to obtain films of the condyle/fossa relationship with the appliance in place and with the patient's teeth occluding without the appliance. In addition to the tomographic views, submentovertex and open mouth Towne projections are usually obtained. These views provide useful information about the relationships of the condyles to each other and to the base of the skull, and they also demonstrate many of the periarticular structures that might be involved with or responsible for the patient's primary complaint.

Tomography and other conventional methods of radiographic examination are able to demonstrate the quality of bony surfaces and the relationship of the bony components of the joint. Unfortunately, the fibrocartilage surfaces, the disc, and the capsule can be evaluated only by inference in these procedures. In some patients the history and clinical evidence point strongly to the existence of joint pathology, but radiographic examination fails to demonstrate an abnormality.

Arthrography

The introduction of opaque fluid into the joint spaces followed by x-ray examination of the joint is a procedure commonly used to evaluate the integrity of larger joints in the body, particularly the knee and shoulder. This technique, arthrography, has been given slight attention in the literature, with varying interpretations of its clinical usefulness. Arthrography of the temporomandibular joint carries with it risks similar to those encountered in arthrographic procedures of other joints. The procedure is contraindicated in the presence of infection in or near the joint and when there is a history of hypersensitivity to the contrast agent or to related compounds. Special risks may exist in patients with impaired renal function, and the accidental introduction of contrast material into the brain through the roof of the glenoid fossa may produce convulsions and possibly fatal reactions. Contrast agents may also cause numerous adverse reactions, which are fortunately infrequent and which can usually be managed with antihistamines. Most patients tolerate the procedure without difficulty. However, insertion of a needle into a small joint and the injection of nonphysiologic fluids can irritate a damaged joint. Patients should be selected for this procedure according to carefully defined criteria after a careful evaluation, and each patient should be fully advised of the possible risks or clinical sequelae.

Arthrography is performed as a sterile procedure. Patients are premedicated with 10 to 20 mg of diazepam approximately 40 minutes before the examination. The skin surface over the condyle is scrubbed with povidone-iodine[5] and draped, and local anesthesia is obtained with lidocaine. Separate injections of contrast agent (Renografin-60) are required for the upper and lower compartments. Although the lower compartment can be approached from the side, there are advantages in directing the needle toward the back of the condyle through the auditory canal. This procedure should be done with direct observation by fluoroscopy in order to reduce the mechanical trauma associated with insertion of the needle and to avoid inappropriate placement of the needle. The upper compartment can be reached by partial withdrawal and reorientation of the needle or by reinserting the needle on the skin surface anterior to the pinna and just below the zygomatic arch.

Injections are observed directly by image-intensified fluoroscopy recorded on videotape. Spot films are obtained at appropriate intervals and positions. When the physical and functional characteristics of a joint have been documented, the procedure is terminated. Patients are given postoperative instructions that include a soft diet, warm packs over the face, and slight exercise for 24 hours.

Arthrographic Findings

A normal lower compartment sits over the condylar head like a cap. The compartment is bordered by the condyle along its inferior aspect and by the capsule and disc at its superior aspect. The lower compartment may be visualized by oblique views during injection (Figure 11-2). Under normal circumstances the configuration of the lower compartment does not change significantly during function. In Figure 11-3 tomograms of a joint are seen with the mouth open and closed and with contrast material in the lower compartment. The dye is redistributed from the anterior to the superior surface as the mouth opens. In this instance a perforation was present in the disc and a small amount of dye was forced into the upper compartment, leaving a streak over the articular eminence when the condyle rested within the fossa.

The upper compartment of the temporomandibular joint is larger in volume than the lower compartment. Dye in the upper compartment dramatically changes its distribution as a result of condylar movement (Figure 11-4). When the condyle is in the fossa, a significant amount of dye lies anterior to the condyle and moves back into the fossa when the condyle is moved. This demonstrates the loose attachments of the upper compartment, which are necessary for normal movement.

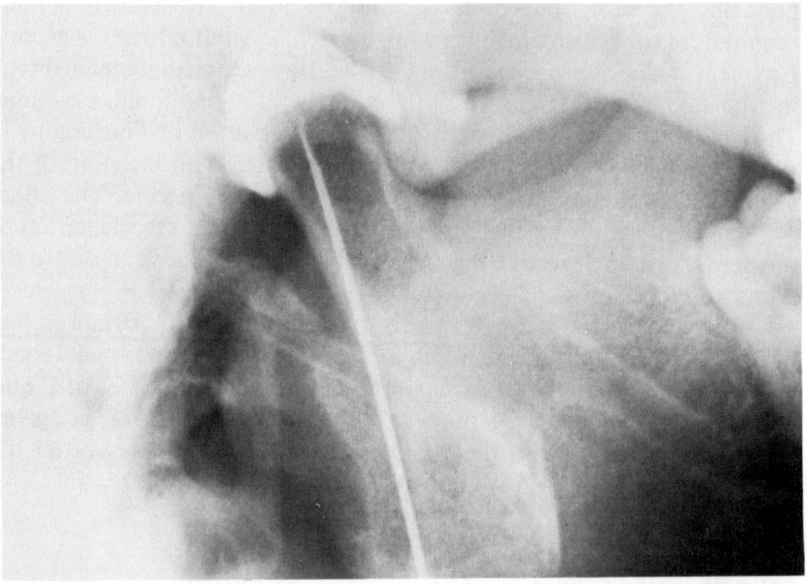

Figure 11-2 The needle is still in place following an injection of contrast media. The lower compartment fits over the condyle like a cap. This space moves with the condyle during function and shows only slight deformity.

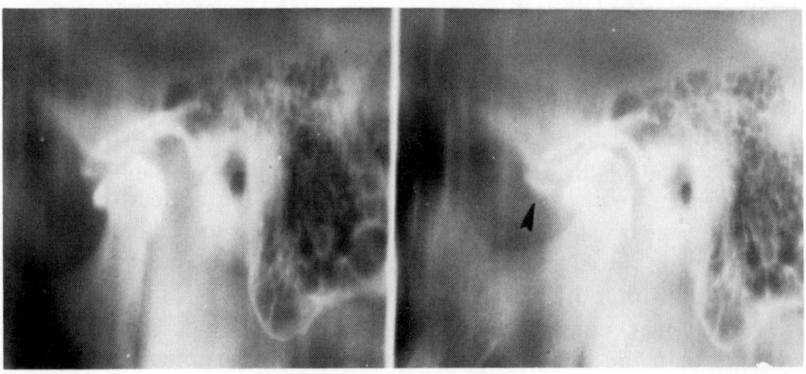

Figure 11-3 When the lower compartment is injected, perforations in the compartment are made obvious by leakage of dye indicated by arrow.

A temporomandibular joint may appear to be radiographically normal in a patient who presents with pain on function. Figure 11-5 shows the result of filling the lower compartment with dye in such a patient. In contrast to the pattern seen in the normal lower compartment, there was evidence of dye trailing behind the condyle as it moved into a protrusive excursion. During surgery this was found to be the result of adhesions between the articular disc and the glenoid fossa that produced tension on the lower compartment when the condyle attempted to move out of the lower fossa.

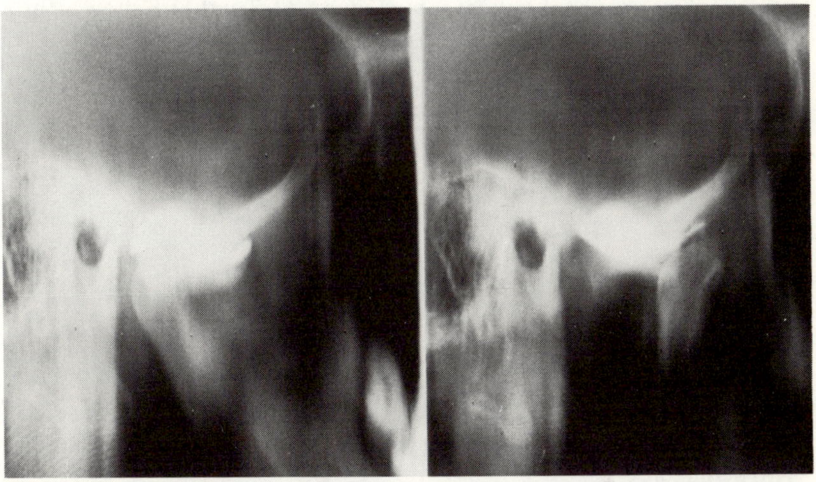

Figure 11-4 The upper compartment is larger and more flexible than the lower compartment. Most joint movement occurs in this space.

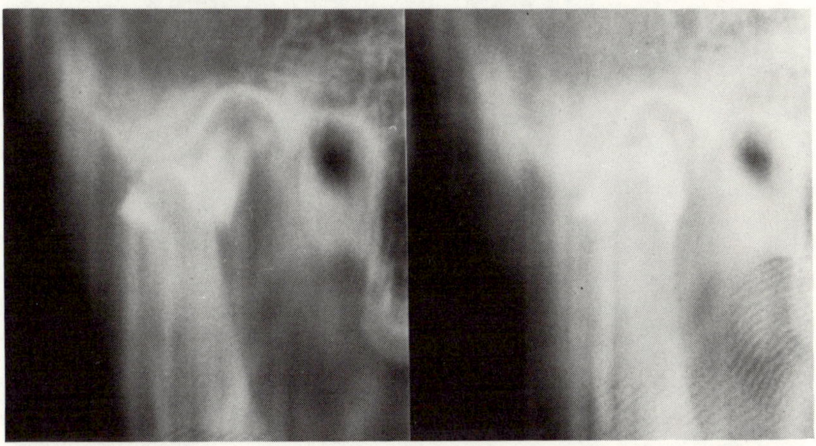

Figure 11-5 Adhesions in the upper compartment are sometimes discovered because of unusual deformity of the lower compartment during function.

Fibrosis and/or adhesions in the upper compartment produce arthrograms in which the normal, regular, well-defined boundaries are obliterated. The patient shown in Figure 11-6 had long-standing pain following a motor vehicle accident. Although there were morphologic changes in the mandibular condyle, the radiographic evidence of joint disease was not impressive.

When destruction of the disc is a component of joint disease or a sequela of surgical treatment, many practitioners place a piece of inert material between the remaining condylar surface and the glenoid fossa to prevent ankylosis. Most of the materials used are radiolucent and cannot be seen on conventional radiographs. Figures 11-7 and 11-8 show arthro-

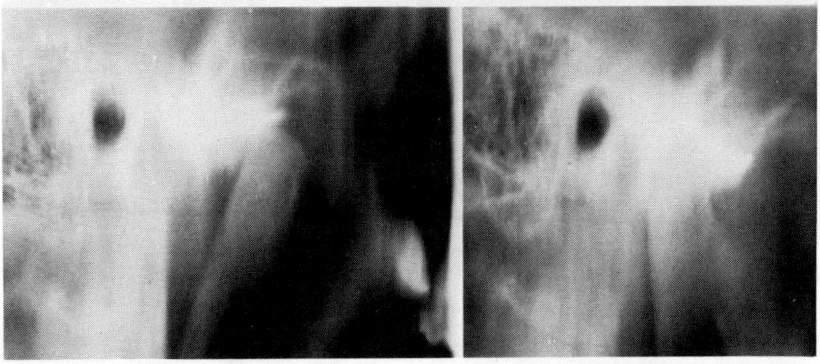

Figure 11-6 When fibrosis is extensive, the margins of the compartment lose their sharp definition.

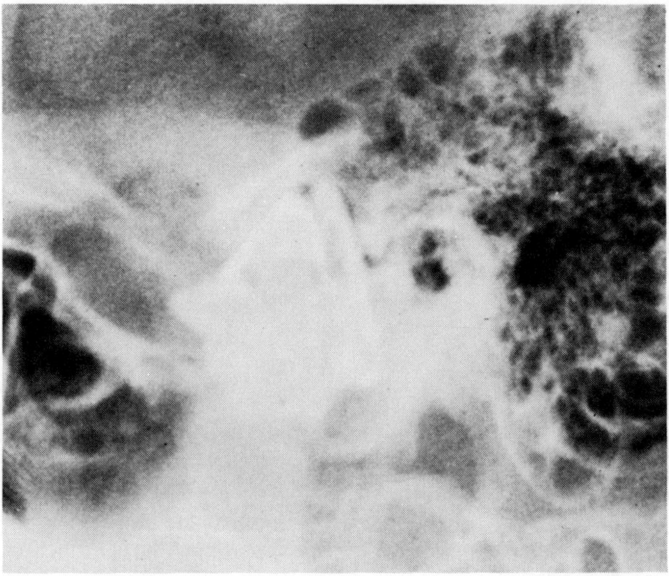

Figure 11-7 The Silastic implant lies between the condyle and the glenoid fossa.

grams of two patients with this type of implant. In one instance, a piece of Silastic has been displaced posteriorly and lies between the condyle and the posterior wall of the fossa. In the second case, the position of the Silastic has been maintained between the articulating surfaces of the joint.

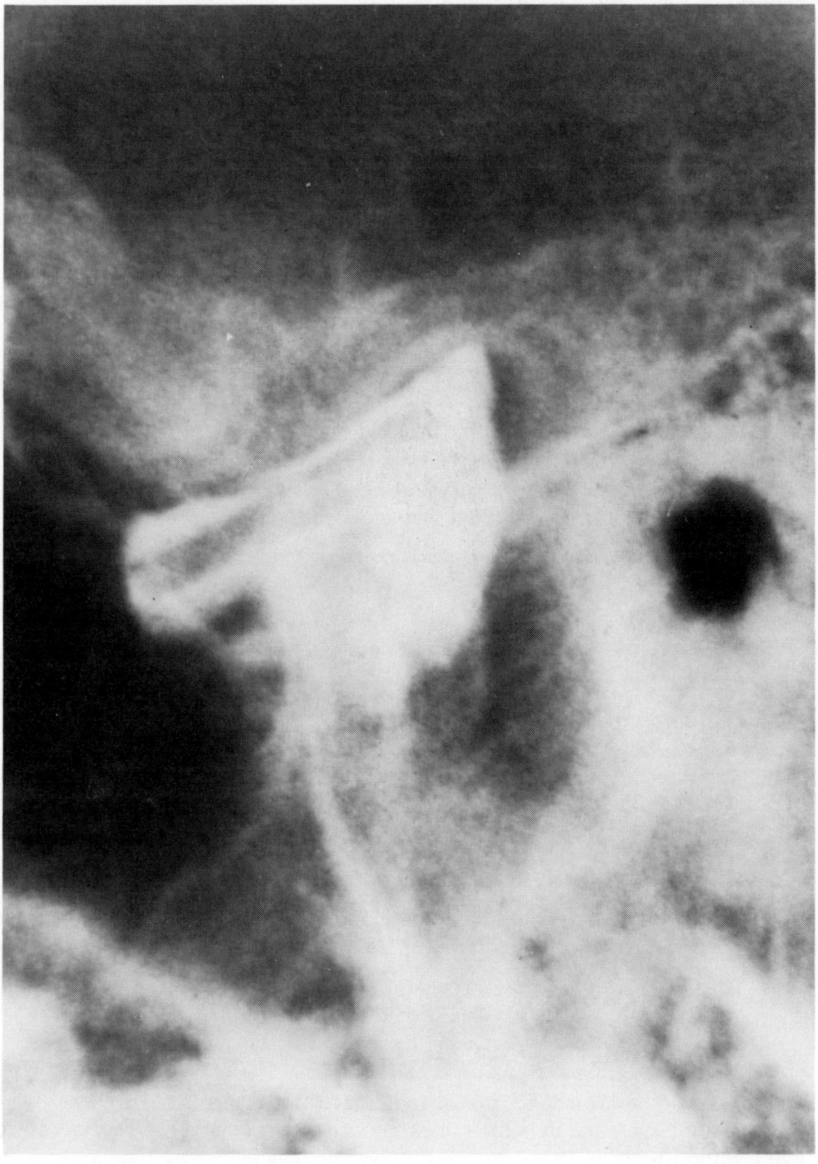

Figure 11-8 A piece of Silastic placed in the joint has slipped behind the condyle and no longer provides separation between condyle and fossa.

RADIOGRAPHIC APPEARANCE OF THE TEMPOROMANDIBULAR JOINT

Normal Joint

Healthy bony surfaces have smooth intact cortical margins. Bony components of the temporomandibular joint are no exception. A radiographically normal temporomandibular joint is shown in Figure 11-9. Margins of the glenoid fossa are smooth and dense except along the posterior surface where the petrotympanic fissure crosses the posterior wall of the fossa. The petrotympanic fissure separates the mandibular fossa into a smooth area anteriorly that is occupied by the mandibular condyle and a posterior-inferior rough portion. Bony surfaces of the mandibular condyle are also smooth and dense. Although the terminal position of the condyle is established by occlusal relationships of the teeth, the distance between the condyle and the anterior surface of the fossa or the articular eminence remains fairly constant during function as a result of interposition of the articular disc.

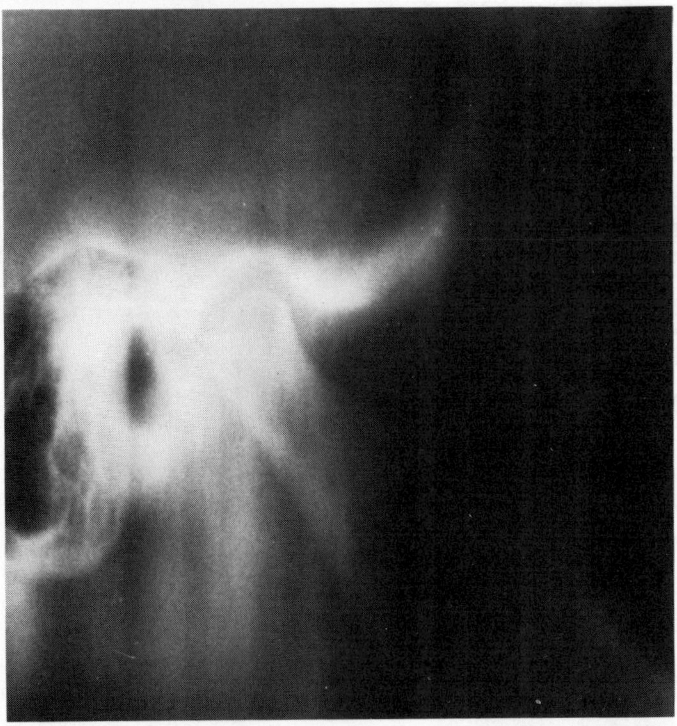

Figure 11-9 The normal temporomandibular joint is characterized by a symmetrical joint space and by well-defined smooth cortical margins on both condyle and glenoid fossa.

In most individuals, the condyle moves to a position anterior and superior to the articular eminence during extreme excursions but returns to the glenoid fossa without difficulty.

The size and shape of the mandibular condyle is extremely variable from one individual to another and even from one side of one individual to another. The orientation of the long axis of the condyle to the midsagittal plane is also variable, but the discrepancy between condyles in a given individual should not be excessive. In some patients the condyles have a medial inclination while in others they lie in a true vertical position or are laterally inclined. In this dimension, however, both condyles normally have the same orientation.

Osteoarthritis

Osteoarthritis or degenerative arthritis is the most commonly observed radiographic change of the temporomandibular joint.[6] It is characterized by roughening of the surfaces of the condyle and articular eminence that may lead to damage or destruction of the articular disc. If the disc perforates or is destroyed, bone-to-bone contact can result and produce further destruction. Radiographically, there is narrowing of the joint space, particularly during function when the condyle moves past the eminence. The articular surfaces become flattened; and attempts at bony repair produce osteophytic lipping, particularly on the anterior and superior surfaces of the mandibular condyle (Figure 11-10). There are often areas of demineralization or surface erosion.

Osteoarthritis is believed to occur primarily at the pressure sites of a joint. Abnormal pressure, stress, or trauma of any sort can result in changes in the cartilaginous surfaces and in bone. As the cartilaginous surfaces become eroded, the joint space may narrow and become asymmetrical. Beneath the bony surfaces, sclerosis and cyst formation may develop.

There is some argument as to whether the pathogenesis of osteoarthritis results from the intrusion of synovium into bone or purely as a result of surface erosion occurring after excessive stress. In the former pathway, synovial fluid may be forced into defects in the cartilaginous surface and into the subsurface bone. In the latter case, it is presumed that the loss of cartilage results in the contact of bony surfaces, which eventually leads to subsurface cyst formation.

The formation of bone spurs appears to be related to the presence of hyperemia and cartilage cells that participate in enchondral bone formation. Abnormal stresses in the joint also lead to buttressing or the production of bony reinforcement beneath the stressed surfaces.

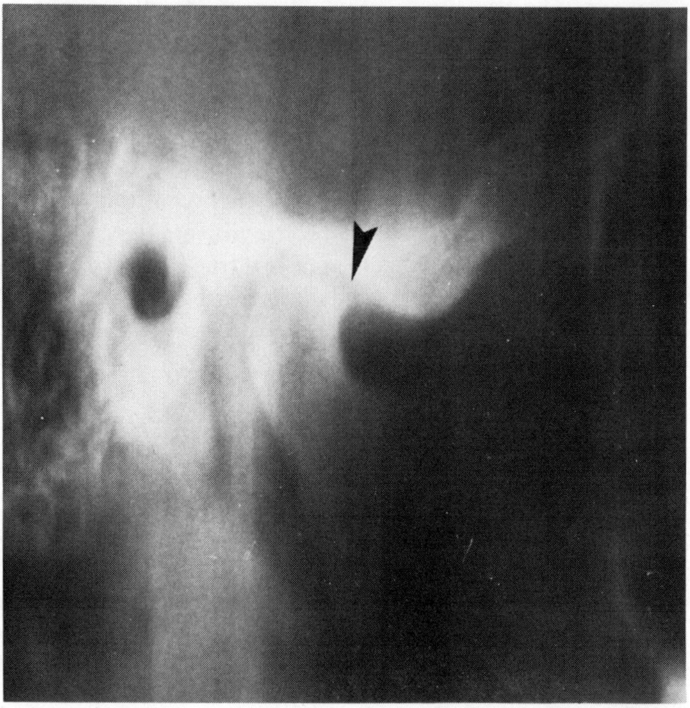

A

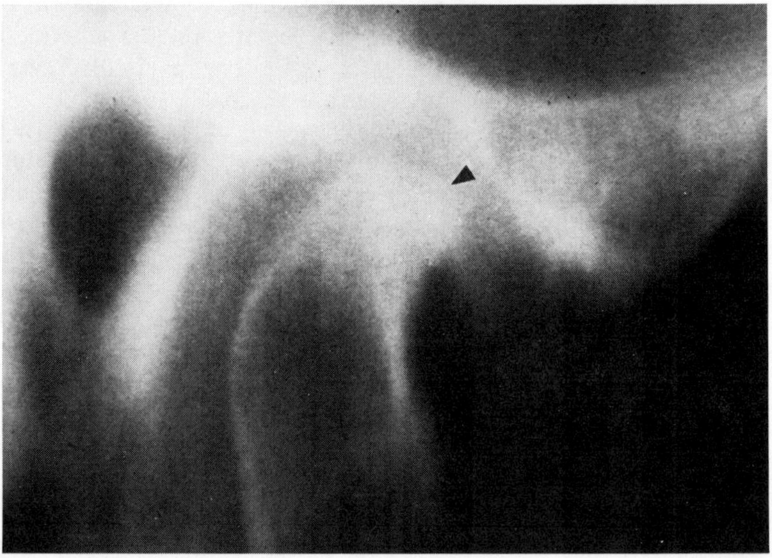

B

Figure 11-10 **A.** The cortex on the anterior surface of the condyle is irregular (arrow) because of bone production occurring in response to stress. **B.** Eventually an osteophyte is produced (arrow).

Osteoarthritis may also reflect bony changes secondary to the development of avascular necrosis. Blockage of small arteries has been demonstrated in subcortical bone. Vascular occlusion is followed by focal bone death, referred to as aseptic necrosis. Trauma, alcoholism, the use of steroids, and a variety of systemic disorders are known to be associated with a high incidence of aseptic or avascular necrosis. Necrotic areas cause structural weakness that may result in collapse of the cortical surface or the production of small fractures. In the healing process, new bone formation around areas of focal necrosis would be indistinguishable from osteoarthritic disease initiated by some other mechanism. Experimentally, avascular necrosis can be caused by physical damage within the joint as well as by the use of systemic agents, making it difficult to determine whether osteoarthritis or avascular necrosis is the primary lesion in any particular instance.

Both avascular necrosis and osteoarthritic damages can occur without the concurrent presence of pain. Radiographically, a distinction between these entities is extremely difficult except at specific stages of the disease process. In large joints the distinction is more easily made.

The clinical signs of osteoarthritic disease are pain and limitation of movement. Pain probably results from vascular changes and irregularities of the bony surfaces, which result from collapse or osteophyte production. Other changes may occur in the capsule and ligaments. Pain is usually relieved by surgically correcting the abnormal bony contours, although the occasional recurrence of symptoms suggests that initial relief may be the result of denervation of the area rather than correction of a mechanical problem.

Rheumatoid Arthritis

Involvement of the temporomandibular joints is common in individuals with rheumatoid arthritis. Radiographically, there is loss of mobility, loss of density due to demineralization, erosion of the cortical surfaces, flattening of the glenoid fossa, and changes in the size of the joint space, depending upon the state of the disease. Rheumatoid disease involving the temporomandibular joints in the absence of systemic disease is uncommon and extremely difficult to diagnose. Patients with localized rheumatoid disease may be seronegative with radiographic changes being the only significant clinical sign of joint involvement.

Bony changes observed in rheumatoid arthritis are presumed to result from involvement of the synovial membrane. At early stages of the disease, the synovium becomes hypertrophied and may fill the articular cavity, producing soft tissue swelling and occasionally a widening of the articular space. The increased fluid and the presence of hyperemia may result in the withdrawal of mineral from bony surfaces. The synovium may invade the cartilaginous surface, causing its destruction (Figure 11-11). At this stage the joint space collapses. Fibrous ankylosis is a common outcome at many sites, but is rare in the temporomandibular joint.

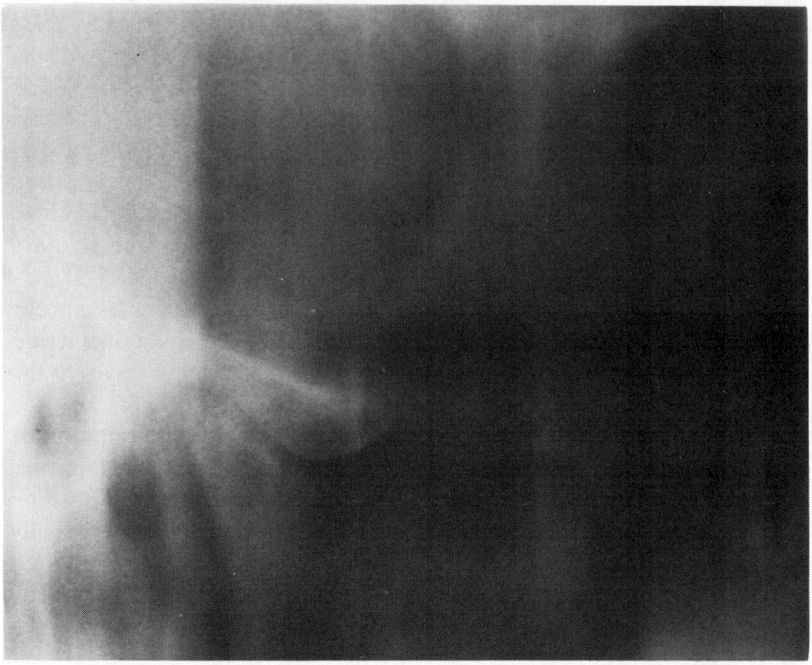

Figure 11-11 Rheumatoid arthritis usually presents as a lytic type of lesion. Bony destruction is evident and the condyles often lack density.

Juvenile Rheumatoid Arthritis

When rheumatoid arthritis occurs before the age of 16 years, it is considered to be a juvenile form. One of the main differences between juvenile and adult rheumatoid disease is that the former may initially affect fewer joints and sometimes presents as monoarticular disease. The incidence of systemic manifestations, including cyclic fever, skin rash, lymphadenopathy, and hepatosplenomegaly, is higher in the juvenile form and precedes evidence of joint involvement. The primary manifestation of this disease in the temporomandibular joints is the destruction of the growth center, resulting in an underdeveloped mandible (Figure 11-12).

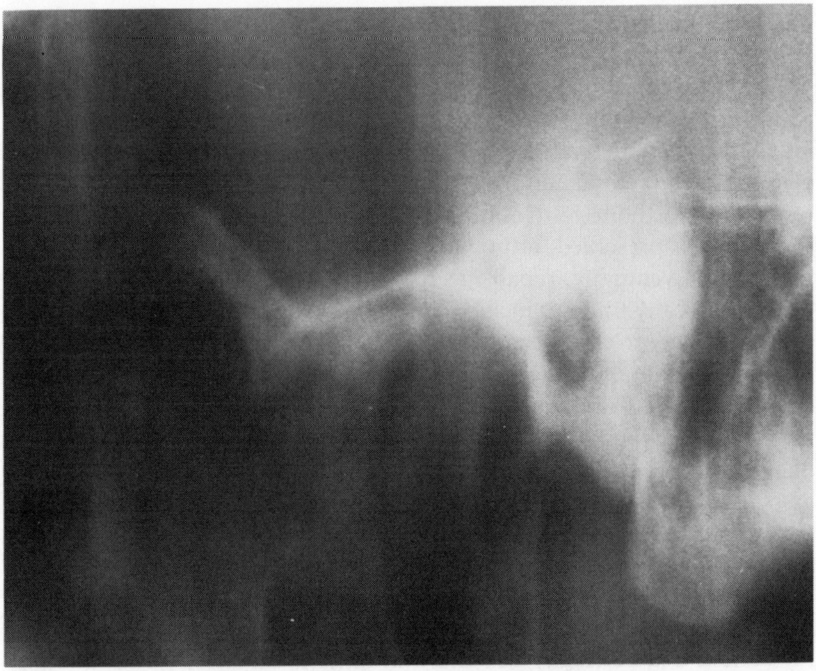

Figure 11-12 In juvenile rheumatoid arthritis the growth center of the condyle may be destroyed, resulting in condylar agenesis or hypoplasia.

Septic Arthritis

Septic arthritis of the temporomandibular joints is extremely rare. As an infection of the articular surfaces and synovium, it should not be confused with osteomyelitis, which is an infection of the underlying bone. Osteomyelitis of the base of the skull is unlikely to present in a dental office although infection of the mandible, including the ramus and condyle, may present.

Septic or infectious arthritis is an acute problem requiring prompt treatment. Joint infection occurs most commonly following surgical procedures, although it is not clear that the surgical site is the portal of entry for microorganisms. Rather, organisms may reach the joint secondary to infections at other sites by extension from infection in adjacent areas.

Radiographically, infected joints often present with enlarged joint spaces, subluxation, or dislocation that is caused by the accumulation of pus and inflammatory exudate. Bony surfaces may show demineralization and eventually erosion or fragmentation. Septic joints often produce deformities that persist after the infection has been eradicated.

Aseptic Necrosis

Aseptic necrosis of bone or osteonecrosis is a condition that occurs when the blood supply to subchondral bone is interrupted. Fibrocartilage lining the joint derives its nutrition from synovial fluid and remains viable, but the small areas of bone surrounding blocked vessels die as the result of inadequate nutrition. In the early stages of aseptic necrosis the joint space is preserved, although lytic lesions may be seen in the subsurface bone. Eventually, repair mechanisms are activated, and new bone is produced. X-ray findings include osteoporosis in the early stages, followed by patchy osteosclerosis, subcortical lucent defects, and in the final stages changes that are indistinguishable from osteoarthritis.

Several factors are believed to contribute to the development of aseptic necrosis. Trauma is a significant etiologic factor that may directly damage local vessels.[7] Aseptic necrosis is also known to occur in association with chronic alcoholism,[8] gout, Gaucher's disease, hypercortisonism, and a variety of hemoglobinopathies. It is conceivable that some of the osteoarthritic changes that are observed in the temporomandibular joints may be secondary to vascular accidents occurring in the condylar bone.

Wang and colleagues[9] found that large doses of cortisone given to growing and adult animals produce avascular necrosis. The cortisone appears to increase serum cholesterol levels with ultimate histologic evidence of fat emboli lodging in bone below articular surfaces. The emboli appear to interfere with the microcirculation of subchondral vessels.

Recently, several cases of aseptic necrosis were reported by Reiskin.[10] The radiographic appearance was extremely variable (Figure 11-13). All of these patients presented with complaints of sudden onset of severe pain that failed to respond to conservative treatment and common analgesics.

Inflammatory Arthritis

Infectious or inflammatory involvement of the temporomandibular joints is unusual. Following trauma, it may result from access to the joint provided by an open wound. It is also possible for infection to spread from the ear, mastoid, or pharynx. In theory, it is also possible for infection to result from the blood-borne transmission of organisms from a distant site.

In the early stages of joint infection, there are likely to be few if any radiographic changes. An effusion into the joint space may cause some enlargement of that space and reflects tenderness of the muscles, which

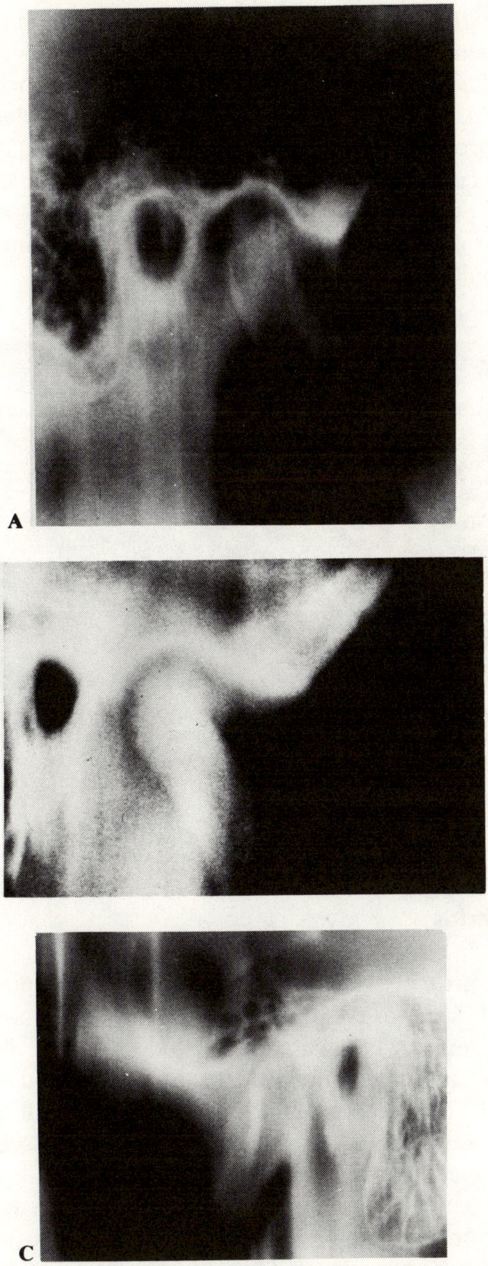

Figure 11-13 The presentation of aseptic necrosis at this site is a function of the age of the lesion and host response. **A.** Portions of the condyle may fracture. **B.** The chalky appearance indicates dead bone. **C.** The cortex fractures over areas of dead bone. In some instances, aseptic necrosis may take on the appearance of osteoarthritis.

may appear radiographically as a limitation of function. The ultimate course of infectious and inflammatory processes depends upon the virulence of the organisms involved and the resistance of the host. Osteomyelitis is an uncommon but recognized problem. A case of histologically proven osteomyelitis is shown in Figure 11-14. The outer cortices of the condyle appear to be intact while the medullary bone is indistinct and deficient. This is not the typical appearance of osteomyelitis at other sites in the body and may sometimes be confused with hypertrophic changes of the condyle.

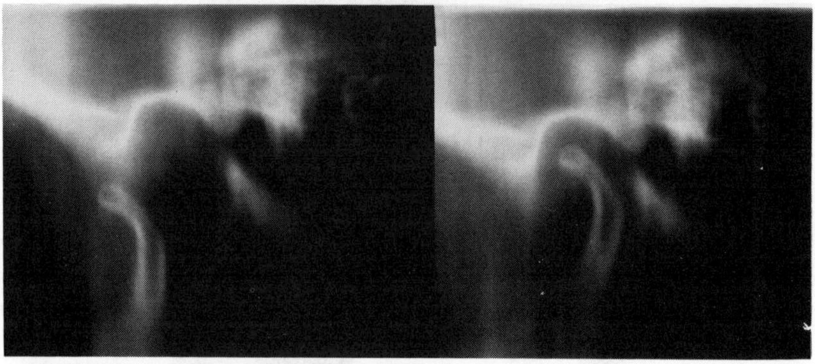

Figure 11-14 Aseptic necrosis and traumatic injuries may heal by a process which is histologically similar to a sterile osteomyelitis.

Traumatic Arthritis

Traumatic arthritis is a diagnosis that usually requires a clear-cut history of direct injury to the joint. In the long term, it may be difficult to distinguish the effects of acute trauma from those that arise from repeated insults caused by abnormal function. Acute and chronic trauma do not always lead to arthritic-type changes of the temporomandibular joints. In some instances, the destruction of blood vessels may cause a hemarthrosis. Stretching or tearing of the capsule and/or ligaments may occur. In some patients the effects of trauma may be demonstrated only by arthrogram, or there may be evidence of hard and soft tissue damage (Figure 11-15). Young individuals may show dramatic changes immediately after a traumatic episode, but subsequent remodeling of the condyle might make evidence of the initial injury obscure. Figure 11-16 shows traumatic arthritis of the temporomandibular joint secondary to a subcondylar fracture.

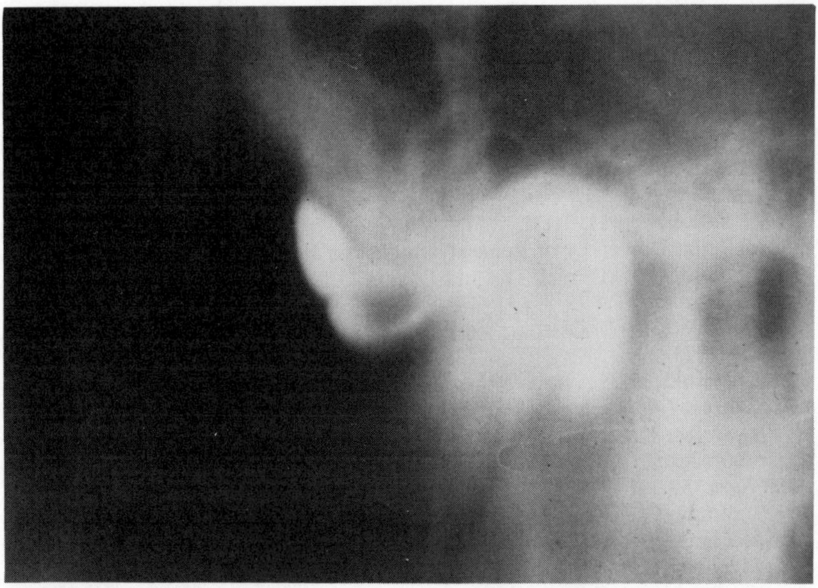

Figure 11-15 Deformity of the condyle and scarring or fibrosis within the capsule may occur following trauma.

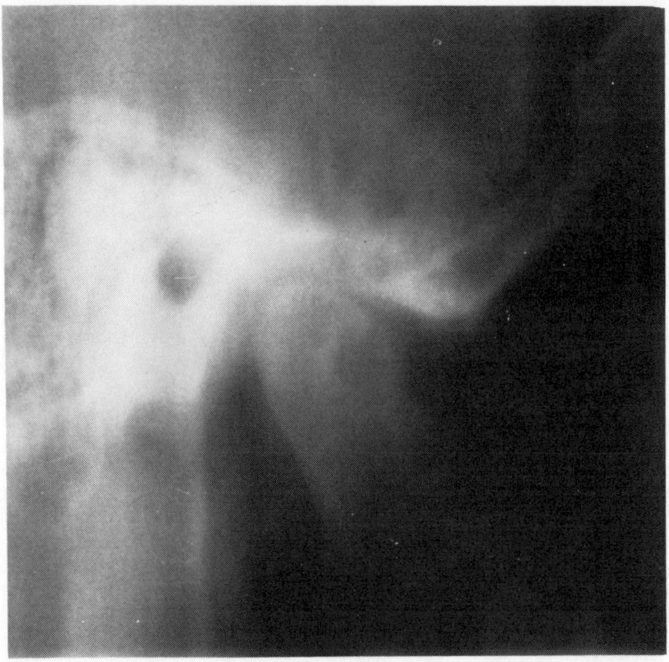

Figure 11-16 Traumatic arthritis of the temporomandibular joint secondary to a subcondylar fracture.

REFERENCES

1. Orban, B.J. (Ed.) *Oral Histology and Embryology.* 4th Ed. St. Louis: C.V. Mosby, 1957.

2. Sicher, H. *Oral Anatomy.* St. Louis: C.V. Mosby, 1960, pp 162–182.

3. Woodburne, R.T. *Essentials of Human Anatomy.* New York: Oxford University Press, 1957.

4. Simon, W.H. (Ed.) *The Human Joint in Health and Disease.* Philadelphia: University of Pennsylvania Press, 1978.

5. Faddis, D., Daniel, D., and Boyer, J. Tissue toxicity of antiseptic solutions. *J Trauma.* 17:895–897, 1977.

6. Toller, P.A. Osteoarthrosis of the mandibular condyle. *Br Dent J.* 134:223, 1973.

7. Herold, H.Z. Avascular necrosis of the femoral head in children under the age of three. *Clin Orthop.* 126:193–195, 1977.

8. Smith, K., Bonfiglio, M., and Dolan, K. Roentgenographic search for avascular necrosis of the head of the femur in alcoholics and normal adults. *J Bone Joint Surg.* 59:391–396, 1977.

9. Wang, G., Sweet, D.E., Reger, S.I. et al. Fat-cell changes as a mechanism of avascular necrosis of the femoral head in cortisone-treated rabbits. *J Bone Joint Surg.* 59:729–735, 1977.

10. Reiskin, A.B. Aseptic necrosis of the mandibular condyle: a common problem? *Quint Int.* 2:1725, 1979.

12 Salivary Gland Disease

The salivary glands are important to dental practitioners who have the responsibility for preventing, diagnosing, and treating diseases of the oral cavity. Salivary secretions play a major role in regulating the oral environment.[1-4] Diseases of the salivary glands may produce symptoms that are indistinguishable from those produced by diseases of the teeth and dental supporting structures and by diseases of the temporomandibular joints. Finally, the salivary glands often reflect abnormalities of the gastrointestinal tract, abnormal function of the immune system, and endocrine dysfunction.[5-7]

Major and minor salivary glands develop as a result of the proliferation of oral epithelium that grows inward as a solid cord of cells into the underlying tissues. The cords ultimately branch and enlarge in diameter until a lumen is developed. Terminal portions of newly formed ducts expand to form secretory acini. Connective tissue surrounding the developing gland separates it into lobules and forms a capsule around the periphery. The parotids are the first salivary glands to develop, followed by the submaxillary glands and the sublingual glands. Among the developmental anomalies which have been described, Stafne's defect[8-10] is of great importance to dentists because it is frequently seen on dental radiographs and can be mistaken for other, more serious conditions. This defect occurs in the mandible near the angle or near the midline and presents as a well-defined radiolucent area (Figure 12-1). Sialography and surgery have demonstrated that this defect in the mandibular bone often contains submandibular gland, muscle, and/or lymphoid tissue.

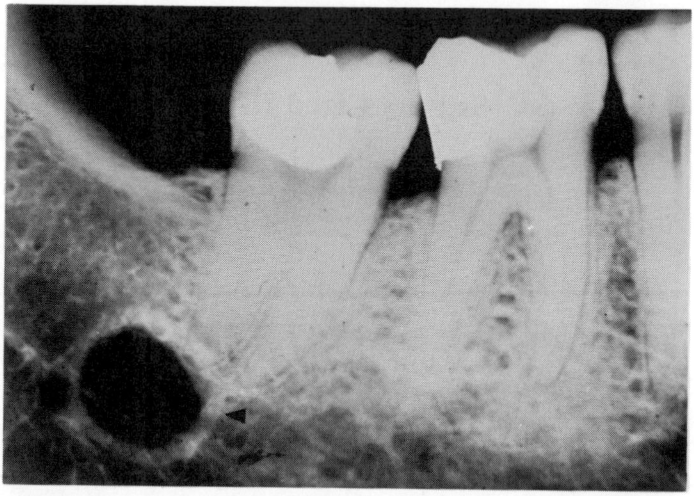

A

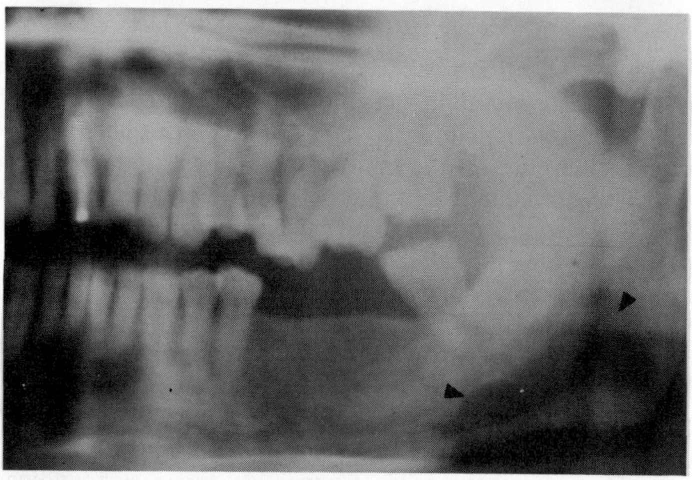

B

Figure 12-1 Areas of relative lucency occur where bone is thin because of pathologic change or normal anatomic variation. **A.** Lucent areas near the mandibular angles or beneath the mandibular molars often represent Stafne's defect, **B.** a nonpathologic entity.

There are several anatomic features of importance for a thorough understanding of the major salivary glands. The parotids lie in a space on the side of the face anterior to the ear. They contain the facial and other nerves as well as blood vessels and lymphatics. The floor of the cavity is formed by the styloid process, the stylomandibular ligaments, the carotid sheath, and the transverse process of the atlas (behind the ramus), which can be mistaken for a tumor of the parotid because it is palpable. The superior boundary of the parotid space is the zygomatic arch. The posterior border is formed by the external auditory canal, the mastoid process, and the sternocleidomastoid. The anterior border follows the form of the masseter muscle. Medially, the parotid closely approximates parts of the pharynx, and neoplastic changes in this portion can give rise to tumors that are visible on intraoral inspection.

The parotid duct (Stensen's duct) arises from the anterior portion of the gland near the zygoma and crosses the masseter muscle, after which it turns to penetrate the buccinator opening in the oral cavity adjacent to the maxillary second molar.

The submandibular gland lies below and in front of the mandibular angle. The upper part of the gland surface lies against the body of the mandible while the lower part is separated from the skin surface by superficial fascia and the platysma muscle. The duct of the submandibular gland (Wharton's duct) travels a distance of approximately 5 cm from the gland to its opening in the oral cavity at the side of the lingual frenum. The hypoglossal and lingual nerves lie in close proximity to the duct.

The sublingual glands lie between the submandibular glands and the opening of Wharton's duct. They may empty directly into the oral cavity through 8 to 20 ducts on the superior surface of the gland. A few of these ducts may join to form Bartholin's duct, which opens directly to Wharton's duct.

The mechanisms of neural regulation of the salivary glands are not fully understood. It is believed that the autonomic nervous system plays a significant role. The parasympathetic innervation appears to be somewhat more important than the sympathetic system.

The composition and flow of saliva is affected by a great many factors. Drugs such as cocaine and reserpine directly stimulate salivary flow while morphine and digitalis are indirect stimulants. Barbiturates and general anesthetics, on the other hand, tend to inhibit salivary gland function. Many of the commonly used tranquilizers and tricyclic antidepressants also inhibit salivary flow.

Although enlargement of the salivary glands may occur in a variety of circumstances, there are few instances in which there is an actual increase in functioning gland substance. The loss of functioning gland substance, however, may occur as a result of chronic inflammation, autoimmune disease, or obstruction of a duct. Systemic diseases, including alcoholism, cystic fibrosis, hypertension, and diabetes, can alter salivary function and size.

Diseases of the salivary glands can be divided into two major and many minor classifications. In the first category, non-neoplastic diseases, are inflammatory processes, metabolic and endocrine diseases, trauma, congenital anomalies, and cysts. Neoplastic diseases of the salivary glands are divided into benign and malignant lesions. A more complete list is shown in Table 12-1.

Table 12-1
Classification of Salivary Gland Diseases*

Non-neoplastic	Neoplastic
Inflammatory	Benign
Acute	Mixed tumor
Mumps	Warthin's tumor
Acute suppurative sialadenitis	Oncocytoma
Acute abscess	Adenoma
Allergy	Lymphoepithelial
Drug-induced	Malignant
Chronic	Carcinoma (multiple types)
Obstructive	Malignant mixed tumor
Allergy	Mucoepidermoid
Drug-induced	
Nonspecific sialadenitis	
Lymphoepithelial disease	
Metabolic-endocrine	
Hypertrophy	
Thyroid	
Diabetes	
Alcoholism	
Menopause	
Starvation	
Atrophy	
Fatty or fibrous replacement	
Chronic obstruction	
Trauma	
Compression	
Penetration	
Congenital	
Dermoids	

*A more complete classification may be found in W.P. Work and J.G. Batgakis. Classification of salivary gland diseases. *Otolaryngol Clin North Am.* 10:287–296, 1977.

SIALOGRAPHY

Sialography is a form of roentgen diagnosis which has the distinction of often being performed in poorly selected patients and with inadequate technique. While radionuclide studies can provide a sensitive index of gland function, sialography provides precise information about the anatomy of the gland and its relation to adjacent structures. Sialography, however, offers significant advantages over other diagnostic techniques only when patients are carefully selected and when the procedure is conducted under optimal conditions.

In 1913, Arcelin[11] injected bismuth into a human salivary gland to provide the first radiographic demonstration of a human salivary gland. Barsony[12] substituted potassium iodide solution and demonstrated dilation of Stensen's duct. According to Rankow and Polyayes,[13] the term "sialography" was first used by Jacobovici[14] to describe the demonstration of salivary glands by radiographic technique.

Since Carlsten[15] and Gullmo[16] described the use of oil-based compounds, the basic technique of sialography has not changed dramatically, although several important refinements have been introduced. Lacrimal probes have been used to find, measure, and dilate the salivary ducts. The introduction of water-soluble contrast agents has significantly reduced the risk of foreign body reactions. Fluoroscopy has made it possible to assess functional characteristics of a gland and to avoid technical errors.

Indications

Sialography has many useful applications. These include: 1) identification of a site for biopsy; 2) demonstration of calculi and foreign bodies whether they are radiopaque or radiolucent; 3) demonstration of fistulae, strictures, and other structural abnormalities; 4) demonstration of a tumor and its size and location; 5) identification of the plane of the facial nerve; and 6) definition of the extent of gland destruction following trauma, surgery, or infection.

It is not uncommon for mucous plugs and small calculi to be dislodged during sialographic procedures. For this reason, studies in well-selected patients often have therapeutic as well as diagnostic value.

Contraindications

Sialography should never be used in the following situations: 1) during acute inflammation, when contrast material may escape through damaged portions of the gland and seep into tissue spaces — some contrast agents, particularly oil-based materials, can be irritating and produce a foreign body reaction; 2) in patients with severe allergies to compounds containing iodine; and 3) immediately before thyroid function tests, since the retention of contrast material may cause spurious results.

Filling of the acini and parenchyma may be seen after the injection of contrast media into the main duct of either the parotid or submandibular gland. The rapid transfer of dye from the acini to the parenchyma may be an indication of pathologic change. This transfer occurs slowly in many normal glands. In absolute terms, the filling or nonfilling of the parenchyma does not in and of itself constitute a positive finding. Considerable pressure is required to fill normal acini, particularly with an oil-based contrast agent. Nonfilling after hand injection is therefore of little significance. In general, submandibular glands fill more rapidly and more easily than parotids.

Large opaque stones in the ducts of either submandibular or parotid glands are easily demonstrated (Figure 12-2). Sialography may be helpful, however, in demonstrating the relative position of these stones in relation to the duct opening (Figures 12-3, 12-4, 12-5). Nonopaque stones, mucous plugs, and small calculi are more difficult to demonstrate (Figure 12-6). These entities may be movable within a duct and may be displaced by the injection of contrast material. The presence of such partial obstructions is most easily demonstrated by fluoroscopic observation. In some instances, small obstructions are fixed and may cause erratic delays in filling or emptying or both. Large stones may occasionally cause perforation of the ductal epithelium, allowing dye to flow into adjacent soft tissue.

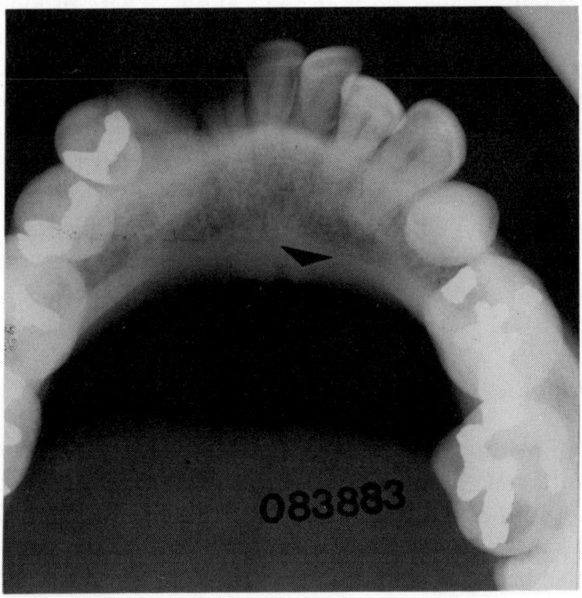

Figure 12-2 A poorly calcified sialolith lying at the orifice of the duct to the submandibular gland (arrow).

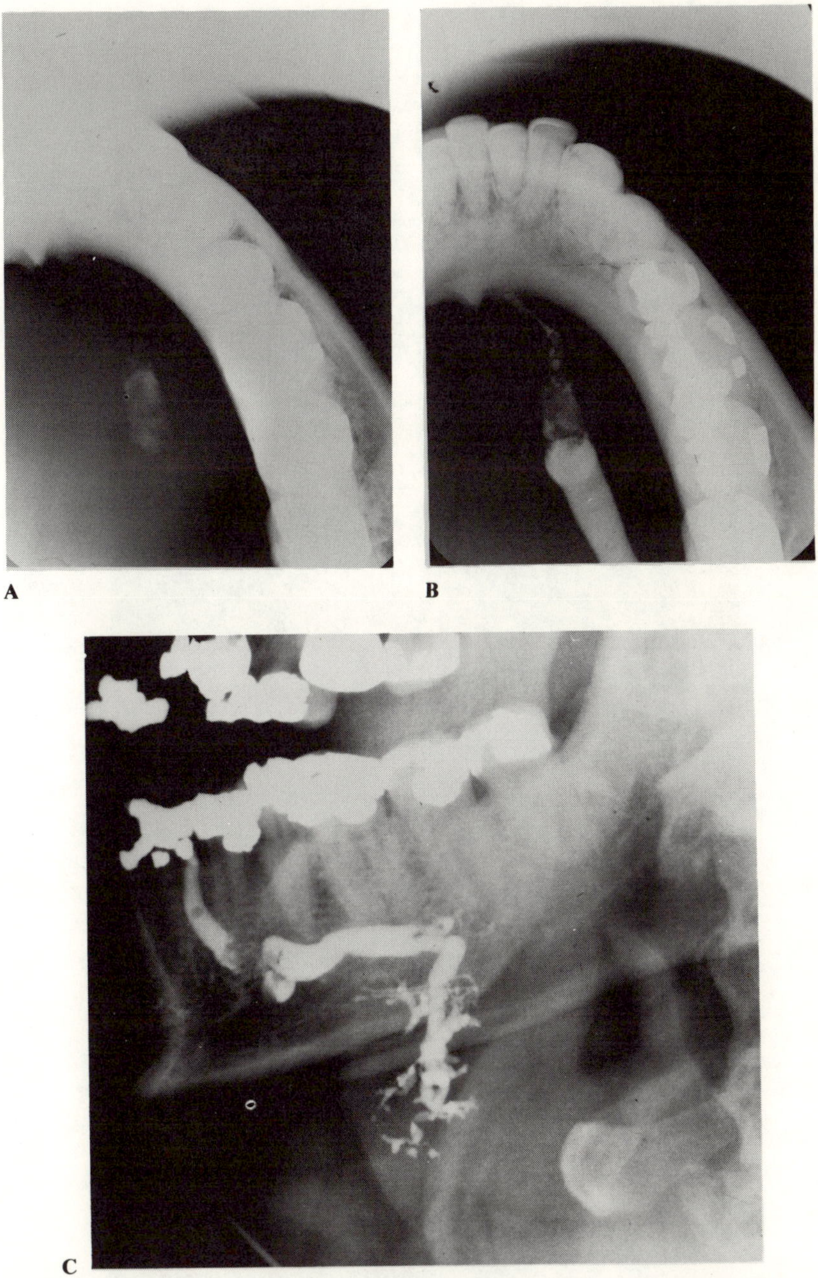

A B C

Figure 12-3 **A.** This sialolith is partially calcified and lies slightly beyond the orifice to the submandibular duct. **B.** When contrast medium is injected into the duct, it becomes clear that the calcification lies within the lumen. **C.** The effects of chronic obstruction are evident. Parts of the gland are atrophied. There is general dilation of the main ducts and segmental dilation of secondary ducts.

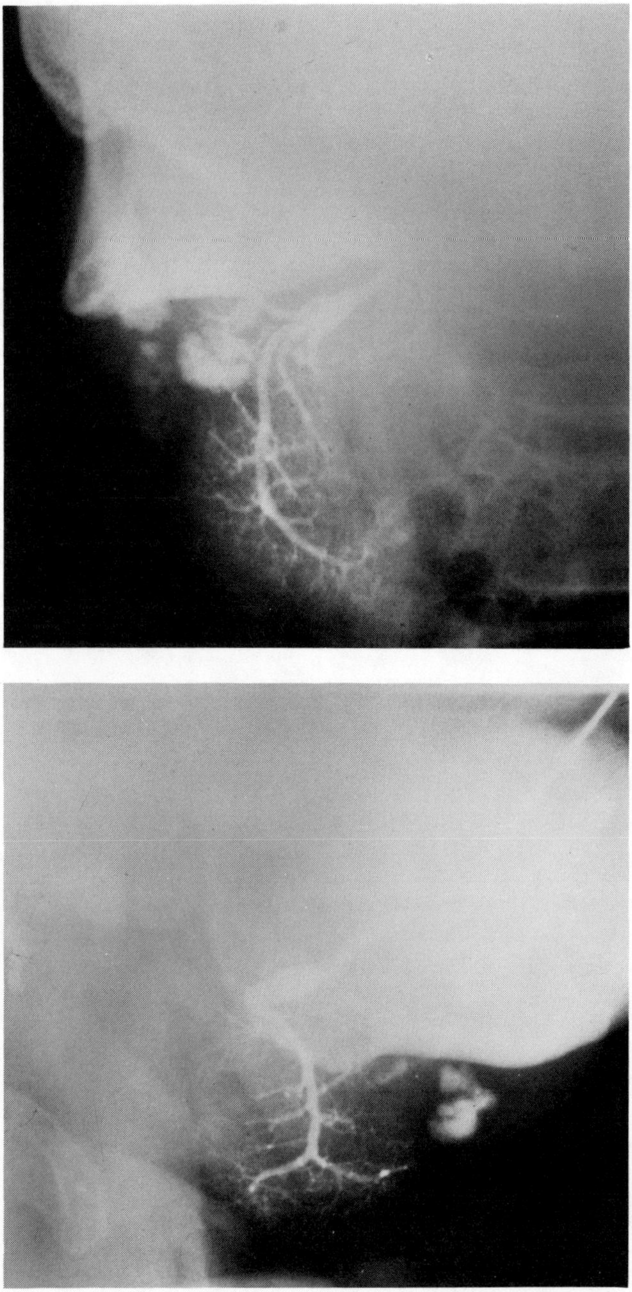

A

B

Figure 12-4 Radiographs are two-dimensional representations of three-dimensional objects. **A.** Calcifications in the submandibular region are superimposed over the gland. **B.** Slight rotation of the patient's head demonstrates that the calcification lies well beyond the boundary of the gland.

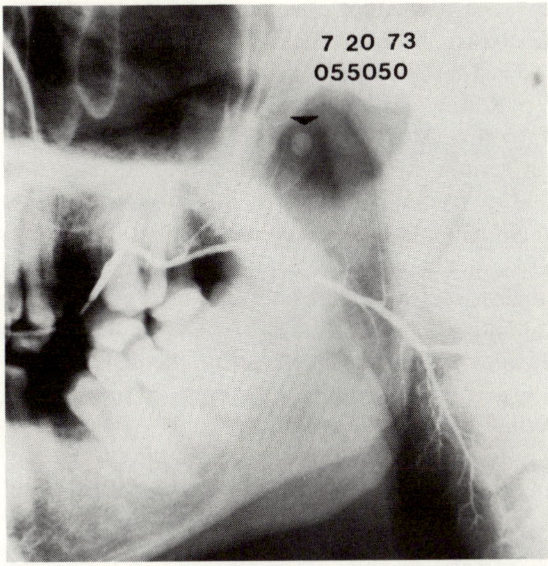

Figure 12-5 Calcifications which lie at the periphery of the gland (arrow) may fail to produce evidence of pathology on a sialogram.

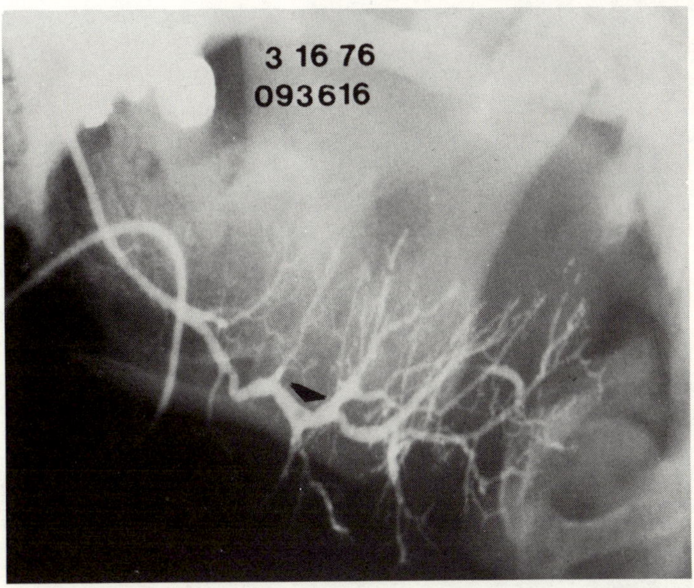

Figure 12-6 A small filling defect caused by a mucous plug or noncalcified stone (arrow). Other smaller obstructions can be recognized by careful observation. The primary obstruction was recognized by direct fluoroscopic observation, which made it possible to distinguish this defect from a bubble in the contrast material. Minor irregularities in the ductal structure indicate that the obstruction has been present for some time.

Salivary stasis, whether the result of obstruction, drug action, autoimmune disease, or mechanical injury, often leads to infection. This may be followed by sialodochitis (segmental construction of ducts), sialadenitis (puddling of dye in the acini and terminal ducts), abscess (seen as areas of focal destruction), and the formation of fistulae. In the absence of infection, atrophy and fibrosis may occur.

Complete or partial obstruction, infection, and sialodochitis often present with clinical and radiographic evidence of soft tissue swelling. A sialogram will often show irregular dilation of the ducts (Figure 12-3C). Terminal portions of the gland may look quite normal. Radiographic evidence of soft tissue swelling may also be evident in sialadenitis and the gland will show evidence of acinar dilation. In such instances, dye may be retained in the acini after the ducts have emptied (Figure 12-7). Table 12-2 summarizes the radiographic evidence of salivary gland disease. As mentioned in a previous section, ultrasonic examinations may be useful in distinguishing between cystic and solid masses within gland tissue.

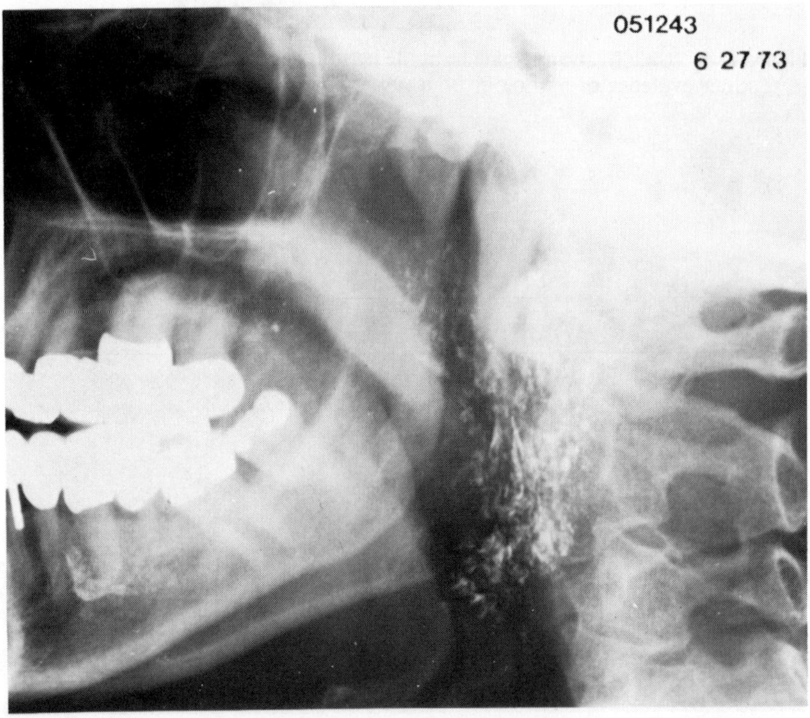

Figure 12-7 Chronic infection or stasis may cause changes in the acini and partial loss of function. These alterations result in the retention of dye for a period of time after the main ducts have emptied.

Table 12-2
Radiographic Evidence of Salivary Gland Disease

Calculus	Sialodochitis	Sialadenitis	Tumor
Opaque or lucent filling defect	Segmental construction of ducts	Dilation of terminal ducts	Large filling defect
Retained contrast	Retained contrast	Retained contrast (in acini)	Compression
Incomplete filling	Slow filling	Normal filling	Displacement

Procedure

Sialographic examinations can be divided into four parts: 1) scout films or initial evaluation; 2) injection; 3) parenchymal filling (water-soluble contrast agents); and 4) evacuation.

The equipment used in the performance of a sialogram includes: 1) a set of lacrimal probes; 2) polyethylene tubing with a tapered or blunt end metallic tip; 3) a syringe; 4) contrast agent (Ethiodol or Renografin-76); and 5) a sialogogue (citric acid 1%) (Figure 12-8).

Although sialograms can be undertaken with any type of x-ray equipment and film, there are distinct advantages in having facilities with specific features. These include a small focal spot x-ray tube (0.3 mm or smaller), an image intensifier, a videotape recorder, automatic exposure

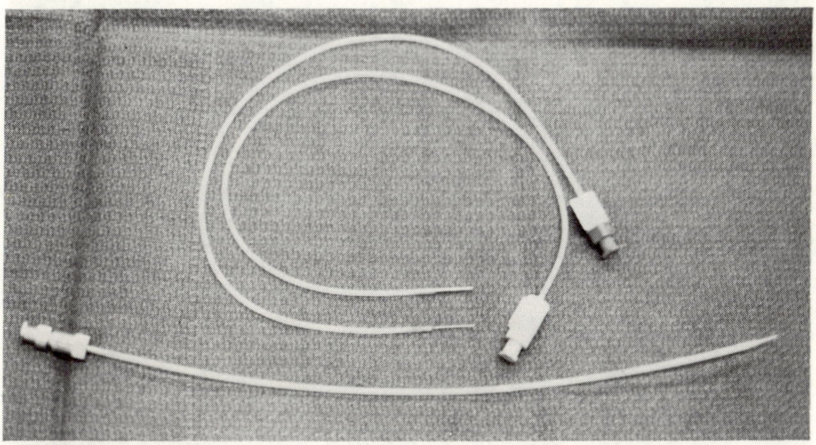

Figure 12-8 Lacrimal probes and disposable catheters and syringes used in sialography.

controls, and high speed film imaging (Figure 12-9). The small focal spot makes it possible to produce magnified views, which are desirable because of the small size of the structures under study. An image intensifier makes it practical to observe the injection or filling phase while remaining within acceptable exposure levels. Direct observation is often the only way to identify some functional abnormalities, errors in technique, or partial obstructions. A videotape of sialographic procedures allows the clinician to review the examination multiple times without re-exposing the patient. High speed imaging systems provide the opportunity for the examination of high resolution hard copy views of critical stages of the examination.

Careful records should be kept of all relevant clinical data, including patient name, age, chief complaint, physical findings and clinical impression, allergy history, history of prior radiographic or radionuclide studies, and the volume and kind of contrast media used in the examination.

It is most convenient for patient and operator when the procedure is carried out with the patient in a supine position. Prosthetic devices should be removed from the mouth since they may overlap radiographic fields of interest. Before starting the procedure, the patient should carefully rinse with an antiseptic solution to minimize the possibility of retrograde infection. After satisfactory anteroposterior, lateral, and/or oblique films have been obtained, the location and size of the duct is determined by the lacrimal probes. A suitable cannula can then be chosen. After the syringe is filled with contrast medium, the cannula is connected and air is flushed

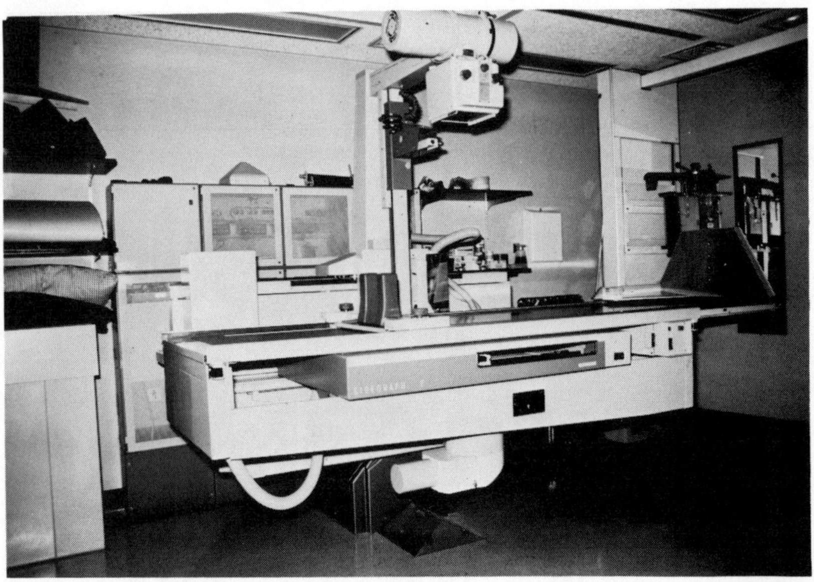

Figure 12-9 Image intensification, small focal spots, and similar features in the x-ray apparatus are desirable.

from the system. The tip of the cannula is then inserted into the opening of the duct and fixed in place. Contrast medium may then be injected under fluoroscopic control by hand, by a mechanical injector, or through the use of a hydrostatic technique. In particular circumstances, occlusal, stereoscopic, subtraction, tomographic,[17] and/or cineradiographic views may be desirable.

Radiographic Interpretation

The first step in a sialographic procedure involves a careful evaluation of plain films taken before the injection of a contrast agent. These views are critical for the identification of calcified stones (Figure 12-10), soft tissue masses, and possible erosion of mandibular bone (Figure 12-11). These initial or scout films usually include posterior-anterior and lateral views and, in the case of the submandibular glands, occlusal views. The scout films also make it possible to identify normal structures which lie adjacent to the salivary glands and may superimpose on gland structure in subsequent films.

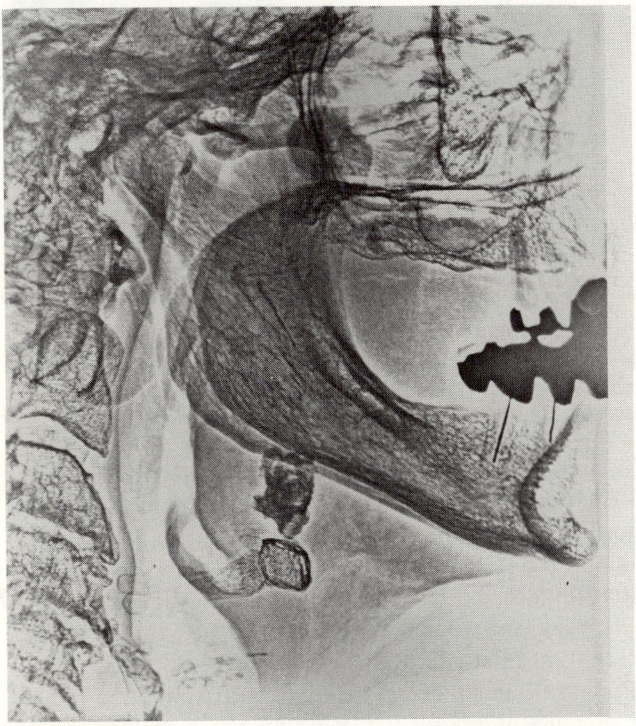

Figure 12-10 Calcifications such as those shown in the submandibular region of this patient may be misinterpreted if they are not evident before the introduction of the contrast agent.

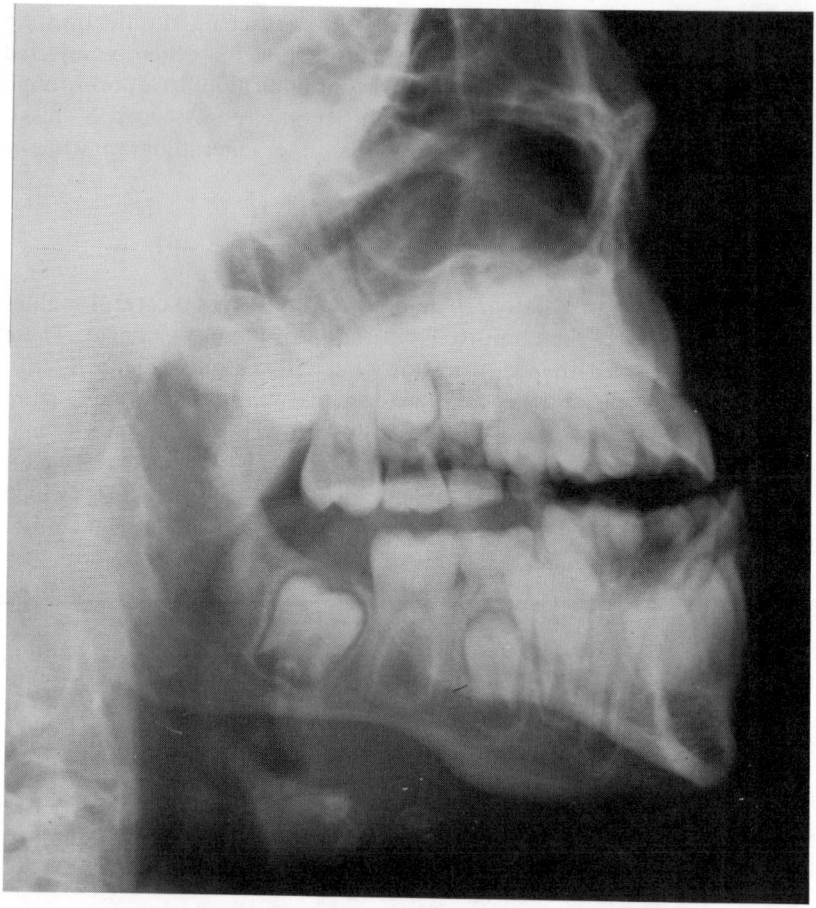

Figure 12-11 In this patient there is clearcut notching of the inferior border of the mandible in addition to evidence of several calcifications. These findings suggest the possibility of vascular and developmental lesions as alternatives to salivary gland disease.

Filling of the ductal system should occur without difficulty and without dilation. The diameter of each duct segment remains constant under normal circumstances, reducing only at the point of branching. A normal gland shows an even pattern of filling without voids or internal interruptions (Figure 12-12). Ducts should be traceable from main branches to the periphery, and when the diameter of a duct changes, as is the case at a bifurcation, at least two branches should be observed.

Failure to fill the ductal system can be attributed to faulty technique or to the presence of an obstructive lesion. Mucous plugs and stones rarely cause complete occlusion of a duct. In many instances, contrast medium will flow around an obstruction, leaving radiolucent gaps which cannot

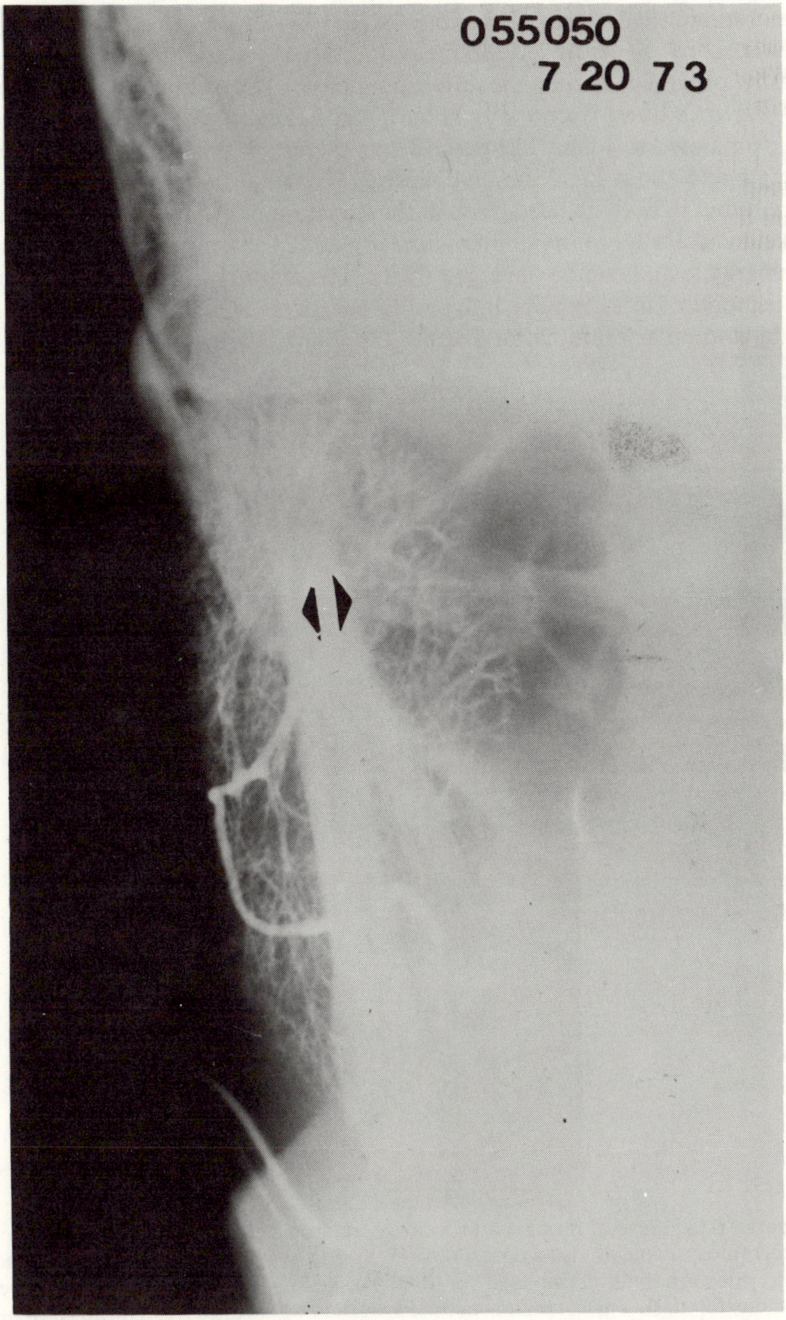

Figure 12-12 A normal gland fills without voids or interruptions. Here, filling of the parotid overlaps the mandibular ramus on its medial and lateral aspects.

be distinguished from air bubbles except by direct observation under fluoroscopy. Strictures in the main duct usually cause dilation which is easily observed during the injection phase. The submandibular duct (Wharton's duct) is normally about 5 cm in length with a lumen of approximately 2 to 4 mm. The parotid duct (Stensen's duct) averages 6 cm in length and about 1 to 3 mm in diameter. Second and third order ductules are found in both glands although the transition is gradual in the parotid gland and abrupt in the submandibular gland. The walls of ducts are thin and fragile and can be damaged by a contrast study (Figure 12-13). The likelihood of injecting dye into soft tissue spaces is slightly greater in the submandibular examination than in the filling of the parotid.

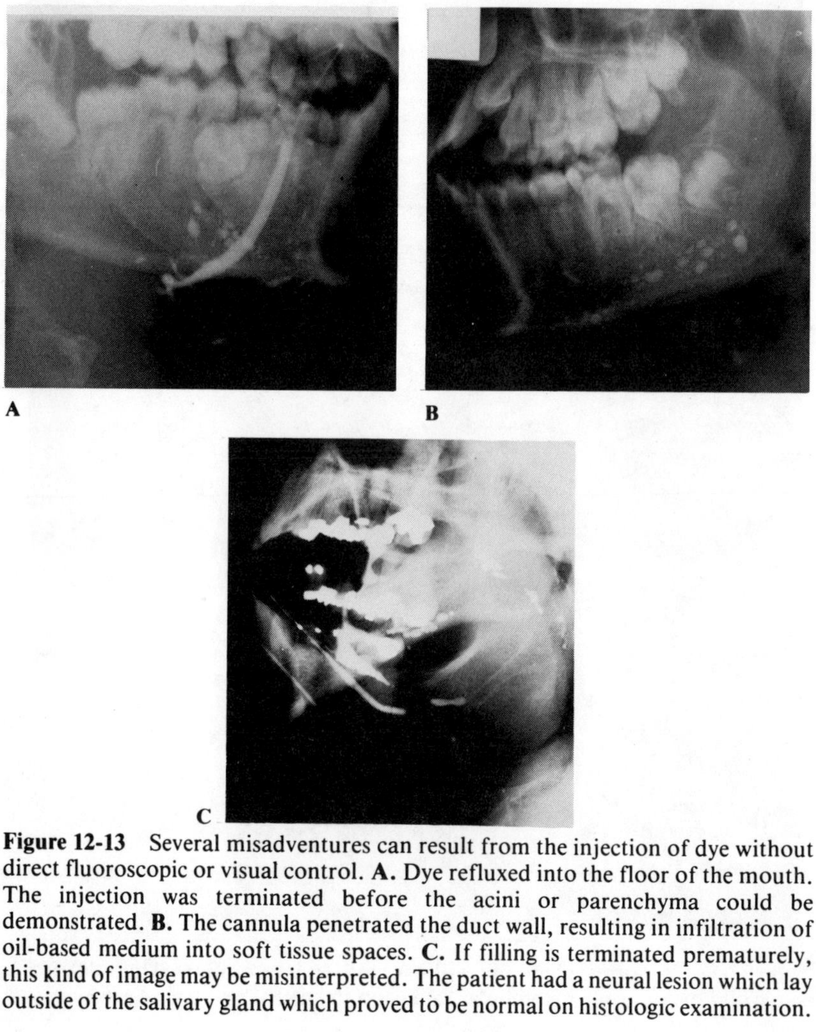

Figure 12-13 Several misadventures can result from the injection of dye without direct fluoroscopic or visual control. **A.** Dye refluxed into the floor of the mouth. The injection was terminated before the acini or parenchyma could be demonstrated. **B.** The cannula penetrated the duct wall, resulting in infiltration of oil-based medium into soft tissue spaces. **C.** If filling is terminated prematurely, this kind of image may be misinterpreted. The patient had a neural lesion which lay outside of the salivary gland which proved to be normal on histologic examination.

As the alveoli are filled, they may assume a cloudlike appearance which can obscure minor changes in the ductal system. Therefore, it is important to obtain films at intermediate stages of filling so that ductal structures can be evaluated in detail.

After a gland has been adequately filled and appropriate films have been obtained, the cannula can be removed. Normal glands will eliminate the contrast agent within a very short period of time (5 to 10 minutes). The retention of contrast for longer intervals should be considered evidence of an abnormality. Retention in isolated segments of the gland strongly suggests the presence of one or more obstructions while diffuse retention is indicative of poor salivary flow. It is common practice to administer a sialogogue to stimulate the evacuation of dye, but in most instances a normal gland will empty without stimulation.

TUMORS

As noted by Shaheen,[18] most (80%) salivary gland tumors are benign. The frequency of malignant disease is higher in the submandibular region than in the parotid. It is therefore predictable that most salivary tumors arise in the parotid region and are most commonly benign.

The most common benign tumors of the parotid gland are pleomorphic adenomas.[19] These tumors occur most commonly in young adults and may be difficult to manage surgically because the tumor mass may surround the facial nerves. Warthin's tumor constitutes approximately 10% of benign parotid tumors. The lesion may be bilateral, and it occurs most commonly in males. Warthin's tumor is easily demonstrated on technetium 99 scans and may be extremely variable in sialographic appearance (Figure 12-14).[20]

A salivary gland mass is often easy to recognize during a contrast study. It may be recognized either as a filling defect or by the accumulation of dye in an area of gland destruction. It is important to distinguish between intrinsic and extrinsic disease. A mass that lies within the gland substance is likely to cause bowing of the duct around the lesion. Intraglandular masses tend to displace isolated ductal segments rather than major segments of the gland. As a tumor mass achieves sufficient size, it may compress ducts, causing obstruction, or it may result in destruction of the ducts, with subsequent leakage of dye into the gland parenchyma. Such leakage will often occur before there is evidence of normal alveolar filling. In contrast to the normal salivary gland, which tends to show a homogeneous blush at the stage of alveolar filling, a gland containing a tumor mass will often show a lack of homogeneity at this stage. Extrinsic tumors or masses are less likely to produce nonuniform distribution of dye during alveolar filling. Masses lying within gland structure will often produce irregular retention of dye because of the compression of intermediate ductal structures. In contrast, extrinsic tumors rarely prevent evacuation of dye from the gland.

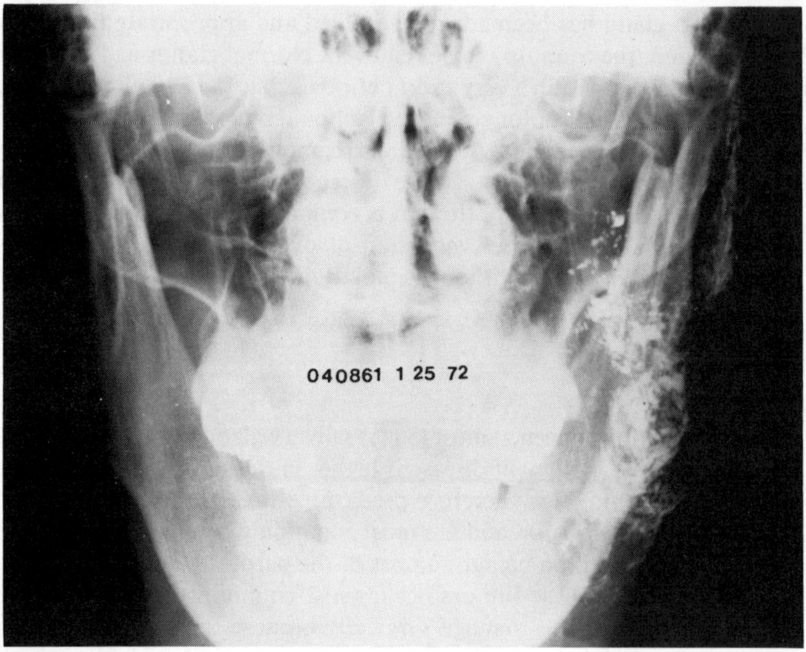

Figure 12-14 In early stages of a Warthin's tumor, there may be no more than a faint blush created by leakage of the dye. In this patient, large cystic cavities caused diffuse leakage of dye into the parenchyma of the gland.

NON-NEOPLASTIC SALIVARY GLAND LESIONS

Non-neoplastic diseases of the salivary glands can be categorized as obstructive or nonobstructive. Obstructive disease is frequently recognized by the presence of a calcified stone or sialolith. In many instances, however, obstruction is caused by a mucous plug, fibrosis, or a stone which lacks sufficient calcium to be recognized on a conventional radiograph. In addition to demonstrating an altered pattern of filling and emptying, the sialogram plays a major role in ruling out the possibility that calcifications observed on plain films lie outside of the salivary gland.

Nonobstructive salivary gland disease is most conveniently divided into several categories, including inflammatory lesions, drug and hypersensitivity reactions, metabolic disease, and autoimmune states.

Inflammatory disease may be the result of infection with a variety of viruses or microbes. It can also occur as a secondary response to other diseases, including sarcoidosis, systemic lupus erythematosus, rheumatoid arthritis, and others. In the case of acute infections, multiple irregular collections of dye may be seen forming within the cavities created by an abscess. In diffuse infections or inflammations, ductal structures assume an irregular pattern which may give the impression of multiple strictures. Involvement of the terminal alveoli can cause areas of puddling in involved segments of the gland (Figure 12-15). In noninfectious inflammatory states, diffuse puddling around the terminal alveoli is a characteristic finding.

Drug reactions or hypersensitivity states may be characterized by inflammatory changes and may also be recognized by functional changes in a gland. The hypersecretion of saliva may cause the formation of bubbles within oil-based contrast agents and the dilution of water-based materials. On the other hand, hyposecretion resulting from a drug reaction will commonly produce an anatomically normal gland which fails to empty within a reasonable period of time.

Autoimmune diseases such as Sjögren's and Mikulicz's syndromes most commonly present as diffuse inflammations on sialography (Figure 12-16). According to Rubin and Holt,[21] Sjögren's syndrome can be

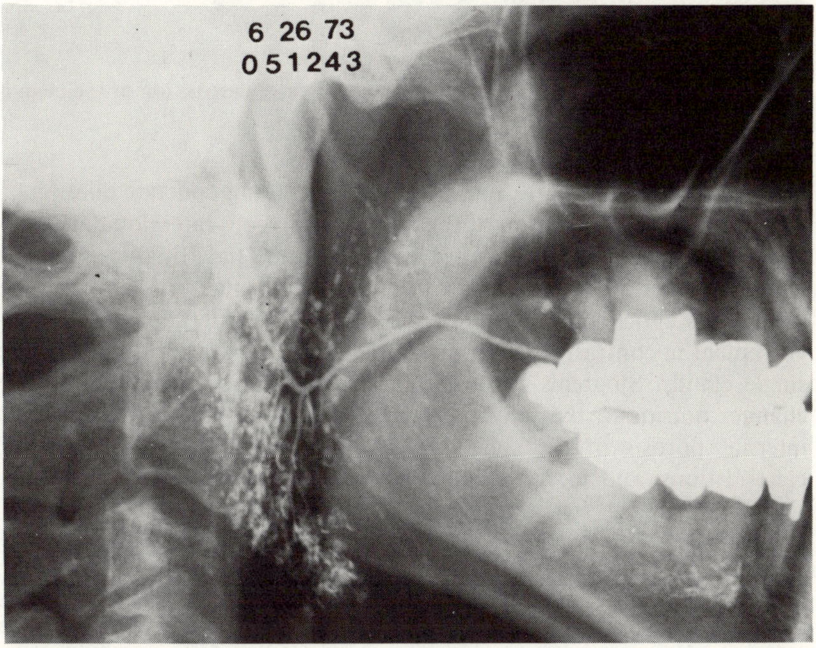

Figure 12-15 Chronic inflammation may result in irregular and diffuse puddling of dye in the acini.

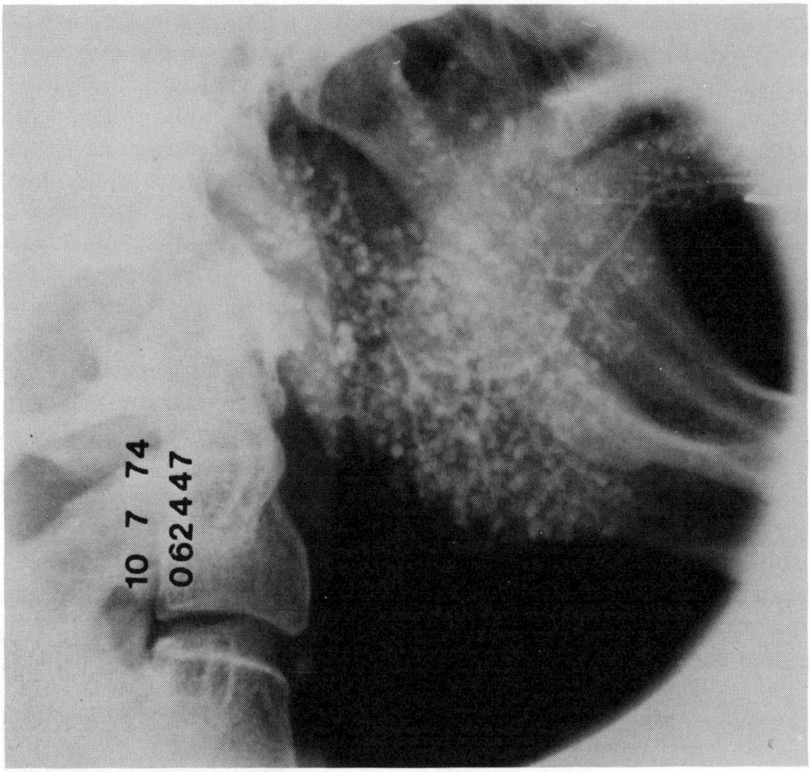

Figure 12-16 In the later stages of Sjögren's disease, destruction of the acini is widespread.

characterized by a progression of changes including punctate dilation of peripheral ducts, expansion of the ducts and alveoli, interglobular structures, cavitation or the coalescence of globules, and, finally, extensive gland destruction reminiscent of neoplastic change. In autoimmune states, it is anticipated that all of the glands will show some level of involvement in contrast to other inflammatory lesions, which may involve single glands. Sjögren's syndrome may also lead to other radiographic changes outside of the salivary glands, including hyperostosis frontalis interna, porosis of the sphenoid, multiple intrasellar and parasellar calcifications, and accentuation of convolutional markings.

CONCLUSION

Any approach to the diagnosis of salivary gland disease must be extremely cautious. Although malignant change is relatively uncommon, the salivary glands are afflicted by a variety of benign neoplasms and cystic lesions. The salivary glands contain lymphoid tissue which can produce symptomatic or asymptomatic enlargement. Autoimmune diseases which involve various tissues in the body, including the thyroid gland, often affect salivary glands as well. When function is altered for physiologic or iatrogenic reasons, there is an increased risk of retrograde infection. The salivary glands are also subject to traumatic injuries and may appear to be diseased when adjacent structures become involved in a variety of pathologic processes. Radionuclide scanning and sialography can be of great assistance to the clinician in ruling out or defining the presence of salivary gland disease when these procedures are performed in patients who have undergone careful and thorough clinical examinations.

REFERENCES

1. Biswas, S.D., and Kleinberg, I. Effect of urea concentration on its utilization, on the pH and the formation of ammonia and carbon dioxide in a human salivary sediment system. *Arch Oral Biol.* 16:759, 1971.
2. Dogon, I.J., and Amdur, B.H. Further characterization of an antibacterial factor in human parotid secretions active against lactobacillus casei. *Arch Oral Biol.* 10:605, 1965.
3. Afonsky, D. *Saliva and Its Relation to Oral Health.* Birmingham: University of Alabama Press, 1961.
4. Mandel, I.D. Relation of saliva and plaque to caries. *J Dent Res.* 53:246, 1974.
5. Wotman, S., and Mandel, I.D. Salivary indication of systemic disease.*Postgrad Med.* 53:73, 1973.
6. Gardner, A.F. *Diseases and Neoplasms of the Salivary Glands.* Chicago: Year Book Medical Publishers, 1966.
7. Ritter, F.N. Salivary gland involvement in systemic diseases. *Otolaryngol Clin North Am.* 10:371-377, 1977.
8. Stafne, E.C. Bone cavities situated near the angle of the mandible. *J Am Dent Assoc.* 29:1969-1972, 1942.
9. Tolman, D.E., and Stafne, E.C. Developmental bone defects of the mandible. *Oral Surg.* 24:488-490, 1967.
10. Uemura, S., Fujishita, M., and Fuchihata, H. Radiographic interpretation of so-called developmental defects of mandible. *Oral Surg.* 41:120-128, 1976.
11. Arcelin. Quoted by A. Berrand. *Rev Pratd d'Electrol et de Radiol Med.* May 3, 1913.
12. Barsony, T. Idiopathische Stenongangdilatation. *Klin Wochenschr.* 4:2500-2501, 1925.
13. Rankow, R.M., and Polyayes, I.M. *Diseases of the Salivary Glands.* Philadelphia: W.B. Saunders, 1976.
14. Jacobovici, Popolitza, and Albu. La sialographie. *Presse Med.* 34:1188, 1926.
15. Carlsten, D.B. Lipiodolinjektion in den Ausführungsgang der Speicheldrüssen. *Acta Radiol.* 6:221, 1926.
16. Gullmo, A., and Book-Hederstrom, G. A method of sialography. *Acta Radiol.* 49:17-24, 1958.

17. Kushner, D.C., and Webber, A.L. Sialography of salivary gland tumors with fluoroscopy and tomography. *Am J Roentgenol.* 130:941–944, 1978.

18. Shaheen, D.H. Salivary gland tumors. *J Laryngol Otol.* 85:1288–1293, 1971.

19. Friedman, E., and Schwartz, A. Diagnosis of salivary gland tumors. *Can J Physicians.* 24:266–273, 1974.

20. Reiskin, A.B., and Puri, S. Radiographic and radionuclide appearance of Warthin's tumors. *Conn Med.* 42:503–506, 1978.

21. Rubin, P., and Holt, J. Secretory sialography in diseases of the major salivary glands. *Am J Roentgenol.* 77:575–598, 1957.

13 Trauma

PRINCIPLES OF THE RADIOGRAPHIC EXAMINATION

In many instances, radiographs do not play an essential part in the primary diagnosis of trauma to the skull.[1-3] Under most circumstances, clinical evidence of both soft tissue injury and fractures is adequate. On the other hand, radiographs play an important role in evaluating trauma to the facial bones and teeth. With injuries to the cranial vault, the major concern involves possible neurologic deficit while injuries to the face and teeth are of cosmetic as well as functional concern. Radiographs are extremely useful in defining the exact location of fracture lines and in determining the number and position of fragments. Radiographs also play an important role in ruling out indirect or contrecoup injuries, and they are valuable in monitoring patients during a course of therapy.

Image quality depends upon an appropriate match between technique factors and the size and density of the structures under examination. In the facial region, the large number of structurally dissimilar bones intermixed with irregular air-containing cavities makes it obligatory to tailor x-ray technique to the exact clinical requirements of each patient.

The use of a routine examination carries with it the risk of missing subtle but important roentgen signs. The clinician designing an examination should take into account the nature of the injuries (blunt or penetrating, contused or crushed, possible missing or distorted structures) and the presence of foreign bodies or noxious agents which may have been ingested, inhaled, absorbed, or forced through some tissue barrier to a body aperture.

Trauma, aside from the fracture or displacement of bones and teeth, produces few characteristic roentgenographic patterns. Most traumatic injuries can produce radiographic pictures similar to those associated with a variety of different nontraumatic diseases or pathologic conditions. Therefore, the interpretation of radiographs must take into account past as well as immediate history, and the individual interpreting the image should be fully aware of the technique used to produce the radiographs.

It must also be stressed that trauma to the face or head which produces clinically detectable damage has a moderately high possibility of having produced injury to the cervical spine, airway, or brain. Extreme caution should be exercised in handling such patients. Manipulation of the head and neck should be postponed until there is firm evidence that such maneuvers can be accomplished without hazard. It should also be recognized that the most superficial structures have the highest probability of being injured. In addition to the teeth, the nasal bones, zygomatic arches, walls of the maxillary sinuses, and the mandible are most likely to be injured. Finally, when a fracture is identified in one structure, careful examination of adjacent structures should be undertaken. It is not unusual for multiple fractures to occur, but they are frequently missed.

FRACTURES OF FACIAL BONES

The dentist may frequently be called upon to deal with patients who suffer from facial fractures. Anatomically, the teeth and the nasal bones are extremely vulnerable and blows to these structures may produce obvious injuries. Fractures of the teeth and the nose may be the only immediate evidence of more serious injury to other parts.

Fractures involving the midface or the nasomaxillary and zygomaticomaxillary structures are difficult to evaluate roentgenographically. The vomer, ethmoid, lacrimal, turbinate, and palatine bones are extremely fine and closely approximated, so that it is almost impossible to demonstrate fractures directly. Injury to these bones is often inferred when there is radiographic evidence of injury to surrounding structures.

The maxilla borders on the orbital, nasal, and oral cavities. The body of the maxilla contains the maxillary antrum, which communicates with the nasal cavity; the frontal process of the maxilla articulates with the frontal, lacrimal, and nasal bones, while the zygomatic extension of the maxilla articulates with the zygomatic bone.

The most common causes of facial bone fractures are automobile and sporting accidents where there are often associated injuries to the skull, with occasional loss of consciousness and/or injury to the neck and cervical spine. Because skull fractures with or without evidence of neurologic damage are assumed to be of utmost importance it is not unusual for facial bone fractures to go undetected. Facial bone fractures are often obscured by soft tissue edema and other injuries which cause patients sufficient distress to overshadow these defects.

Facial bone fractures may be suspected clinically by the presence of an asymmetry, a step sign or displacement of a bony margin, bleeding into the soft tissues around the face, subcutaneous emphysema which may be detected clinically or by x-ray, mobility or crepitus associated with one portion of the face, trismus, malocclusion, altered sensation, and lucent or missing teeth.

Fractures of the nasomaxillary complex are often the result of blows delivered to or to one side of the facial midline. The force of the blow will usually determine the extent of the injury. Radiographic examination of the nasomaxillary complex should include occlusal views of the maxilla, occlusal and lateral views of the nasal bones, a Waters' view of the maxillary sinus, and lateral views of the maxillary sinus.

Blows to the side of the face more commonly cause fractures of the zygomaticomaxillary complex. Depressed fractures of the zygomatic arch create major cosmetic defects and may impinge on the coronoid process of the mandible, causing loss of function. Sufficiently forceful blows may cause fractures in the wall of the maxillary sinus so that evidence of antral opacification or a fluid level following trauma should lead to the suspicion of a fracture. In addition to Waters' and lateral views of the maxillary sinuses, submentovertex or axial views and occlusal views are often of value when fractures of the zygomaticomaxillary complex are suspected. Care should be taken not to mistake sutures between the zygomatic bone and the zygomatic extension of the maxillary or temporal bones for fracture lines.

MANDIBULAR FRACTURES

Posteroanterior views and right and left lateral oblique views of the mandible are often sufficient to demonstrate fractures in this area. Because of its ring-like structure, mandibular fractures are often paired; when they occur as single fractures, they may occur on the side opposite to which a blow was delivered. Mandibular fractures should be suspected if there is clinical evidence of swelling, deformity, loss of mandibular mobility, or malocclusion. Panoramic views may lead to both false positive and false negative diagnoses in trauma patients. When mandibular fractures are encountered, the dentist should always examine the maxillary teeth because of the high likelihood that they have been involved in the impact (Figure 13-1). It is also of particular importance to establish whether or not fracture lines pass through the periodontal ligament spaces of teeth or developing tooth follicles, particularly if there is evidence of periodontal disease or infection. Such fractures result in communications between injured bone and the oral cavity, thereby increasing the risks of infection.

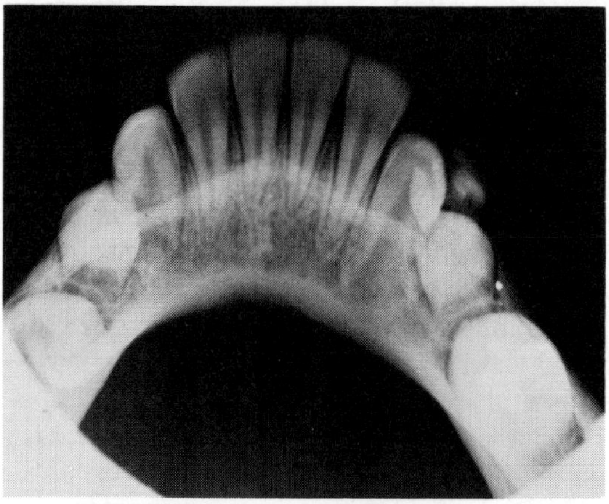

A

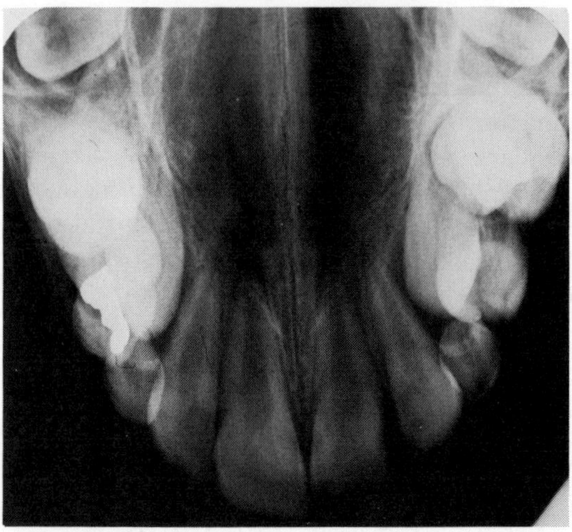

B

Figure 13-1 This young boy flew over the handlebars of his bike, landing on his chin. Clinically, the primary injury appeared to involve skin, lip, and tongue. **A.** Intact mandibular incisor teeth and anterior bony mandible. **B.** Subluxation of the maxillary central incisors with fracture of one crown.

C
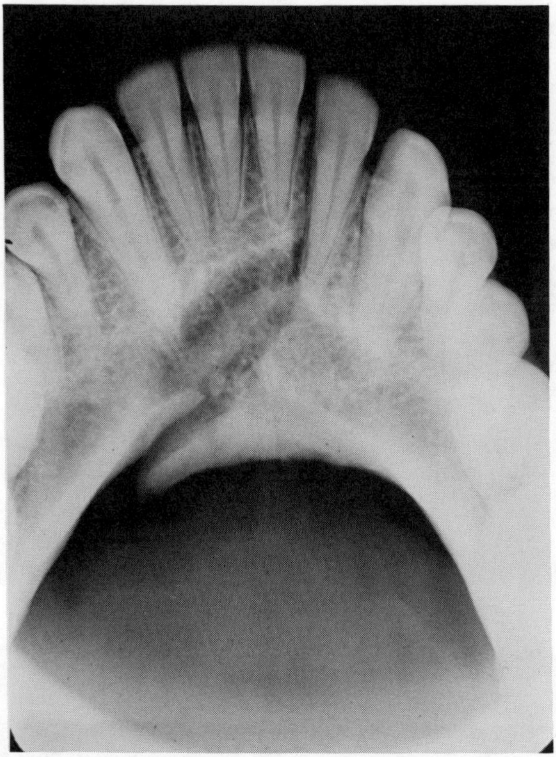

Figure 13-1 **C.** Fracture involves periodontal ligament space.

Trauma to the mandible may result in radiographically inapparent fractures or other injuries which are not recognized at the time of the initial insult. Subsequent alterations in condylar morphology, including hypertrophy and/or remodeling, may provide indirect evidence of severe injury at a later date (Figure 13-2).

Radiographically, a primary concern in trauma to soft tissues is the recognition of foreign bodies and/or generalized increases in density which result from the accumulation of blood or other fluids within tissue. Under ideal circumstances, special soft tissue techniques such as xeroradiography should be used since conventional x-ray techniques may fail to demonstrate the presence of radiolucent foreign bodies and early signs of tissue swelling. The presence of air or air spaces within soft tissues also provides evidence of the loss of surface integrity and should prompt an intensified search for the site of primary injury and for possible foreign bodies.

Radiographic evidence of trauma in hard tissues is most often recognized as fracture lines which are sharp and irregular and which generally extend through bony cortices or margins.

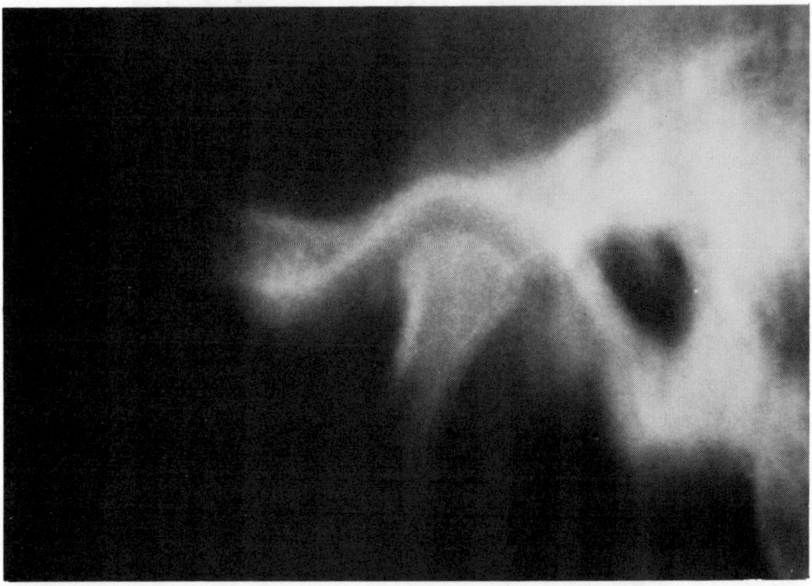

A

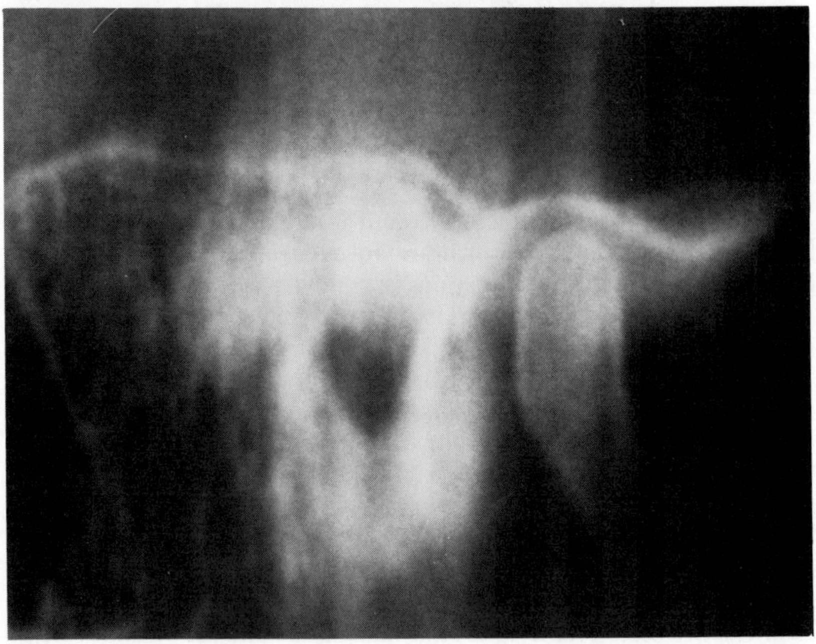

B

Figure 13-2 **A.** Morphology of the condyle and glenoid fossa are atypical. The condyle and fossa are flattened and the anterior border of the condyle is sclerotic. **B.** On the opposite side, there is evidence of condylar hypertrophy.

It should be remembered that fractures can occur without displacement of adjacent bony segments. In such cases, fracture lines may be difficult to visualize on conventional radiographs (Figures 13-3, 13-4, 13-5). Again, the use of xeroradiography, tomography, or high resolution techniques may be a useful adjunct in the examination of traumatized patients. Often, by waiting approximately 10 days to 2 weeks a nondisplaced fracture will become visible on x-ray because reaction of the injured periosteum produces layers of new bone or callus.

Examination of radiographs obtained during the evaluation of traumatic injuries should be thorough. In many instances, evidence of trauma is indirect. Fluid in the maxillary sinus may be the only radiographic clue to a fracture through the maxilla or the orbit. Similarly, air trapped within the soft tissues of the face or the neck may provide the only evidence of more extensive injuries or fractures to the jaws and facial bones. The characteristic roentgen findings in acute injuries include 1) discontinuity of a bony surface, 2) dislocation or displacement of a joint, 3) swelling of soft tissues, 4) altered vascular response, 5) abnormal or lost function, and 6) the presence of a foreign body.[4]

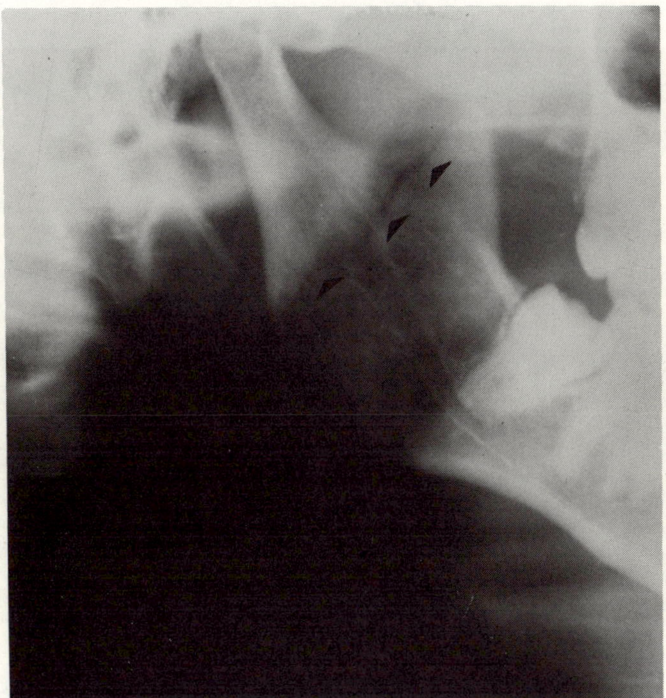

Figure 13-3 Fractures which run between the angle and the sigmoid notch are often obscured by superimposition of the airway, particularly if the fractures are nondisplaced.

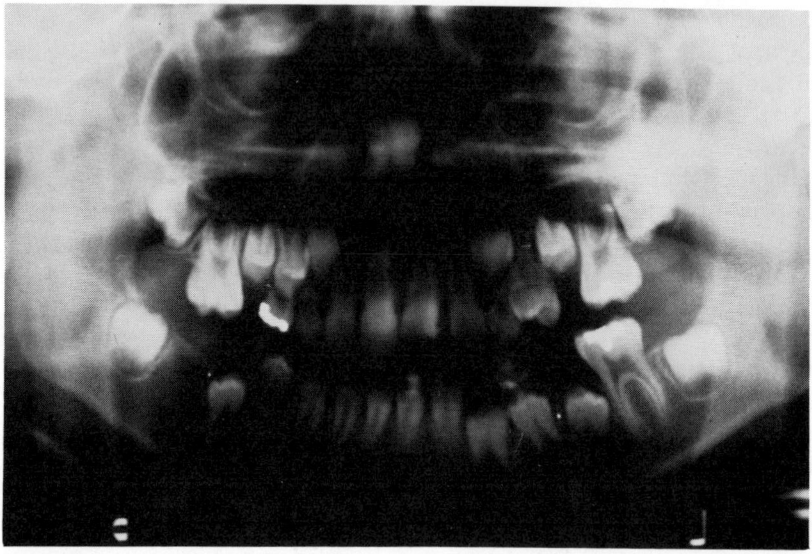

A

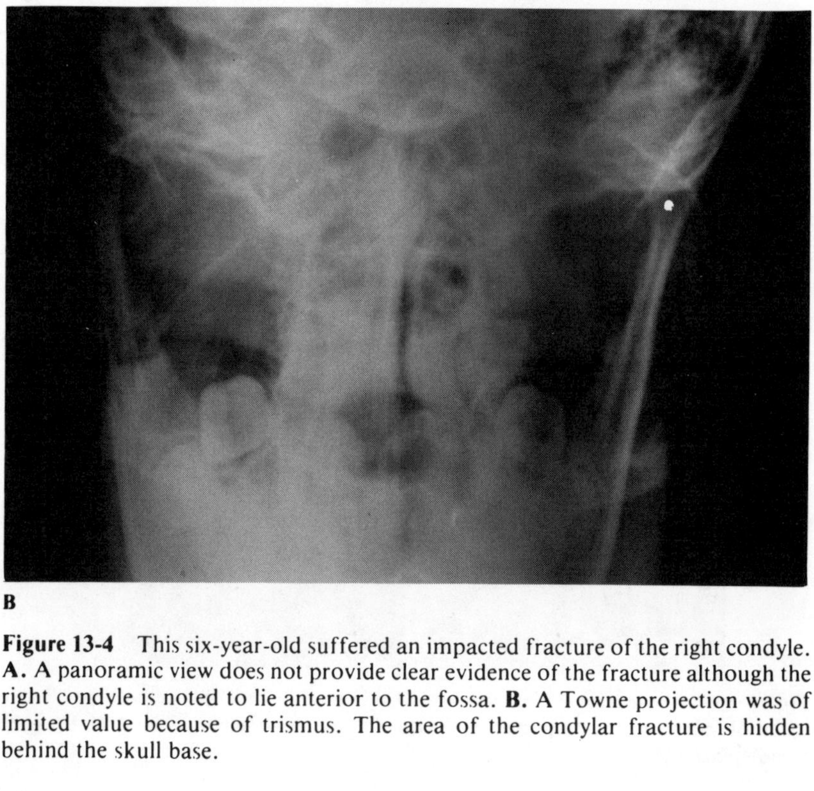

B

Figure 13-4 This six-year-old suffered an impacted fracture of the right condyle. **A.** A panoramic view does not provide clear evidence of the fracture although the right condyle is noted to lie anterior to the fossa. **B.** A Towne projection was of limited value because of trismus. The area of the condylar fracture is hidden behind the skull base.

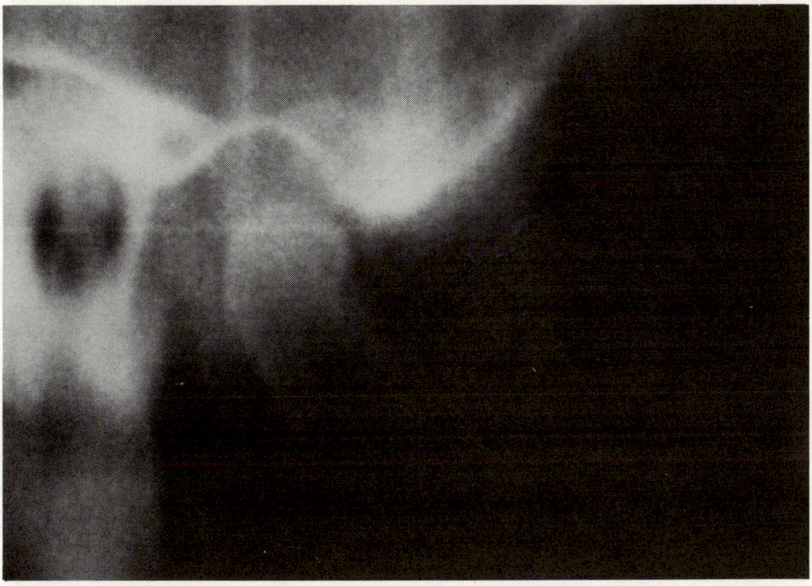

C

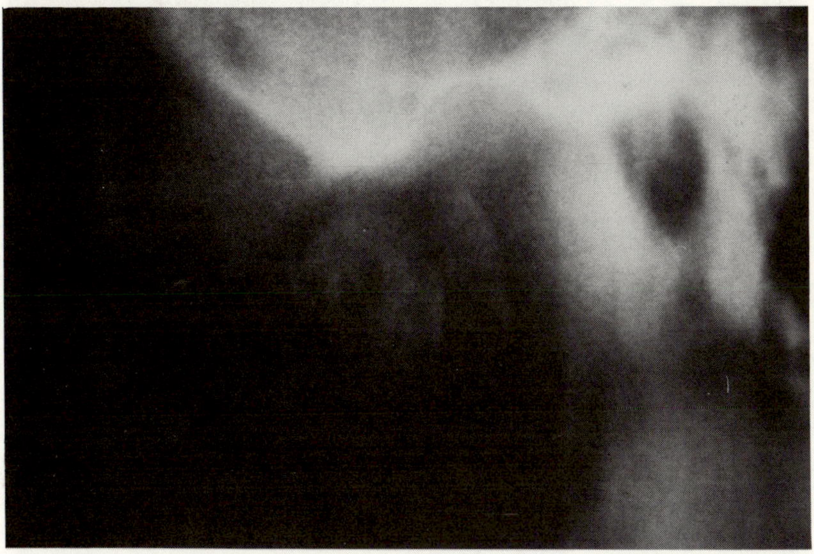

D

Figure 13-4 **C.** A lateral tomogram of the unaffected side shows an enlarged joint space which may result from altered occlusion or intra-articular edema. **D.** The fragmented condyle is clearly illustrated in a lateral tomogram through the right temporomandibular joint.

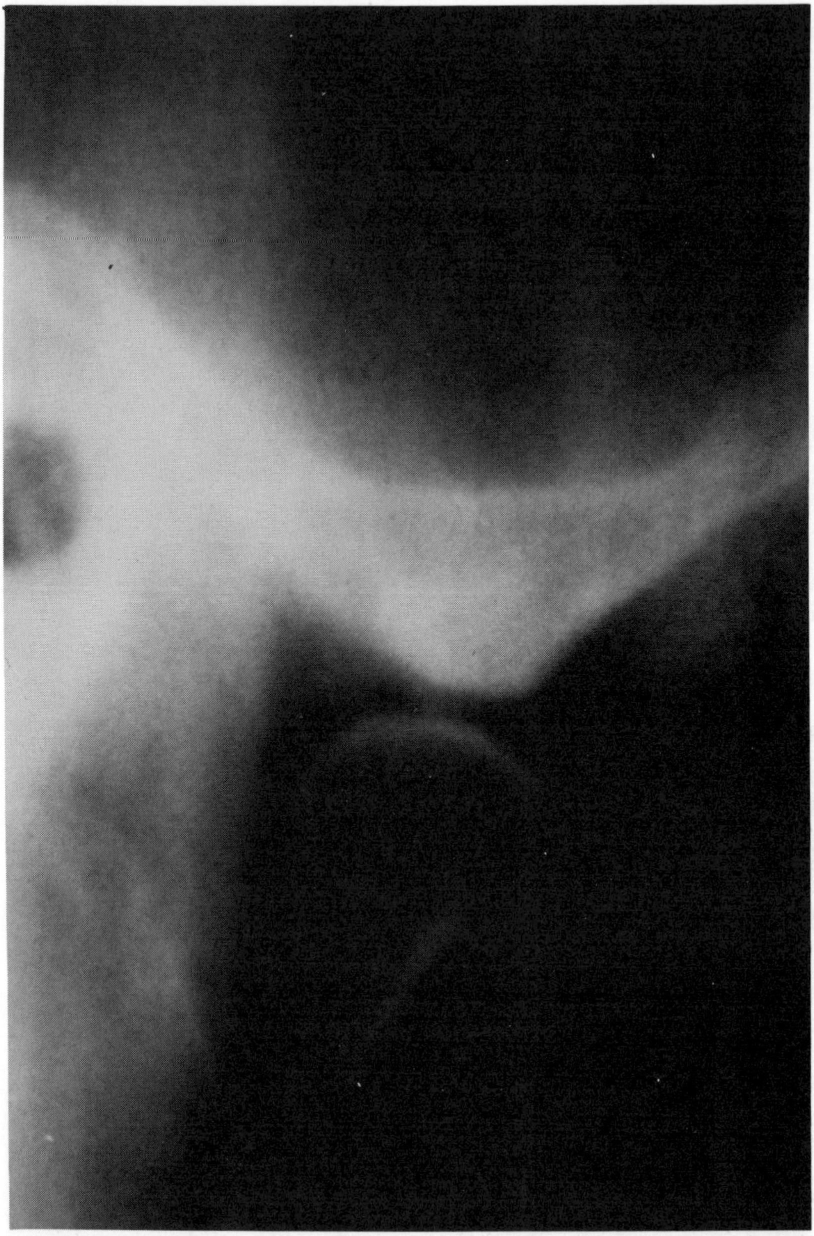

Figure 13-5 A middle-aged male was kicked in the face after having been thrown from a horse. After a significant time interval, he developed a facial asymmetry. **A.** A lateral tomogram through one temporomandibular joint. Condylar morphology is severely altered and a bony projection can be seen on the anterior surface of the condyle.

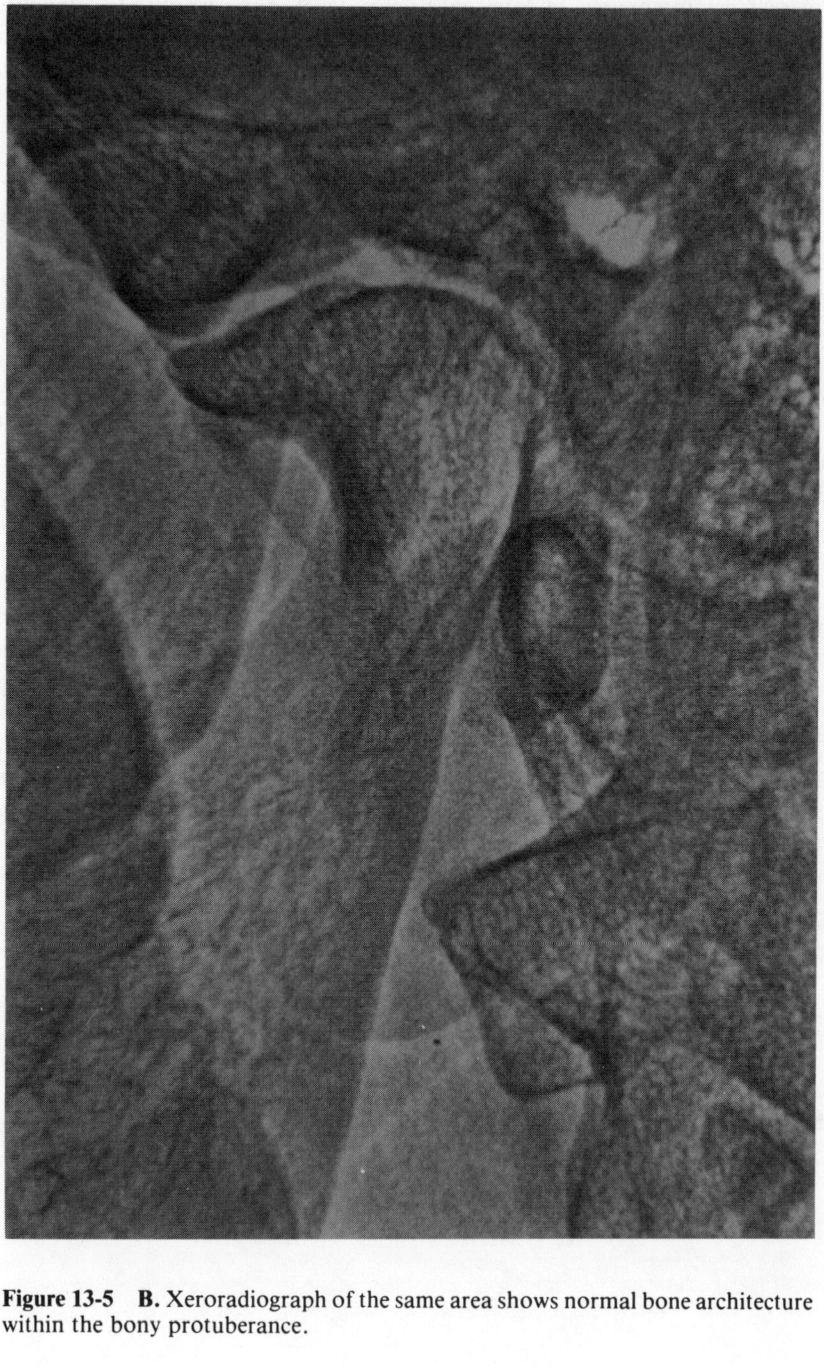

Figure 13-5 **B.** Xeroradiograph of the same area shows normal bone architecture within the bony protuberance.

SUBCLINICAL CHANGES

Certain changes in calcified tissues develop in response to subacute trauma or as late effects of acute trauma and may therefore be overlooked during a radiographic examination. Included in these late and subclinical changes are atrophy, infarction, necrosis, infection, altered growth, and atypical calcification.

Bone Atrophy

Atrophic changes may be anticipated when loss of function results from an injury. In the jaws, such changes may be secondary to the loss or displacement of teeth, to injury of the temporomandibular joints, or to intermaxillary fixation required for the immobilization of fractures. The radiographic signs of atrophy include overall loss of bone density and thinning of associated cortical margins.

Infarction

Many injuries result in a disturbance of the circulatory system supplying a traumatized bone or bone segment. Loss of the blood supply results in necrosis within the marrow spaces. Bone infarctions cannot be recognized radiographically at the time of their occurrence but are demarcated as the result of secondary changes. They often appear as lucent shadows, often occurring in clusters. Because the infarcted areas may be structurally weakened, they may be more susceptible to injuries from what would otherwise be inconsequential trauma.

Aseptic Necrosis

The exact etiology of aseptic necrosis is controversial but it is known to occur in association with traumas of various types, including freezing, eating, poisoning, fracture, thrombosis, and other traumatic and non-traumatic events. In the early stages of aseptic necrosis, the involved areas are recognized by their increased radiodensity. Areas of lytic change may appear with subsequent fragmentation of devitalized bone. As the repair process is initiated in areas of aseptic necrosis, the region becomes indistinguishable from other types of reactive bone lesions.

INJURIES TO THE TEETH

Although trauma to the teeth can occur at any age and under variable circumstances, fractures are most common in children between the ages of 8 and 11 years.[5] The anterior teeth are most vulnerable because of their position. Since the management of trauma is related to the extent of injury, it is helpful to use terminology which is based on the treatment needs of a specific injury. According to Bennett,[6] trauma is classified in the following manner:

Class I: trauma to a tooth without evidence of fracture
- (a) no displacement
- (b) subluxation

Class II: fracture of the crown
- (a) enamel
- (b) enamel and dentin

Class III: fracture of the crown with pulpal exposure

Class IV: root fracture
- (a) without fracture of the crown
- (b) with fracture of the crown

Class V: avulsion of the tooth

Radiographic changes associated with injuries in Classes II through V are conspicuous and immediate. Roentgen changes associated with Class I injuries may be obscure and late in their development. In either instance, radiographic surveillance is of value. Since it is unlikely for any but the most severe changes to occur within a period of less than two weeks, radiographs taken to follow the progress of treatment should be widely spaced unless there are extenuating clinical circumstances. A close association may exist between an injured primary tooth and its developing permanent successor (Figure 13-6). Close attention must be paid to the possible involvement of the permanent successor, which may not become evident for some time after the initial injury.

Not all fractures lead to pulpal necrosis or loss of the tooth. In some instances, clinical and radiographic surveillance suggest that healing of root fractures by scarring or some other mechanism may occur (Figure 13-7).

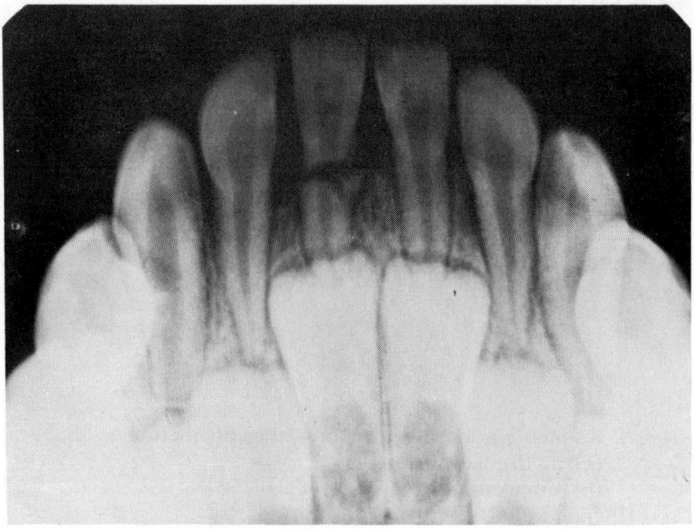

Figure 13-6 The injury to the deciduous incisor is of considerably less consequence than the potential injury to its permanent successor.

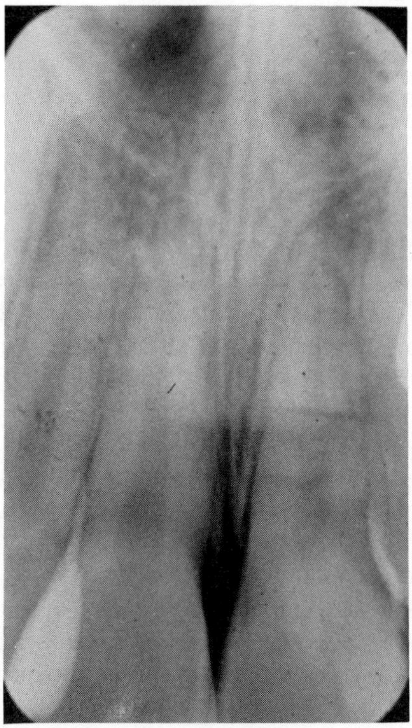

Figure 13-7 Multiple fractures are seen through the root of the central incisor. The fragments are not displaced and the root is vital.

COMMENTS

The radiographic presentation of trauma is similar in different body parts. In the course of dental practice, radiographs of the hand and wrist may be taken for purposes of skeletal aging. Careful scrutiny may result in the detection of hitherto unsuspected injuries. Figure 13-8 reveals a small chip fracture which apparently resulted from minor athletic injury.

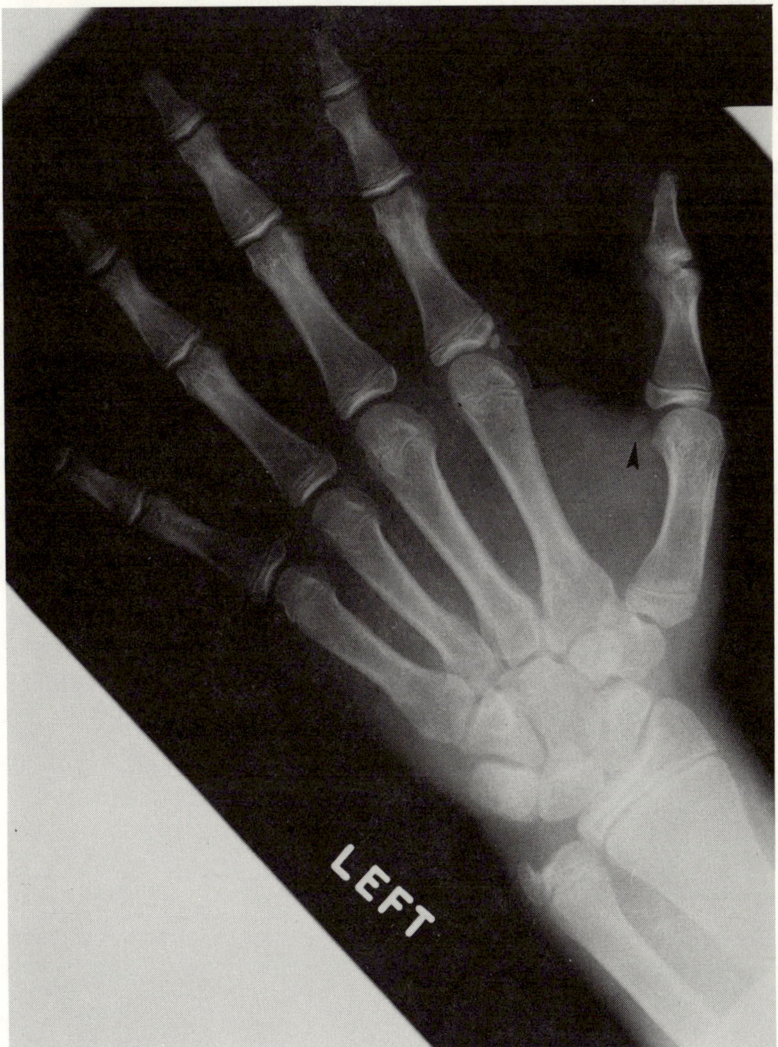

Figure 13-8 Routine examination for skeletal aging. A straight arrow points to a bone fragment which is a normal sesamoid. The curved arrow illustrates a small chip fracture at the edge of the proximal phalanx of the second digit.

Radiographs taken for any reason should be carefully scrutinized so that information retrieval is optimal.

Since an understanding of the etiology of traumatic lesions of the teeth and supporting structures is important to the rational use of radiology, brief reviews by Killey[7,8] and Schultz[9] may be useful.

REFERENCES

1. Boulis, Z.F., Dick, R., and Barnes, N.R. Head injuries on children—aetiology, symptoms, physical findings and x-ray wastage. *Br J Radiol.* 51:851–854, 1978.

2. Webber, R.L., and Folio, J. Radiographic detectability of occipital and temporal-parietal fractures induced in cadaver heads. *J Trauma.* 16:115–124, 1976.

3. Eyes, B., and Evans, A.F. Post-traumatic skull radiographs: a time for a reappraisal. *Lancet* 2(8080):85–86, 1978.

4. Zatzkin, H.R. *The Roentgen Diagnosis of Trauma.* Chicago: Year Book Medical Publishers, 1965.

5. Hallett, G.E.M. Cited in Bennett, D.T. Traumatized anterior teeth. *Br Dent J.* 115:309–311, 1963.

6. Bennett, D.T. Traumatized anterior teeth. *Br Dent J.* 115:309–311, 1963.

7. Killey, H.C. *Fractures of the Mandible.* Dental Practitioner Handbook No. 5. Bristol: John Wright & Sons, Ltd., 1974.

8. Killey, H.C. *Fractures of the Middle Third of the Facial Skeleton.* Dental Practitioner Handbook No. 3. Bristol: John Wright & Sons, Ltd., 1974.

9. Schultz, R.C. *Facial Injuries.* Chicago: Year Book Medical Publishers, 1970.

SECTION III

RADIATION SAFETY

14 Radiobiologic Considerations

The production of x-ray images is based on the differential absorption by or transmission of x-ray photons through an object or body part. Photons which are absorbed by biologic structures transmit their kinetic energy to those structures. This energy is often enough to disrupt the anatomic structure of the absorber, producing both chemical and biologic changes.

The process by which x-ray photons are absorbed by matter is complex and depends upon the energy of the photons and the chemical and physical nature of the absorber. The exact mechanism of interaction is unimportant for our purposes. It is the net result, namely, the breakage of chemical bonds which can be expressed as different types of biologic damage, that is significant.

When biologic tissues are exposed to x-rays, the effect of exposure can be divided into three categories, depending upon the amount of x-ray involved and the rate of exposure. At high doses and high dose rates, *early* or *short-term effects* become apparent. Early effects usually occur after exposures of 100 R or more to most or all of the body. These effects include depression of the bone marrow, intestinal damage, and, at sufficiently high doses, neurologic damage.

Secondary effects, which also occur at high doses, include the premature aging or atrophy of tissues, ulceration, and epilation. In ordinary usage, diagnostic x-rays should not produce early effects or secondary effects although carelessness and/or neglect may result in these changes.

The major concern involved in diagnostic uses of x-rays is the production of *late effects.* These can be subdivided into two categories, genetic and somatic. Both are considered to have no threshold and a linear dose reponse to x-ray exposure. Somatic effects include nonspecific aging or life-shortening, cataract production, and the induction of a variety of neoplasms. The latent period between exposure to x-rays and the appearance of biologic damage may vary from a few years to several decades. Because of the difficulty in associating late effects with specific episodes of exposure, these late effects are of considerable significance from a public health point of view.

The problem of identifying and measuring radiation effects is particularly difficult because exposure to x-rays does not induce any unique disease. The effects are expressed as statistical increases in the incidence of diseases already existing within the population. In most instances, the incidence of a referenced disease is normally low, making it necessary to observe very large populations of irradiated individuals in order to establish a significant increase as the result of radiation exposure.

RISKS ASSOCIATED WITH EXPOSURE TO IONIZING RADIATION

Prior to the 1970s the major focus of radiation protection policy was the occupationally exposed worker. It was tacitly assumed that other individuals would not be exposed without pressing need and that small exposures to isolated body parts were unimportant. Allowable exposure limits were established for occupationally exposed individuals based on the concept of acceptable risk.[1] Although unproven at that time, a no-threshold concept, that is, no exposure free from some degree of risk, was balanced against the potential benefit which might accrue from exposure. In the case of radiation workers, the benefit included personal satisfaction and financial reward in return for a slightly increased risk of neoplastic disease or nonspecific life-shortening. The bulk of the data upon which risk estimates were based came from several different sources.

A large body of data involved experiments with laboratory animals (mostly rodents) and tissue culture systems. Some of these studies were able to demonstrate that even low level exposures were capable of damaging chromosomes[2-4] and/or causing mutations in somatic cells. The significance of these observations is still uncertain. Other studies have shown that exposure to small amounts of radiation can enhance the cancer-inducing potential of viruses and chemicals which are commonly found in the oral cavity and upper respiratory tract.[5,6]

Evidence related to the induction of cancer in humans was available from several sources. In the early part of the century, luminous numerals made of radium-containing phosphorescent paint were applied to watches and instruments by workers who often tipped their brushes on their lips or tongue. These workers ingested significant quantities of radium and in later years developed a high incidence of bone sarcomas and other malignancies related to the radiation emanating from the radium.[7,8]

Physicians and dentists who used x-rays for diagnostic purposes were, in the early part of this century, unaware of the hazards associated with exposure, and they accumulated large doses of radiation. As early as 1910 there were reports of cancer deaths attributed to x-ray exposure. Among dentists, carcinoma of the fingers which were used to hold the film in place was common.[9] Subsequent studies by Lewis[10] also found an increased incidence of cancer in radiologists.

Many European mines which were worked for pitchblende in the early part of this century contained sizable quantities of uranium. Uranium dust was inhaled by mine workers who subsequently developed a high incidence of lung cancer.[11]

Other data have come from the experience of atom-bomb survivors at Hiroshima and Nagasaki.[12] These populations showed significant increases in leukemia and cancer of the thyroid and breast.

Other human populations have been irradiated for therapeutic purposes.[13,14] Included in this group are individuals suffering from ankylosing spondylitis, children with enlargement of the thymus, and children with ringworm of the scalp. Patients with ankylosing spondylitis showed significant increases in the incidence of leukemia while the children treated for thymus enlargement or ringworm had dramatic increases in the incidence of thyroid carcinoma although the thyroid was usually located outside of the primary field of irradiation and received a comparatively small dose.[15]

Still more data are available from groups of women who had multiple fluoroscopic examinations while being treated for tuberculosis. The fluoroscopies were performed to establish the effectiveness of artificially induced pneumothorax. The incidence of breast cancer in these individuals was up to eight times higher than the rate for unexposed women.[16]

Other individuals were irradiated in utero as a result of pelvic x-ray examination of the mother. Retrospective studies of the mothers of leukemic and nonleukemic children suggested a meaningful correlation between in utero irradiation and the risk of childhood leukemia.[17]

In each of these instances the validity of the data as a basis for extrapolation was uncertain. All of the animal and human populations were exposed to relatively high doses of radiation delivered at high dose rates. This is in contrast to most diagnostic situations where the dose rate may be high but the total dose is comparatively small. Some of the study populations received whole body exposures whereas patients and occupational workers usually receive partial body exposures. At Hiroshima and Nagasaki, many individuals suffered and/or died from the effects of heat and blast, starvation, and other factors so that many individuals who might have contributed to an increase in the incidence of late effects were removed from the population. In humans who were therapeutically irradiated, it is extremely difficult to evaluate the effect of the disease for which therapy was required in spite of attempts to use control populations.

Nevertheless, some of the data were evaluated and summarized in a report by the Advisory Committee on the Biological Effects of Ionizing Radiation.[18] The BEIR Report called attention to many important issues and focused on the need to consider somatic as well as genetic effects in the development of risk estimates related to radiation exposure. The assumption that genetic risks from low level exposure were of greater importance than somatic risks was rejected on several accounts. Using the available data, the BEIR Committee calculated that exposures of 5 rem per 30 years could cause between 3000 to 15,000 cancer deaths annually, approximately a 2% increase in the spontaneous cancer death rate.

The BEIR Committee was formed primarily as a result of the concern over the increased use of nuclear energy but the assessment also considered exposures from medical and dental applications. Medical and dental exposures have traditionally been excluded from any control, guidance, regulation, or law. The BEIR Committee, recognizing that radiation exposure from medical applications would constitute the major contribution to population exposure, recommended that these exposures should be evaluated according to the same criteria used for other types of manmade exposures.

It is difficult to assign any precise level of risk to the radiation exposure which results from dental examinations. The most sensitive tissues likely to be exposed during dental procedures are the eye, the bone marrow and the thyroid, in order of increasing sensitivity. An analysis of epidemiologic data on the dose response of radiation-induced tumors in the thyroid gland and blood forming tissues may be helpful in providing a perspective from which the hazards of dental x-ray can be assessed.

Hemplemann and colleagues,[19,20] and Modan and colleagues,[21,22] studied the incidence of carcinoma of the thyroid in individuals who had received radiation therapy as children. In this study population, the thyroid gland was at the periphery of the therapeutic field. Detailed studies[22] showed that the thyroid in these patients should have received average doses ranging from approximately 6 to 7 rad. Although the risk of developing carcinoma of the thyroid varied within different subgroups, the risk of cancer was found to be proportional to thyroid dose with a linear response beginning from as low as 1 rad. The risk of thyroid cancer in some irradiated subgroups was found to be 17 times higher than in the rest of the population.

Within the last few years, additional data have been collected on the relationship between radiation exposure and the induction of leukemia. Mancuso, Stewart, and Kneale[23] examined the lifetime health and mortality experience of employees at the Hanford Works in Richland, Washington, one of the largest atomic facilities in the United States. The workers, who are primarily white males, had complete records of sex, date of birth, date of hire, dates of entering and leaving specified occupations, external and internal radiation exposures, and the date and cause of death. The radiation exposure records were obtained from radiation badges which were obligatory in all workshops and laboratories and which were read at frequent intervals. From the available data it was possible to calculate doubling doses for radiation associated cancers. The calculations suggest that exposures as low as 12.2 rad could double the normal risk of dying from any type of cancer while doses as low as 0.8 rad could conceivably double the risk of leukemias or cancers of the bone marrow.

A similar study by Najarian and Colton[24] reviewed the death certificates among former workers at the Portsmouth Naval Shipyard, New Hampshire where nuclear submarines are repaired and refueled. Their study indicated that occupationally exposed shipyard workers had six times the proportional mortality of leukemia and twice the proportional mortality for all cancers expected for United States white males of the same age groups. It appeared that the total lifetime exposure of these workers averaged less than 10 rad.

These most recent studies indicate that exposure levels well within the range of those used in diagnostic procedures are capable of increasing the spontaneous incidence of cancer. It has been estimated that under ideal conditions some dental examinations may expose the bone marrow to one-tenth or more of the estimated doubling dose for leukemia. Public Health Surveys conducted in 1964[25] and 1970[26,27] suggest that exposure levels in actual practice could be in excess of ten times higher than this ideal.

Block, Goepp, and Mason[28] reported thyroid exposures of approximately 600 to 800 milliroentgens resulting from poor positioning during panoramic examinations with lower but significant doses measured in cephalometric radiography. These exposure levels also were obtained using appropriate technique factors and film processing and are in the range of 10% or more of doses which have been shown to have a carcinogenic effect. Again, there is reason to suspect that the actual doses used in many clinical settings are considerably higher. Furthermore, it is not unusual for individuals to undergo frequent re-examination during certain types of treatments, including orthodontics.

Bross and Natarajan[29,30] have estimated that exposure to all levels of ionizing radiation may account for drastically increased risk of leukemia and other disease in children (up to fiftyfold increase). Pochin[31] has also concluded that the induction of malignancies in man occurs at doses of less than 10 rad. In experimental systems, fractionation of low doses of radiation were found to enhance transformation of cells in vitro. In oral mucosa, Lurie[5] reported a significant increase in the yield of tumors resulting from a chemical carcinogen when animals were exposed to low level x-rays. Exposure to x-rays alone failed to produce any tumors. Lurie also found that tumors induced by the combined effects of chemical carcinogens and x-ray exposure were larger and developed after a shorter latent period than tumors produced by the chemical carcinogen alone.

Incomplete data based on studies by Commoner[32] of servicemen exposed to radiation from hydrogen-bomb tests in Nevada suggest that there is an increased incidence of leukemia in these individuals. The same study also evaluated workers associated with various aspects of the uranium industry and found that they, too, have a higher cancer death rate than nonirradiated individuals in the population.

The perspective of radiation safety has changed dramatically in the last decade. The assumption that only large exposures are of consequence can no longer be supported. Although it remains important to implement effective controls to protect individuals who are occupationally exposed to x-rays, it is equally important to develop thoughtful guidelines to minimize the exposure of patients. Patient exposure is most effectively minimized by assuring that x-ray examinations are performed only when necessary, that they are performed by well-trained individuals, and that they employ only state-of-the-art techniques with built-in quality assurance measures.

UTILIZATION

In 1964 and again in 1970, the Public Health Service conducted studies of population exposures to x-rays.[25-27] The resulting reports described patterns of utilization in dentistry as well as in other health care areas. In 1970, 59.2 million persons were x-rayed for dental purposes, and dental exposures occurred at a peak rate in younger populations. The rate of exposure also varied according to geographical location and social and economic status. Even educational background affected the frequency of x-ray exposure.

Although dental x-rays may not contribute significantly more than 3% of the total adult per capita bone marrow dose, the dental x-ray is one of the most common types of radiographic examination in use. While good data are not available, there is reason to believe that the growth of use of dental x-rays may be exceeding the growth patterns for other types of examinations. It is currently estimated that there are more than 143,000 dental x-ray units in use in the United States. A recent survey of practices in American dental schools indicated that x-ray examinations were conducted routinely and without prior determination of need.[33] As a matter of experience rather than mandate, dental students become accustomed to the concept of routine x-ray examination.

Inappropriate utilization of x-ray examinations can have important implications for the well-being of the patient. One of the most serious concerns has to do with the generation of false negatives which may lead to unnecessary delays in treatment. In a previous section, several examples of false negative diagnoses resulting from the inappropriate use of panoramic examinations were cited. There are numerous other examples in the literature. Burns[34] pointed out that false negative mammograms obtained during screening examinations led to significant delays in the diagnosis of breast cancer because clinicians came to rely too heavily on the radiographs. Bell and Loop[35] found that $15 million a year could be saved by eliminating x-ray examination of patients who had suffered head injuries when clinical examination suggested that x-ray studies would be unproductive.

The dental literature contains statistics which could be used for the development of so-called high yield criteria to help in determining when examinations were appropriate. For example, Morris and Jerman[36] studied the frequency of embedded third molars in United States Air Force recruits and found that 65.5% of individuals ranging in age from 17 to 24 years presented with impactions. Follicular cysts occurred with a frequency of just over 4%. While such data constitute an adequate justification for the examination of third molar regions in young adults, consideration can be given to the use of periapical examinations or limited panoramic views (Figure 14-1) as a means of reducing the volume of tissue exposed to x-rays.

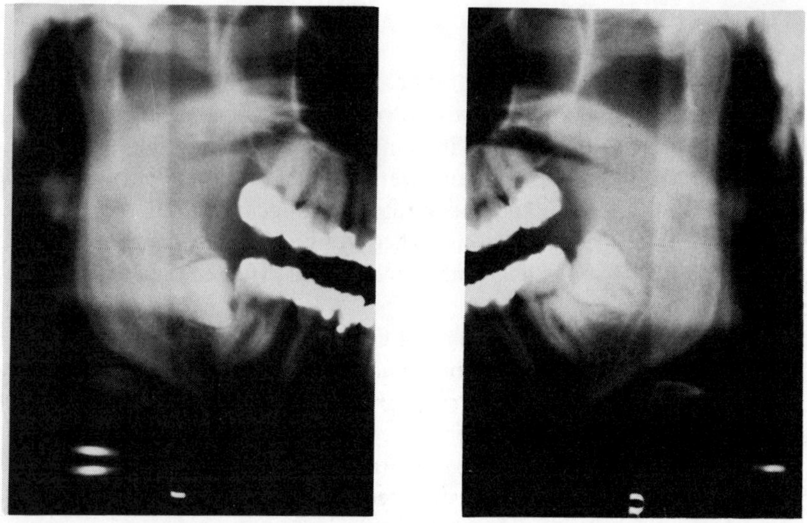

Figure 14-1 It has become common practice to use panoramic machines for the evaluation of the third molars, because of their convenience or because candidates for extraction suffer from trismus. Many panoramic machines can be operated from either direction and/or over limited segments of their cycle. It is possible to demonstrate the third molar regions without exposing the rest of the facial bones and cranium. The radiograph shown above was produced on a G.E. Panelipse and results in approximately one-third of the exposure required for a full panoramic view.

RECOMMENDATIONS

In March of 1978 the American Dental Association's Council on Dental Materials and Devices published its recommendations in radiographic practices.[33] The recommendations were prefaced by a statement that, "The American Dental Association has consistently stated that the use of x-radiation for diagnostic purposes should be made only after consideration of both the dental and general health needs of the patient." It was further stated that, "Diagnostic radiology should be limited to those instances in which the dentist anticipates that the information he is likely to obtain will contribute materially to proper diagnosis, treatment, or prevention of disease, or all of these." As the American Dental Association points out, "Use of professional judgement to determine the frequency and extent of each radiographic examination" is essential. It would be impossible to provide a comprehensive list of criteria qualifying as indications for x-ray examination, but it is possible to identify many issues which should be taken into account.

Evidence of Disease

Clinical signs or symptoms constitute the most obvious indications for radiographic examination of dental structures. Evidence of carious lesions, periodontal disease, swellings or discolorations of oral soft tissues, fistulae, ulcerations, pain, or altered sensation requires examination of underlying structures. The type and extent of examination should be determined by the specific findings in each individual.

Growth and Development

During development of the primary and permanent dentition, a number of treatable abnormalities occur with a sufficiently high frequency to warrant radiographic examination of the jaws. These abnormalities include congenitally missing and supernumerary teeth, impacted teeth, malpositioned teeth, and developmental cysts occurring in association with a tooth follicle or bony suture. The radiographic examination of symptom-free developing individuals should be based on a thorough knowledge of the most common sites and times of occurrence of these abnormalities and should also take into account the most effective time for therapeutic intervention. Since most of these abnormalities cease to be issues in the adult, they also cease to be justifications for periodic re-examination.

Dental Therapy

Certain types of dental treatments are in and of themselves indications for periodic x-ray re-examination of dental structures. For example, the likelihood of pathologic changes occurring in pulpal or periodontal tissues of teeth which have been traumatized, endodontically treated, or extensively resorbed is considerably higher than in teeth which are clinically sound. In many of these circumstances, however, pulpal and periodontal pathology develop very slowly so that frequent radiographic examination in the absence of symptoms is inappropriate because it may produce a false sense of security by examining structures before sufficient time has elapsed for changes to become apparent in an x-ray image.

Caries Attack Rate

The frequency of radiographic examination, particularly bitewings, should be determined by the caries attack rate of the patient. Individuals who have been raised in fluoridated areas and who have good oral hygiene and a reasonable diet will require less frequent examination than individuals with less favorable backgrounds. The number and type of restorations must also be considered in determining the frequency with which bitewing films should be taken. Full coverage of crowns with metallic restoration will limit the value of radiographs. The margins of such crowns can be checked more effectively by clinical examination than by x-ray.

PROTECTION OF THE PATIENT

A significant reduction in patient exposure can be achieved without compromising the efficiency with which diagnostic data are collected and without significant increments in expense.[37] Dental radiography is of particular interest because its use is so widespread, because it often involves young people, and because it is often performed by auxiliaries with little or no training.

The development of recommendations for reducing the size and frequency of exposures is most easily approached by reviewing some of the more readily recognized abuses.[38] Overexposure can be related to problems in the areas of prescription of x-ray studies, equipment, and technique.

Prescription of X-Ray Examinations

One of the most effective ways of reducing exposures to x-rays is to eliminate clinically unproductive examinations. The justification for x-ray examinations is varied and should be based on the need for diagnostic information determined by history and clinical examination. Many if not most x-ray examinations are, however, prescribed as a routine matter. Frequent explanations for the examinations include inexperience on the part of the clinician, intellectual curiosity, defense against peer criticism and legal action, administrative convenience, and public health screening. These latter excuses for patient exposure are likely to be unproductive since they are not sufficiently specific to form the basis for deciding on the number and types of views which are required in accordance with the principles of good practice. In many instances, radiographs taken for legal purposes become a liability rather than an asset since they place on record the clinician's decision that the examination was necessary and lay open to examination his judgement related to the need for appropriateness and quality of the examination as well as his skill in interpreting the data produced by the exposure.

X-ray examinations should be prescribed only by properly trained clinicians who have established the patient's need and who can appropriately weigh the anticipated benefit against the potential risk. Individuals who order x-ray examinations must be familiar with the type of examination which is to be performed and its probable yield. X-ray examinations should not be initiated by auxiliaries with limited health care training.

Practitioners who accept the responsibility for ordering x-ray examinations should, from time to time, review the criteria which they use in their decision-making process. A periodic review of patient records may establish that adequate information can be obtained without radiographs or with fewer numbers of radiographs. Only when the yield of diagnostic information is high can the risk of radiation exposure be offset.

X-Ray Equipment

The performance characteristics of x-ray units can be an important factor in limiting patient and operator exposure. The same technique factors set on different x-ray machines result in widely varying x-ray exposures. In 1974 federal performance standards came into effect and required manufacturers to certify that equipment sold after that date met specific requirements. Equipment assembled and sold prior to 1974 was, for all practical purposes, uncontrolled and unregulated.

Many older machines are capable of adequate performance and some new x-ray units operate at substandard levels. The evaluation of machine performance is relatively simple, and in most instances, substandard performance can be corrected simply and inexpensively. All certified and noncertified dental x-ray machines should meet the following standards,[38] prepared by the U.S. Atomic Energy Commission, the U.S. Public Health Service, and the Conference of Radiation Control Program Directors in cooperation with the Council of State Governments:

A. *Source-to-Skin Distance.* X-ray systems designed for use with an intraoral image receptor shall be provided with means to limit source-to-skin distance to not less than:
   (1) 18 centimeters if operable above 50 kilovolts peak, or
   (2) 10 centimeters if not operable above 50 kilovolts peak.

B. *Field Limitation.*
   (1) Radiographic systems designed for use with an intraoral image receptor shall be provided with means to limit the x-ray beam such that:
      (a) If the minimum source-to-skin distance (SSD) is 18 centimeters or more, the x-ray field, at the minimum SSD, shall be containable in a circle having a diameter of no more than 7 centimeters; and

(b) If the minimum SSD is less than 18 centimeters, the x-ray field, at the minimum SSD, shall be containable in a circle having a diameter of no more than 6 centimeters.

(2) An open ended shielded position indicating device shall be used.

C. *Timers.* Means shall be provided to terminate the exposure at a preset time interval, preset product of current and time, a preset number of pulses, or a preset radiation exposure to the image receptor. In addition,

(1) Termination of exposure shall cause automatic resetting of the timer to its initial setting or to zero.

(2) It shall not be possible to make an exposure when the timer is set to a zero or off position if either position is provided.

(3) *Reproducibility.* When four timer tests taken at identical timer settings are performed the average time period ($\overline{T}$) shall be greater than five times the maximum period (T_{max}) less the minimum period (T_{min}). $\overline{T}$ shall be less than or equal to 5 seconds.

$$\overline{T} > 5\,(T_{max} - T_{min})$$

D. *X-Ray Control (Exposure Switch).*

(1) A control shall be incorporated into each x-ray system such that an exposure can be terminated at any time, except for exposures of one-half second or less.

(2) Each x-ray control shall be located in such a way as to meet the following criteria:

(a) For stationary x-ray systems, it shall be required that the control switch be permanently mounted in a protected area (e.g., corridor outside the room) so that the operator is required to remain in that protected area during the entire exposure.

(b) For mobile and portable x-ray systems which are:

(i) used for greater than 1 week in 1 location (1 room or suite) shall meet the requirements of D2a above.

(ii) used for more than 1 hour and less than 1 week at 1 location (1 room, or suite) shall meet the requirements of D2b(i) or be provided with a 6.5-foot-high protective barrier which is placed at least 6 feet from the tube housing assembly and at least 6 feet from the patient.

(iii) used to make an exposure(s) of only 1 patient at the use location shall meet the requirement of D2b(i) or (ii) or be provided with a method of control which will permit the operator to be at least 12 feet from the tube head assembly during an exposure.

(3) The x-ray control shall provide visual indication observable at or from the operator's protected position whenever x-rays are produced. In addition, a signal audible to the operator shall indicate that the exposure has terminated.

E. *Exposure Reproducibility.* The *exposure* produced shall be reproducible to within the following criteria:

When all technique factors are held constant, the coefficient of variation shall not exceed 0.10. This shall be deemed to have been met if when four *exposures* at identical technique factors are made that the value of the average *exposure* ($\bar{E}$) is greater than five times the maximum *exposure* (E_{max}) minus the minimum *exposure* (E_{min}).

$$\bar{E} > 5\,(E_{max} - E_{min})$$

F. *Operating Controls.*

(1) Patient and film holding devices shall be used when the techniques permit.

(2) Neither the tube housing nor the position indicating device shall be hand held during an exposure.

(3) The x-ray system shall be arranged and operated in such a manner that the useful beam at the patient's skin does not exceed the dimensions specified in B1.

(4) Dental fluoroscopy without image intensification shall be prohibited.

G. *Additional Requirements Applicable to Certified Systems Only.* Only diagnostic x-ray systems incorporating one or more certified component(s) shall be required to comply with the following requirement(s) which relate to that certified component in addition to other applicable requirements of these regulations.

(1) *Reproducibility.* The following requirement shall apply when the equipment is operated on an adequate power supply as specified by the manufacturer.

(2) *Coefficient of Variation.* For any specific combination of selected technique factors, the estimated coefficient of variation of radiation *exposures* shall be no greater than 0.05.

(3) *Linearity.* The following requirement applies when the equipment allows a choice of x-ray tube current settings and is operated on a power supply as specified by the manufacturer in accordance with the requirements of applicable Federal standards for any fixed x-ray tube potential within the range of 40 percent to 100 percent of the maximum rated.

(4) *Average Exposure Ratios.* The average ratios of *exposure* to the indicated milliampere-seconds product (mR/mAs) obtained at any two consecutive tube current settings shall not differ by more than 0.10 times their sum. This is:

$$|\bar{X}_1 - \bar{X}_2| \leqslant 0.10\,(\bar{X}_1 + \bar{X}_2)$$

where $\bar{X}_1$ and $\bar{X}_2$ are the average mR/mAs values obtained at each of two consecutive tube current settings.

(5) *Accuracy.* Deviation of technique factors from indicated values shall not exceed the limit provided for that system by its manufacturer.

Technique

Poor quality radiographs are of little use to patient or dentist. The acquisition of a maximum amount of information with minimum patient exposure requires the development of appropriate technique factors.

Consistent results also require the implementation of a quality assurance program to establish before the fact that high quality images are obtainable.

Operating Procedures

Before each examination the operator must establish that equipment is operating correctly and that the appropriate kilovoltage, milliamperage, and time are set on the x-ray control. Packets containing fresh, properly stored film of the correct size and number should be selected. Film holders which exteriorize the position of the film and assure correct alignment and collimation should be used except in situations where their use would cause unreasonable discomfort or compromise the geometry of the examination.

Processing facilities should be checked prior to use to determine that solutions are fresh and present in adequate quantities. All radiographs should be processed according to the manufacturer's instructions, taking into account both time and temperature.

All inadequate examinations should be recorded and evaluated in order to determine the nature of the error so that corrective action can be taken.

Operators should be aware of the way in which technique factors can be used to minimize patient exposure. Operators should be adequately trained and should be periodically tested to demonstrate continuing competence. In general, neither dentist nor dental auxiliaries should use x-ray equipment unless they have received minimal training such as that recommended by the American Academy of Dental Radiology and the Oral Radiology Section of the American Association of Dental Schools.

Patient exposures in dental examinations should never exceed 700 mR and should ideally be kept to 200 mR per film.

REFERENCES

1. National Council on Radiation Protection and Measurements. *Basic Radiation Protection Criteria.* Report No. 39. Washington, DC: US Government Printing Office, 1971.

2. White, S. Effects of low level x-radiation on chromosomes. *J Dent Res.* 46:1177–1181, 1967.

3. Bloom, A.D., and Tjio, J.H. *In vivo* effects of diagnostic x-irradiation on human chromosomes. *N Engl J Med.* 270:1341–1344, 1964.

4. Langlands, A.O., Smith, P.G., Buckton, K.E. et al. Chromosome damage induced by radiation. *Nature* 218:1133–1135, 1968.

5. Lurie, A.G. Enhancement of DMBA tumorigenesis in hamster cheek pouch epithelium by repeated exposures to low-level x-radiation. *Radiat Res.* 72:499–511, 1977.

6. Yang, T.C.H., Tobias, C.A., Howard, J. et al. Effect of radiation and high temperature on the viral transformation of cells *in vitro. Radiat Res.* 74:538, 1978.

7. Looney, W.B. Late effects (25–40 years) of the early medical and industrial use of radioactive materials. *J Bone Joint Surg.* 37:1269, 1955.

8. Martland, H.S. Occupational poisoning in manufacture of luminous watch dials. *JAMA*. 92:466, 1929.

9. Mohs, F.E. Roentgen ray cancer of the hands in dentists. *J Am Dent Assoc.* 45:160, 1952.

10. Lewis, E.B. Leukemia, multiple myeloma and aplastic anemia in American radiologists. *Science* 142:1492–1494, 1963.

11. Peller, S. Lung cancer among mine workers in Joachimsthal. *Hum Biol.* 11:130, 1939.

12. Beebe, G.W., Kato, H., and Land, C.E. Studies of the mortality of A-bomb survivors. *Radiat Res.* 75:138–201, 1978.

13. Court-Brown, W.M., and Doll, R. Leukemia and aplastic anemia in patients irradiated for ankylosing spondylitis. *Medical Research Council Special Report Series* No. 295:1–135, 1957.

14. Court-Brown, W.M., and Doll, R. Mortality from cancer and other causes after radiotherapy for ankylosing spondylitis. *Br Med J.* 2:1327–1332, 1965.

15. Barnett, M.H. *The Biological Effects of Ionizing Radiation: An Overview.* DHEW Publ. No.(FDA) 77-8004. Washington, DC: US Government Printing Office, 1976.

16. Mole, R.H. The sensitivity of the human breast to cancer induction by ionizing radiation. *Br J Radiol.* 51:401–405, 1978.

17. Stewart, A., Webb, J., Giles, D. et al. Malignant disease in childhood and diagnostic irradiation in utero. *Lancet* 2:447, 1956.

18. Advisory Committee on the Biological Effects of Ionizing Radiations. *The Effects on Populations of Exposure to Low Levels of Ionizing Radiation.* Washington, DC: National Academy of Sciences, National Research Council, 1972.

19. Hemplemann, L.H. Risk of thyroid neoplasms after irradiation in childhood. *Science* 160:159–163, 1968.

20. Hemplemann, L.H., Hall, W.J., Phillips, M. et al. Neoplasms in persons treated with x-rays in infancy: fourth survey in 20 years. *J Natl Cancer Inst.* 55:519–530, 1975.

21. Modan, B., Baidatz, D., Mort, H. et al. Radiation-induced head and neck tumours. *Lancet* 1:277–279, 1974.

22. Werner, A., Modan, B., and Davidoff, D. Doses to brain, skull and thyroid, following X-ray therapy for Tinea Capitis. *Phys Med Biol.* 13:247–258, 1968.

23. Mancuso, T.F., Stewart, A., and Kneale, G.F. Radiation exposures of Hanford workers dying from cancer and other causes. *Health Phys.* 33:369–385, 1977.

24. Najarian, T., and Colton, T. Mortality from leukemia and cancer in shipyard nuclear workers. *Lancet* 1:1018–1020, 1978.

25. US Public Health Service. *Population Exposure to X-Rays U.S. 1964. A Report on the Public Health Service X-Ray Exposure Study.* DHEW Publ. No. (PHS) 1519. Washington, DC: US Government Printing Office, 1964.

26. Brown, R., White, E.L., and Gitlin, J.N. Preliminary Estimates from the U.S. Public Health Service 1970 X-Ray Exposure Study. Paper presented at the Roentgen Ray Society Meeting, Boston, September 29, 1971.

27. Brown, R., Fuchsberg, R.R., and Gitlin, J.N. Preliminary Dose Estimates from the U.S. Public Health Service 1970 X-Ray Exposure Study. Paper presented at the 49th Annual Meeting of the American College of Radiology, Miami Beach, April 6, 1972.

28. Block, A.J., Goepp, R.A., and Mason, E.W. Thyroid radiation dose during panoramic and cephalometric dental x-ray examinations. *Angle Orthod.* 47:17–24, 1977.

29. Bross, I.D., and Natarajan, N. Leukemia from low-level radiation. *N Engl J Med.* 287:107–110, 1972.

30. Bross, I.D., and Natarajan, N. Genetic damage from diagnostic radiation. *JAMA.* 237:2399–2401, 1977.

31. Pochin, E.E. Radiology now: malignancies following low radiation exposures in man. *Br J Radiol.* 49:577–579, 1976.

32. Commoner, B. Hiroshima at home. *Hosp Prac.* 13:58–63, 1978.

33. Council on Dental Materials and Devices. Recommendations in radiographic practices—March 1978. *J Am Dent Assoc.* 96:485–486, 1978.

34. Burns, P.E. False-negative mammograms delay diagnosis of breast cancer. *N Engl J Med.* 299:201–202, 1978.

35. Bell, R.S., and Loop, J.W. The utility and futility of radiographic skull examination for trauma. *N Engl J Med.* 284:236–239, 1971.

36. Morris, C.R., and Jerman, A.C. Panoramic radiographic study of embedded third molars. *J Oral Surg.* 29:122–125, 1971.

37. International Commission on Radiological Protection. *Protection of the Patient in X-Ray Diagnosis.* ICRP Publication No. 16. New York: Pergamon Press, 1969.

38. US Environmental Protection Agency. *Radiation Protection Guidance for Diagnostic X-Rays.* Federal Guidance Report No. 9, EPA 520/4-76-019. Washington, DC: US Government Printing Office, 1976.

15 Quality Assurance

On May 7, 1976, the *Federal Register* contained a notice by the Food and Drug Administration of its intent to propose recommendations related to quality assurance programs for diagnostic x-ray facilities. Quality assurance was defined as the planned and systematic actions that provide adequate confidence that a diagnostic x-ray facility will produce consistently high quality radiographs at minimum cost and minimum patient exposure. Quality assurance actions were divided into quality control procedures and quality administration procedures, the former involving physical techniques for testing the components of an x-ray system, and the latter referring to owner or management actions which guarantee that monitoring is properly performed and evaluated.

Several types of data led to the conclusion that quality assurance programs were necessary. One indication of need came from a study of radiographs submitted to the National Institute of Occupational Safety and Health. This unit operated a pneumoconiosis compensation program in which participants were required to have their facilities certified as being competent. Certification was based on data that included the evaluation of sample radiographs. The competence of individuals reading films was also assessed. Trout et al[1] found that 44% of the certified facilities had from 10% to 40% of their radiographs rejected because they were of inadequate quality for the diagnosis of pneumoconiosis.

In dentistry, image quality was studied by Beideman, Johnson, and Alcox.[2] These investigators surveyed preauthorization radiographs submitted to Pennsylvania Blue Shield. Between one-half and three-quarters of the films were considered to be inadequate for determining the efficacy of a proposed treatment plan. Other investigators[3-5] found that electrical and mechanical problems that lead to poor image quality exist in a large percentage of x-ray units.

Concern for radiographic quality has many components. First, if image quality is poor, the clinician is at greater risk of arriving at an erroneous conclusion. Second, if radiographic quality is sufficiently poor, the examination will be repeated and the patient will have been unnecessarily exposed by the first examination. Finally, the time and materials involved in repeating examinations add an unnecessary financial burden to the health care system. The Food and Drug Administration estimated that by reducing the number of repeated radiographs in hospitals alone, the population could be spared from approximately 209,000 to 333,000 rem to the active bone marrow and that many institutions could save from $10,000 to $100,000 annually.

RECOMMENDATIONS

On April 28, 1978, specific recommendations for quality assurance programs appeared in the *Federal Register.* These quality assurance programs were recommended for *all diagnostic radiology facilities.* It was anticipated that each facility in which an x-ray system was used for diagnosis or visualization would establish guidelines for the extent to which a quality assurance program should be implemented, based on an analysis of that facility's resources and objectives.

It was recommended that, within each facility, the responsibility and authority for quality assurance should be specified and recorded in a quality assurance manual developed for the facility. It was assumed that the practitioner in charge of the facility would have the primary responsibility for implementing the program, although day-to-day execution might be delegated to auxiliary personnel. Individuals performing quality assurance procedures, however, were expected to be qualified to carry out these duties.

In addition, it was recommended that the purchase of new equipment should be preceded by a careful definition of performance specifications by the individuals who would ultimately use the facility.

The Food and Drug Administration recommended that quality control monitoring be conducted on a formalized and regular schedule. The monitoring systems were expected to employ state-of-the-art procedures and devices. The system parameters monitored and the frequency of monitoring were to be based on an analysis of needs. Included in the parameters to be considered for monitoring were film processing, radiographic x-ray units, cassettes, view boxes, and tomographic systems.

FILM PROCESSING

Processing is one of the most variable procedures in radiography. The chemical reactions which result in development are highly dependent upon the concentration of ingredients in the developer, temperature, pH, and the time of development. All of these factors must be checked and controlled if there is to be a satisfactory and a consistent result. Under ideal circumstances, the processing system (tank or machine) should be evaluated on a daily basis and the results compared to the standard established when the processing facility was cleaned and set up with fresh chemicals.

The test procedure requires the exposure of a film by a sensitometer (calibrated light source) or by x-ray transmitted through a step wedge (Figure 15-1). The step wedge is placed on top of a periapical film and exposed with factors normally used for molar teeth. The step wedge and film should be centered under the x-ray tube and the cone should be no more than one inch from the surface of the step wedge.

The exposed test film is then processed at the exact temperature and for the precise amount of time specified by the manufacturer of the processing chemistry. The developed film should show a clear area, a dark grey area, and a black area. The test film should also be compared to a standard.

When the x-ray chemistry is fresh, the test film is helpful in establishing the correct exposure factors. If the middle third of the test film is dark, the x-ray exposure is too great and the time should be decreased. If the middle step is too light, an increase in the exposure time is necessary.

A fogged test film exposed with normal factors may result from the use of outdated film, exposure of the film by scattered radiation, inadequate lighting, contaminated developer, light leaks, improper film storage, and other less likely factors.

When correct exposure factors have been established but the middle step of the test film is too light, the activity of the developer may be low as the result of excessive use, oxidation, or contamination. If the test films are not completely transparent in unexposed areas, depletion of the fixer is likely.

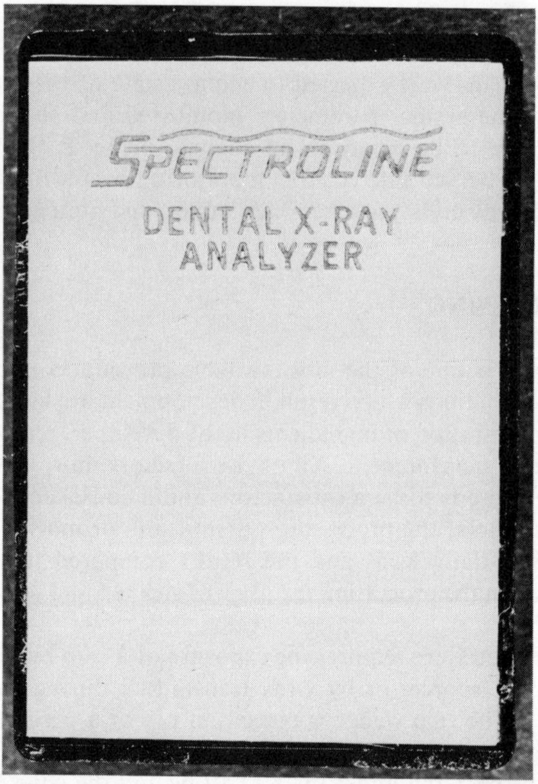

A

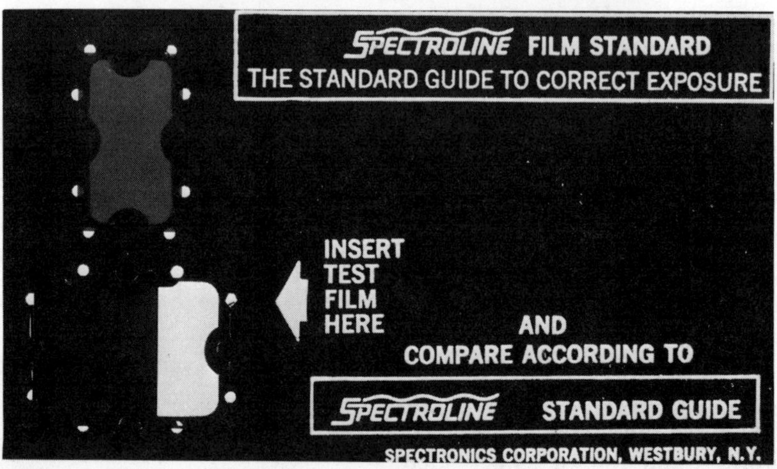

B

Figure 15-1 **A.** A small, three-step aluminum wedge suitable for use in a quality assurance program (Spectronics Corp., Westbury, New York). The step wedge is the same size as a No. 2 periapical film. **B.** A radiograph exposed through the step wedge with factors commonly used for periapical views uses the complete density range of the film. One step is clear, one is grey, and one is black.

It is desirable to keep a tally of the number of films processed each day so that the solutions can be replenished in a reasonable way. Figures 15-2 and 15-3 are graphs of the rates of replenishment required by machines using Kodak RP chemistry. The computation is based on a requirement for 120 ml of developer and 200 ml of fixer for 238 square inches of film (14 × 17). A number 2 dental film is 2.5 square inches. Although the emulsion on a dental film is thicker than that on medical screen films, these rates of replenishment have proven to be adequate.

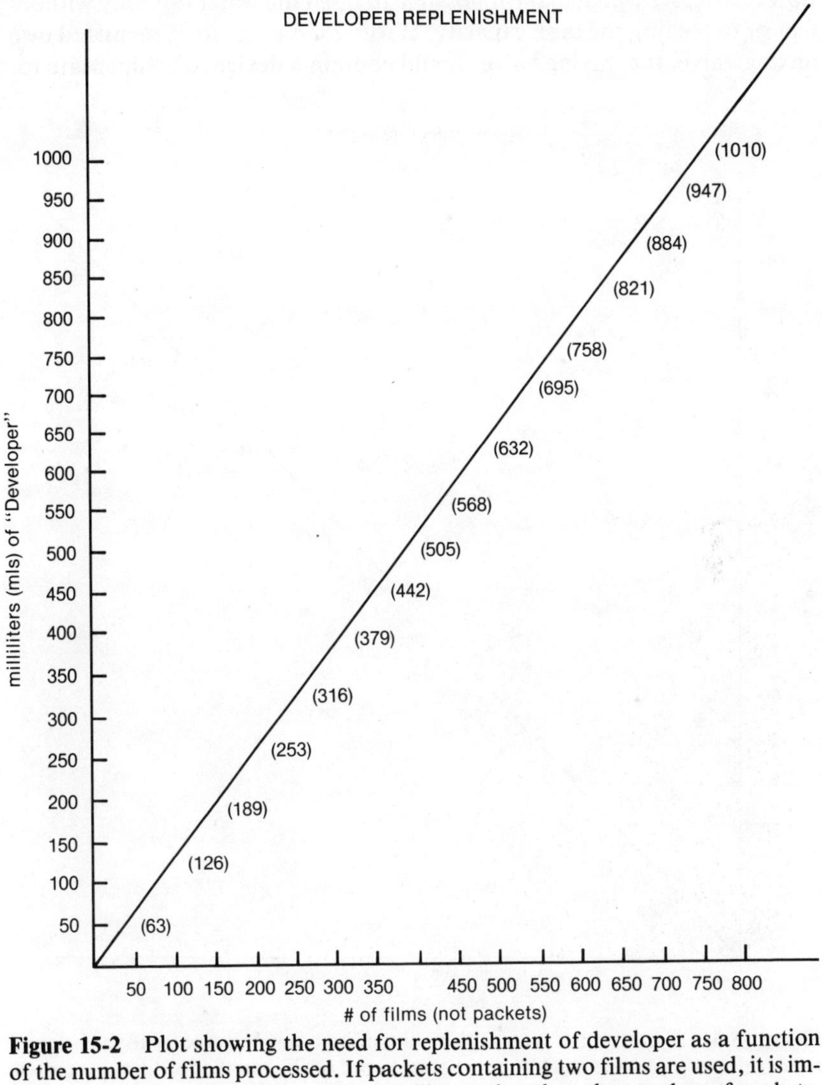

Figure 15-2 Plot showing the need for replenishment of developer as a function of the number of films processed. If packets containing two films are used, it is important to keep track of the number of films rather than the number of packets.

A few tips on the maintenance of the processing facility may be helpful. The surfaces of mechanical processors or chemical tanks should be kept clean. Acid cleaning solutions may be used in the developer compartment and alkaline materials in the fixer section. These compounds must be completely removed by careful rinsing before the processing facility is refilled. Abrasive materials should not be used. Scratched surfaces tend to collect precipitates and make cleaning more difficult.

The flow of water should be carefully regulated. Inadequate washing will result in stained films. Processors which are plumbed should contain flow restrictors which make it possible to open the water tap fully without fear of exceeding the tank capacity. If water temperature is regulated by a mixing valve, the mixing valve should contain a device to compensate for

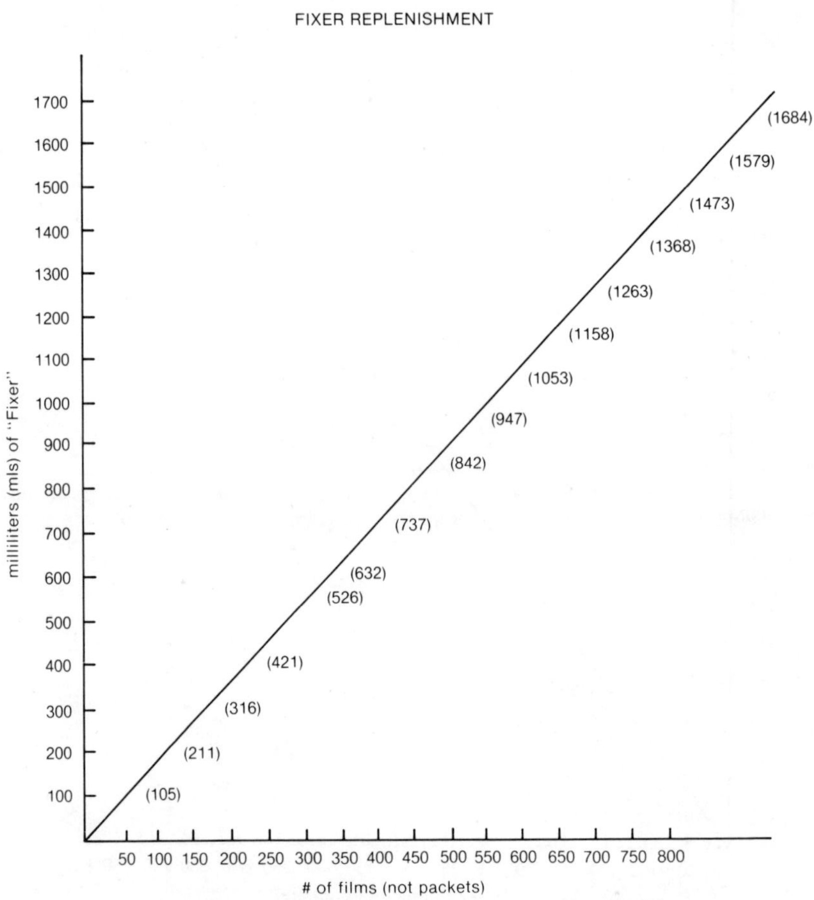

Figure 15-3 The need for fixer replenishment is somewhat greater than the need for developer replenishment. Again, some record of the number of films processed is essential for proper replenishment.

fluctuations in water pressure. Mixing valves without such devices are subject to more frequent failure. Mixing valves of all types require periodic cleaning. The frequency of cleaning will vary, depending upon the quality of the water and the extent of its use. Periodical turning of the mixing valve to its hot and cold extremes may help to prevent the accumulation of deposits which interfere with the free action of the valve.

Darkrooms should be kept clean and well ventilated. Chemical fumes accumulate and can cause deposits on surfaces where film or other sensitive materials are handled.

THE X-RAY UNIT

There are three major parameters in the x-ray machine which should be checked at least yearly. These include the functions of time, milliamperage, and kilovoltage.

The accuracy of the timer can be checked in two relatively simple ways. An electronic impulse counter can be attached to the tube so that the number of electronic pulses reaching the tube can be measured directly (Figure 15-4). Other devices using ionization chambers can be placed in the x-ray beam where they measure the number of x-ray pulses emitted

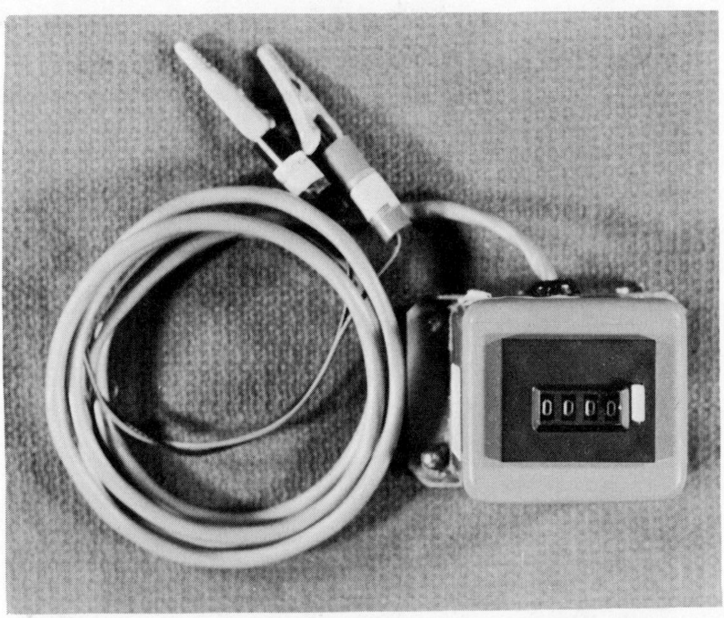

Figure 15-4 This electronic impulse counter can be attached to leads on the tube head where it directly measures the number of electronic pulses reaching the tube. The device can be reset after each exposure.

during the course of an exposure. Perhaps the easiest device for testing the accuracy of the timer is the spin top (Figure 15-5). The top has a notch cut at one point in its circumference which will allow x-rays to reach a film placed below the top. If the top is spinning during an x-ray exposure, a number of exposed dots equal to the number of impulses coming from the timer will appear on the film (Figure 15-6).

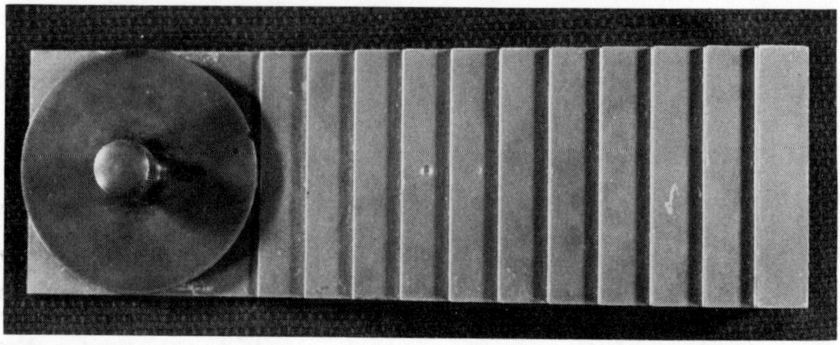

Figure 15-5 This combination step wedge and spin top can be used for a variety of test purposes.

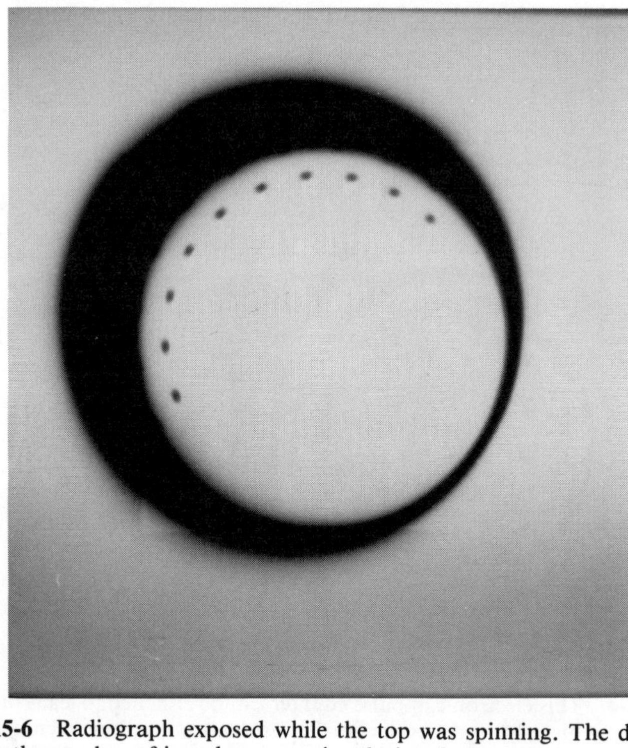

Figure 15-6 Radiograph exposed while the top was spinning. The dots correspond to the number of impulses occurring during the exposure.

Although the kilovoltage or power supply to the tube can be measured electronically, the energy distribution of the x-ray beam is best measured with a step wedge or a device known commercially as a Wisconsin Test Cassette (Figure 15-7).[6] With a step wedge, the number of grey levels from clear to black should remain constant for any particular kilovoltage setting. Changes in the number of grey levels indicate either a change in the amount of filtration in the x-ray beam or a change in the performance of the x-ray generator and tube. The Wisconsin Test Cassette uses one intensifying screen which is covered by material that attenuates light in five separate areas. The front of the cassette contains a lead mask with five pairs of columns with ten holes in each column. This mask is positioned so that one line in each column is aligned with the device which attenuates the light. Different thicknesses of copper are placed over the holes in the left hand column. Four of the pairs of columns are used for kilovoltage measurement while the last pair is used to measure the half value layer. Use of the Wisconsin Test Cassette is complicated and may be impractical in offices that do not have automatic processing. The simple step wedge will generally provide an adequate estimate of the consistency of the x-ray beam quality.

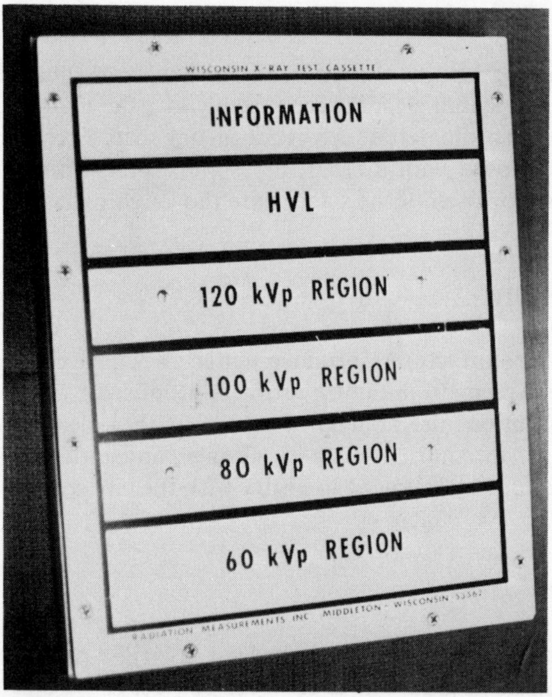

Figure 15-7 The Wisconsin Test Cassette has become a standard item for checking the kilovoltage setting on an x-ray machine.

The third function, milliamperage, can also be measured electronically within the x-ray generator or indirectly by examining the density of a test film. Assuming that the timer is of proven accuracy and the chemicals are fresh, increases or decreases in density of a test film can be attributed most logically to changes in the milliamperage or tube current.

Variations in beam quality, intensity, or the x-ray timer should be investigated by a competent service technician. X-ray machines and processing units that do not pass simple quality assurance tests should not be used for patient care until appropriate repairs have been effected.

CASSETTES

There are three main reasons for the failure of optimum performance from cassettes: dirt, static electricity, and poor contact between screen and film. Films exposed in cassettes containing intensifying screens should be inspected carefully for artifacts which can be attributable to these problem areas.

Dirt

Intensifying screens should be cleaned regularly, based on the frequency of use, with a cleaner recommended by the manufacturer of the screen, using a soft material such as cotton or gauze. Excess screen cleaner should be removed with a clean, dry sponge or cotton wad. Cassettes should be left open until the screens are thoroughly dry.

Static Electricity

Several manufacturers produce materials which can be applied to intensifying screens to minimize artifacts produced by static electricity. Antistatic solutions are applied to screens with a clean cotton wad or gauze sponge. In contrast to screen cleaner, antistatic solutions should not be wiped dry but allowed to airdry with the cassettes open.

Film-Screen Contact

Test patterns of wire mesh imbedded in a rigid plastic are available for assessing the adequacy of film-screen contact (Figure 15-8). The wire mesh is laid directly over a loaded cassette and exposed with the x-ray tube at a distance of 40 inches. If film-screen contact is uniform, a sharp

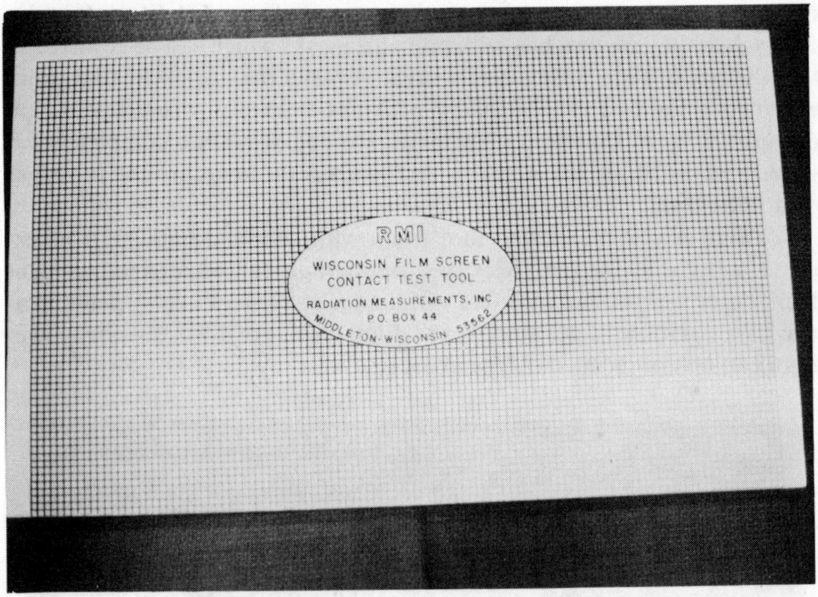

Figure 15-8 Test patterns of wire mesh. These devices are particularly helpful for testing film-screen contact. Since cassettes and screens can be damaged in use, periodic checks are essential.

uniform image will be produced on the processed film. Nonuniformities in alignment of the wire mesh or in its sharpness indicate poor film-screen contact, and the cassette should be discarded unless appropriate repairs can be made.

VIEW BOX

The view box is a frequently neglected component of the x-ray system. Most view boxes contain multiple light sources which can deteriorate unevenly with time. The surface of the view box is usually an opalescent glass or plastic material that may become scratched, dirty, or discolored with use. To avoid the possibility of interpretive errors resulting from uneven or deceptive illumination, view boxes should be cleaned regularly and the light sources changed at intervals slightly shorter than their rated lifetime. Additionally, if a densitometer is available, the uniformity of illumination should be checked over the surface of the view box at monthly intervals.

Since film density may vary in spite of quality assurance procedures, it is desirable to have view boxes with variable intensity light sources so that it is possible to compensate for unusually light or dark films. It is also desirable to have a view box with movable masks which can be adjusted so that the size of the viewing field is no larger than the size of the film, since extraneous light at the periphery provides a serious visual distraction (Figure 15-9). If shuttered view boxes are not available, completely exposed and processed films can be used to mask the areas around the edges of a radiograph.

Films should be viewed in a room with subdued light. Just as extraneous light at the periphery of a radiograph can be distracting, light from other sources can interfere with image analysis. Finally, magnification is a useful adjunct since many films have greater resolving power than can be appreciated by the unaided eye.

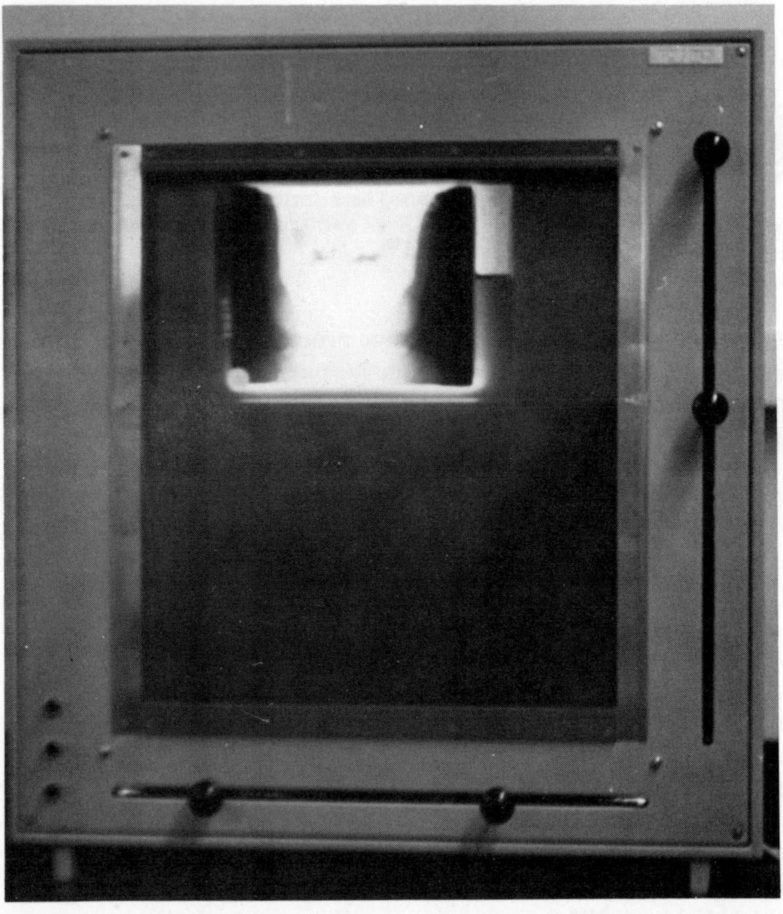

Figure 15-9 Shuttered view boxes are considerably more expensive than conventional units but provide added convenience and greater effectiveness for film interpretation.

TOMOGRAPHIC EQUIPMENT

Pantomography is the most common type of tomography used in dental practice. The devices needed to measure the alignment of the tomographic image layer with the patient positioning device vary from machine to machine. Under ordinary circumstances, the positioning device is used by the service man when a machine is installed and rarely reevaluated unless there is a conspicuous malfunction. Test devices can be purchased from the manufacturer so that periodic tests can be made in the office. The alternative is testing by a qualified service technician (Figures 15-10, 15-11, 15-12).

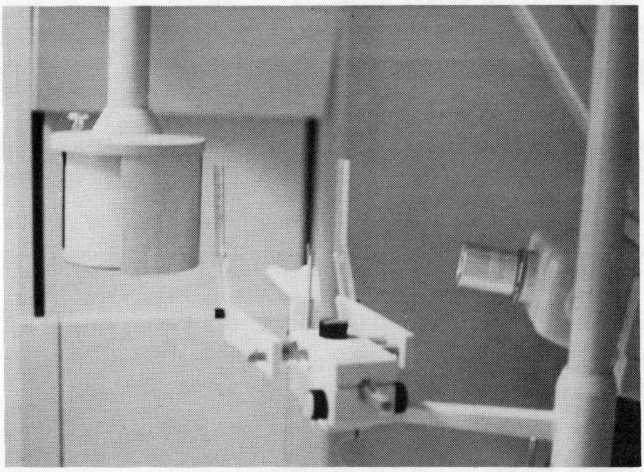

Figure 15-10 General Electric Panelipse with the chin rest and bite guide in the operating position.

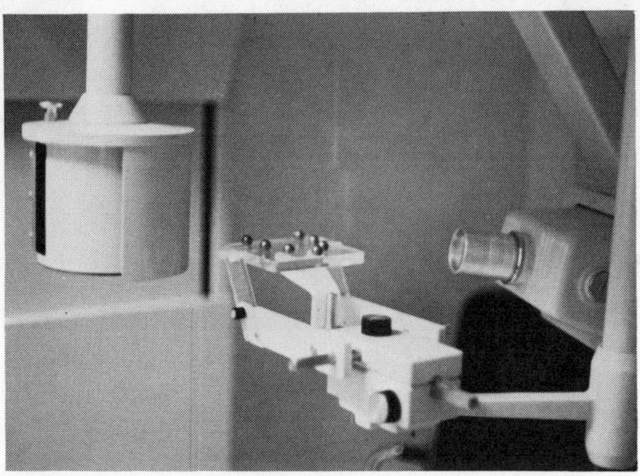

Figure 15-11 Panelipse with bite guide and chin rest replaced by a tomographic phantom containing three steel balls.

For other types of tomographic devices, a number of test tools are available. The unit shown in Figure 15-13 can be used for assessing linear or pluridirectional tomographic systems.

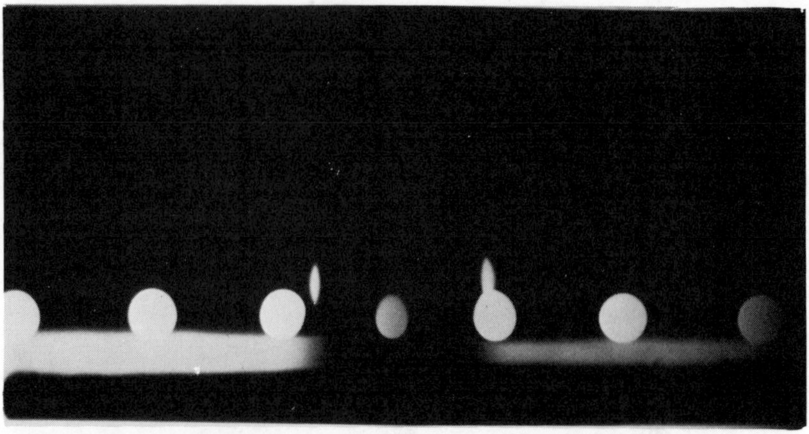

Figure 15-12 A radiographic image of the phantom is used to verify adjustments in the Panelipse. Similar devices are available for other tomographic units.

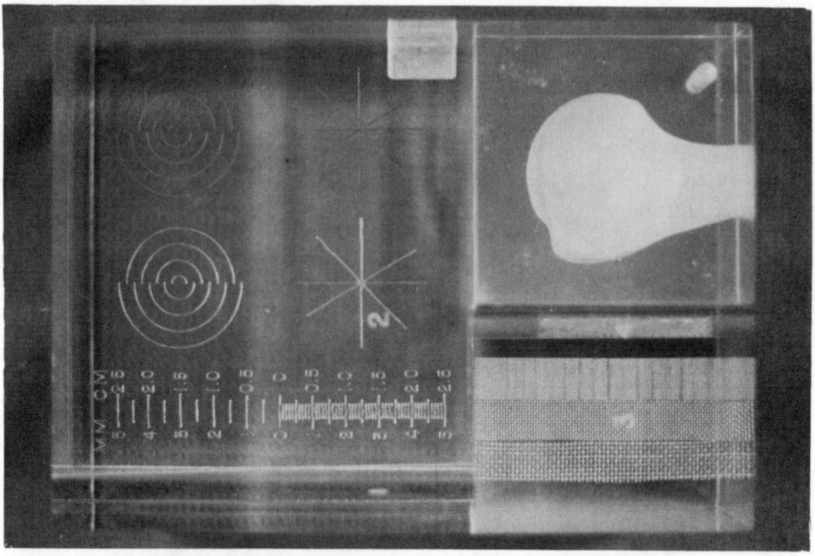

Figure 15-13 The tomographic phantom shown here has multiple components and can be used for nonpanoramic tomographic units. It can measure the thickness of the image layer, resolution, and the location of the image layer.

IMAGE INTENSIFIERS

Although image intensification is not commonly used in dental practice, this valuable tool is likely to experience greater popularity in the coming years. Image intensifiers generally lack the high resolution obtainable on film and are rarely used for studies requiring extreme precision.

Because the image is comparatively coarse, deterioration of the image often goes unrecognized. Periodic checks of an image intensifier are, therefore, of great importance. A simple test device is made up of pieshaped segments of wire mesh with different size holes. The test object is placed as close as possible to the input phosphor of the intensifier. The image of the test plate should be examined under fluoroscopic conditions similar to those used in patient examinations. The resolution is assessed by reporting the smallest mesh visible on the screen. Because the image may not be uniform over the entire field, it is desirable to rotate the test objects several times during the process of testing.

The same test object can be used to measure the resolution of videotape recorders and spot film devices. However, it should be remembered that the human eye has a limited capacity to integrate visual signals and deceptively high estimates of resolution may be obtained if long exposure times are used with different recording devices.

A step wedge placed in the x-ray field can be used to establish the contrast characteristics of an image intensification system. It is helpful, however, to place some scattering material around the step wedge since the system may not be adequate to deal with low contrast images when the relative amount of scattered radiation is high.

FOCAL SPOT

The resolving power of an x-ray tube is primarily a function of the size of its target or focal spot. Performance standards require the labeling of each x-ray tube with the effective focal spot measured at the time of manufacture. As an x-ray tube ages the effective focal spot may change as a result of partial destruction of the anode or changes of the electrical fields in the tube. Several devices are available for measuring resolution, focal spot size, and focal spot position. Figure 15-14 illustrates a device containing a test pattern whose image is projected onto a film using a predetermined geometry. By determining the smallest group of bars which can be distinguished from each other, both the resolution and the approximate size of the focal spot can be established.

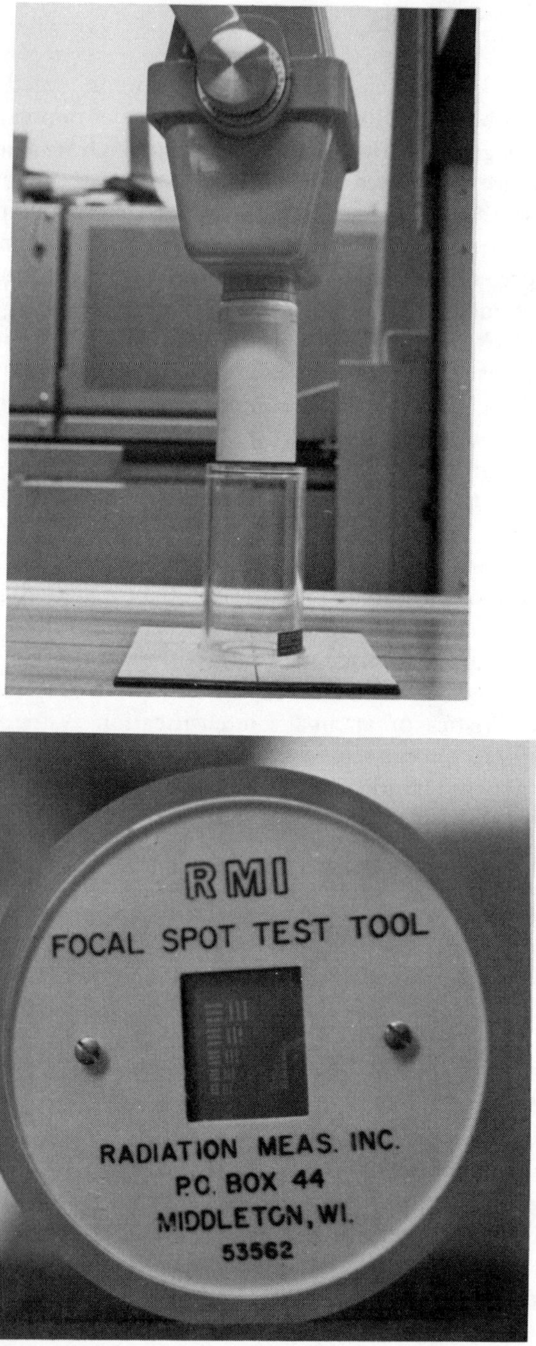

A

B

Figure 15-14 **A.** Unit used to measure focal spot size and position. **B.** One end of the unit contains a metal test pattern which is imaged on a radiographic film.

REFERENCES

1. Trout, E.D., Jacobsen, R.T., Moore, R.T. et al. Analysis of the rejection rate of chest radiographs obtained during the coal mine black lung program. *Radiology* 109:25–27, 1973.

2. Beideman, R.W., Johnson, O.N., and Alcox, R.W. A study to develop a rating system and evaluate dental radiographs submitted to a third party carrier. *J Am Dent Assoc.* 93:1010–1013, 1976.

3. Brown, M.R. Preventive maintenance reduces x-ray equipment costs. *Dimens Health Serv.* 51:3, 1974.

4. Starchman, D.E., Johnson, R.G., and Howland, W.J. Linearity of exposure with indicated time and current for diagnostic radiography units. *Radiology* 122:489–492, 1977.

5. Starchman, D.E., Johnson, R.G., Hykes, D.L. et al. The role of kVp accuracy of diagnostic x-ray units and other performance parameters in quality assurance. Application of Optical Instrumentation in Medicine. V. *Proc Soc Photo-Optical Instrumentation Eng.* 96:31–36, 1976.

6. Ardran, G.M., and Crooks, H.E. Checking diagnostic x-ray beam quality. *Br J Radiol.* 41:193–195, 1968.

16 Legal Aspects of Radiologic Practice

In dentistry, the use of x-rays raises several legal issues. This chapter is intended to provide limited background information, not definitive guidelines for the practitioner. Laws and their interpretations vary from state to state and sometimes from city to city. Practitioners are strongly urged to make themselves aware of relevant laws and legal precedence which may affect their practice of dentistry.

RETENTION OF RADIOGRAPHIC RECORDS, DISCLOSURE, PRIVACY, AND MALPRACTICE

Retention

There is little or no evidence to indicate that a dentist is obliged to retain radiographs in his file for a finite period of time. We have found neither federal nor state statute containing such a requirement. However, some states have regulations which require the retention of written records and in those instances it is presumed that a verbal description of pertinent radiographic findings would be entered into the patient's chart.

The guiding rule with regard to retention should be common sense. A single policy should apply to all patients in a given practice, and records, including radiographs, should be retained for as long as they may influence the well-being of the patient.

The federal government thus far has chosen not to regulate the retention of x-ray films. It does, however, require the accreditation of federally supported hospitals and thereby indirectly requires the acceptance of standards established by the Joint Commission on the Accreditation of Hospitals. The Joint Commission itself does not specifically require the retention of x-ray films for a particular length of time, but does mandate the retention of a radiologist's report as a part of the patient's medical record. In many states, the patient's records must be retained for 25 years.

Access

In some states, of which Connecticut is an example, there is specific legislation which defines a patient's right to access to his own records. In most instances, records can be withheld only if there is evidence that their release would cause harm to the patient. The patient is usually given the right to have the information contained within the record rather than to have ownership of the record itself. As a practical matter, particularly in the case of radiographs, the most reasonable means of transmitting the information from doctor to patient is through an acceptable copy.

Since statutes rarely require that the patient be given a copy of a radiograph, it may even be legitimate to charge a fee for the provision of copies or to require examination of records in the doctor's office.

Disclosure

Under ordinary circumstances there is little information contained in a patient's dental radiograph which could prove to be an embarrassment. Nevertheless, many states have enacted statutes to protect the privacy of all individuals; therefore, the transmission of radiographs from one practitioner to another may require the written consent of the patient. From a practical point of view, the provision of copies is a useful way of minimizing the need for re-exposure but a patient's consent to be referred to a specialist does not imply that the patient also agrees to give the specialist access to all of his or her health records.

Radiographs, or the information contained on radiographs, may not be disclosed to insurance companies or state agencies without consent of the patient.

In several cases, including *McGarry vs J.A. Mercier Company,* 272 Mich. 510, 262 N.W. 296 (1936), and *Hyat, Hyat, and Groeshel, Law of Hospital, Physician and Patient,* 772 (1972), the courts found that x-ray films belonged to the practitioner in the absence of any specific agreement to the contrary. It must be remembered, however, that ownership of the film does not necessarily carry with it the right to withhold the information contained in that film.

Malpractice

In any allegation of malpractice, an x-ray film can be a valuable piece of evidence. Likewise, the destruction of an x-ray film can constitute malpractice. The role of x-ray films in malpractice suits is often used to determine the length of time during which a radiograph should be retained as a part of the patient's record. Since most states have statutes of limitations which apply to malpractice, it is often presumed that records can be destroyed once a patient can no longer bring suit. Many practitioners fail to recognize that the statute of limitations usually applies to the time of discovery of an injury and not to the time of its occurrence. Therefore, a suit can be initiated at any point subsequent to treatment that injury resulting from treatment is first detected.

It is not uncommon to hear colleagues discuss the fact that many x-ray examinations are undertaken for medicolegal purposes. The data to support this notion that radiography is an effective means of defensive practice are difficult to find. X-ray films are diagnostic tools and the most likely suits involving x-rays will usually result from an allegation of misdiagnosis and improper treatment. The ordering or exposing of a radiograph places a practitioner on record as suspecting a particular disease or disease process. The failure to recognize that or any other problem on the resulting radiograph, the production of a radiograph of unacceptable quality, or the failure to institute other supporting procedures places the practitioner in a compromised position.

Recommendation

If possible, radiographs should be retained indefinitely. These records would have value in the maintenance of an individual's health during his lifetime and as a source of identification following death. Although the storage of medical films is expensive because they are bulky, this problem is not a significant factor with dental radiographs. Policies shoud be made explicit and applied uniformly to all records. If there were evidence that normal office routines had been violated, the loss of a radiograph or a radiographic report could be interpreted as an attempt to cover up wrongdoing. If a normal period of retention is defined, it should not be excessively short. Prolonged retention of radiographs is likely to be of benefit to the patient and is unlikely to be regarded as suspicious by courts involved with malpractice suits. Records designated for destruction should be doublechecked to avoid the potential for erroneously discarding the wrong record. Provisions should be made for visibly identifying radiographs and records which are or have been involved in litigation.

SALE, PURCHASE, AND USE OF X-RAY MACHINES

It would be extremely difficult to provide readers with a comprehensive description of all of the laws and regulations which apply to the purchase, installation, operation, and relocation of x-ray machines. Until recently, there was relatively little regulation in this area. It was tacitly assumed that any graduate of an accredited health care institution possessed adequate training to allow the safe and effective use of x-ray diagnosis.

At the present time, however, such assumptions are no longer accepted. Considerable consumer pressure has been brought to bear on governmental agencies at all levels. As a result, one may find city, state, and federal regulations in force in many localities.

In concept, the thrust of regulation and/or legislation is directed at three separate but overlapping domains: machine performance; prescription; and operator competence.

X-Ray Equipment Standards

Many state regulations concerning equipment standards, structural shielding, and operating procedures, are summarized in a report by the Councils on Legislation, Dental Research, and Dental Materials and Devices of the American Dental Association.[1] In most instances, the regulations were based on recommendations contained in the National Bureau of Standards Handbook No. 76.[2] Table 16-1 is a revised version of the original report and contains several interesting points. First, state regulations are still based on federal regulations although in many instances the National Council on Radiation Protection and Measurements Report No. 35[3] has superseded the National Bureau of Standards Handbook No. 76 with regard to dental x-ray matters. Second, many states have already or are currently in the process of revising their regulations.

In general, revision means more stringent control. Third, the focus of state regulations is slowly changing from protection of the x-ray operator to protection of the patient as well as the operator. Fourth, in general, state regulations are less rigorous in establishing equipment standards than are newly enacted federal regulations. Fifth, state regulations tend to be advisory and in only a few instances does noncompliance constitute a felonious act. Sixth, states recommending operating procedures are largely out-of-date and are likely to be modified in the near future.

An x-ray equipment standard was issued by the Food and Drug Administration under the authority of the Radiation Control for Health and Safety Act (Public Law 90-602). Under the terms of this act, the Secretary of Health, Education and Welfare is required to conduct a radiation control program which includes the development and administration of standards to reduce human exposure to electronic (x-ray) product radiation. Technically, this responsibility has been delegated to the Bureau of Radiological Health, which is a subdivision of the Food and Drug Administration.

The Radiation Control for Health and Safety Act, often referred to as the Diagnostic X-ray Equipment Standard, was put into effect in August of 1974. The new regulations set standards for manufacturers and were not intended to regulate the use of diagnostic x-ray users. Until 1974 an individual purchasing an x-ray machine had no assurance that the machine would satisfy reasonable operating requirements. Although the federal performance standards are directed toward manufacturers, the purchaser has responsibility for assembly and maintenance and for uses which vary from the prescribed indications established by the manufacturer.

Applicability

The federal performance standard applies primarily to equipment that was manufactured on or after August 1, 1974. The standard does not require the modification of x-ray machines which were manufactured or put into use before 1974. The regulations do require that the repair of x-ray systems manufactured before August 1, 1974, with certified components will thereafter be required to use only certified replacement components. The standard further required that any equipment sold or assembled after August 1, 1974, would necessarily meet certification standards.

The standards affect the reliability of x-ray systems and are aimed at minimizing the risk of operator error. X-ray systems are required to perform in a linear manner; that is, x-ray output must vary in direct proportion to changes in tube current setting. The standard also requires the permanent installation of minimal amounts of filtration and requires a high degree of reproducibility from one exposure to the next.

Table 16-1
State Regulations Concerning Radiographic Equipment

State	Specific legislation	General radiation codes	Regulations for dentistry mand. recom.	Administering agency	Inspection	Operating* procedures	Other specific* dental regulations
AL	Yes	Yes	Yes	State Board of Health	Yes	a,b,c,d,e	
AK							
AZ	Yes	Yes	Yes	State Atomic Energy Comm.	Yes	a,b,c,d,e, f,g,h,i	a,b,c,d,e,f,g,h,i, j,k; prescription
AR	Yes	Yes	Yes	State Dept. of Health	Yes	a,b,c,d,e,g	a,b,c,d
CA	Yes	Yes	Yes	Board of Dental Examiners	Yes	a,b,c,d,e,f	a,c,i,j
CO	Yes	Yes	Yes	State Board of Health	Yes	a,b,c,d,e,g	a,b,c,d,i
CT							
DE	Yes	Yes	Yes	Dept. Health Social Serv.		a,b,c,d,e	
DC							
FL				Dept. Health/ Rehab. Serv.		prescription	
GA	Yes	Yes	Yes	Dept. Human Resources	Yes	a,b,c,d,e, g,i,j,l	a,b,c,d

HI							
ID				Dept. Health and Welfare			
IL	Yes	Yes	Yes	Dept. Public Health	Yes	a,b,c,d,e,g	
IN							
IA							
KS	Yes	Yes	Yes	Dept. Health/ Environment	Yes	a,b,c,d,i	a,c,d
KY	Yes	Yes	Yes	Dept. Human Resources	Yes	a,b,c,d,e, f,g,h	a,i,j
LA							
ME	Yes	Yes	Yes	Dept. Health/ Welfare; Bur. of Health	Yes	a,b,c,d,e,g	a
MD				Dept. Health and Mental Hygiene	Yes		
MA							
MI							
MN	Yes	Yes	Yes	State Board of Health	Yes		b,c
MS	Yes	Yes	Yes	State Board of Health	Yes	a,b,c,d,e,g	a,c,d
MO							

*See pages 306–307

Table 16-1 *(continued)*

State	Specific legislation	General radiation codes	Regulations for dentistry mand. recom.	Administering agency	Inspection	Operating* procedures	Other specific* dental regulations
MT	Yes	Yes	Yes	Dept. Health/ Environmental Services	Yes	a,b,c,d,e,g	a,c,d,g,i
NE	Yes	Yes	Yes	Dept. Health/ Div. Rad. Health	Yes	a,b,c,d,e	a,c,d,k
NV	Yes	Yes	Yes	Board of Health Bureau Consumer Services	Yes	a,b,c,d,e	a,c,d
NH	Yes	Yes	Yes	Dept. Health/ Welfare; Rad. Control Agcy.	Yes	a,b,c,d,e	a,b,c,d,i
NJ							
NM	Yes	Yes	Yes	Dept. Health Environment	Yes	a,b,c,d,e,g	a,c,g,i
NY	Yes	Yes	Yes	Dept. Health	Yes	a,c,d,g,h,i	a,c,i
NC							
ND							
OH	Yes	Yes	Yes	Dept. Health	Yes	a,b,c,d,e	a,c,d
OK	Yes	Yes	Yes	Dept. Health		a,b,c,d,e	a,c,d

OR	Yes			Health Div. Rad. Control Section	Yes	a,b,c,d,e,g	a,c,d
PA	Yes	Yes	Yes			a,c,d,e	a,c,d,g,i
PR	Yes	Yes	Yes	Dept. Health	Yes	a,b,c,d,e	a,c,d,e,g,i
RI	Yes	Yes	Yes	Rad. Control Agency	Yes	a,b,c,d,f, g,h,i,j	a,c,d,i,j
SC				Dept Health; Sanitation and Safety			
SD		Yes		Dept. Health; Sanitation and Safety			a
TN	Yes	Yes	Yes		Yes	a,b,c,d,e,h	a,c,d,i,j,k
TX	Yes	Yes	Yes	Dept. Health	Yes	a,b,c,d,e,g	a,c,d,i,j
UT							
VT	Yes	Yes	Yes	Dept. Health	Yes		
VA							
WA	Yes	Yes	Yes	Dept. Social and Health Serv.	Yes	a,b,c,d,e	a,c,d,i,j
WV				Dept. Health			
WI	Yes	Yes	Yes	Board of Health	Yes	a,b,c,d,e,g	a,c,i
WY							

*See pages 306–307

OPERATING PROCEDURES:

a. Neither the dentist nor his assistant shall be permitted to hold patients or films during exposure, nor shall any individual be regularly used for this service.
b. During each exposure, the operator shall stand at least six (6) feet from the patient or behind a protective barrier.
c. Only the patient shall be in the useful beam.
d. Neither the tube housing nor the pointer cone shall be hand-held during exposure.
e. Fluoroscopy shall not be used in dental examinations.
f. Each patient undergoing dental radiography shall be draped with a protective apron of not less than 0.25 mm lead-equivalent to cover the gonadal area.
g. Personnel monitoring equipment shall be used as required by (these RAD regulations).
h. Whenever possible, fast film shall be used for diagnostic work.
i. The gonads of children and persons who have not passed the reproductive age shall be protected from the useful beam either by the use of shielding (0.5 mm Pb equivalent) collimation or special gonad shields when this will not impair the value of the examination.
j. A protective leaded apron shall be worn.
k. Protective leaded apron is recommended but not required.

OTHER SPECIFIC DENTAL REGULATIONS:

a. The registrant shall assure that all x-ray equipment under his jurisdiction is operated only by individuals adequately instructed in safe operating procedures and competent in safe use of the equipment.
b. The registrant shall make available to each individual operating x-ray equipment under his jurisdiction a copy of the current recommendations of the National Committee on Radiation Protection pertaining to x-rays, such as National Bureau of Standards Handbook 76.
c. The registrant shall provide to the individuals operating x-ray equipment under his jurisdiction safety rules, including any restrictions of the operating technique required for the safe operation of the particular x-ray apparatus, and require that the operators demonstrate familiarity with these rules.
d. The registrant shall be responsible for assuring that all requirements (of this part) are met.
e. He (the registrant) shall insure beyond reasonable doubt that no radioactive material (including that in patients, animals, and equipment) is allowed to leave the jurisdiction of the radiation user under circumstances that may subject other persons to radiation in amounts in excess of those indicated...in these regulations.
f. (The Director) may require the user to provide protective clothing suitable to work carried on in each radiation installation.

g. There shall be a responsible person in charge of radiation protection in each radiation installation. He shall be cognizant of the radiation hazards associated with the use of radiation equipment or material and when necessary obtain the services of a qualified engineering and/or radiation expert to furnish such information as is necessary for the safe handling and use of such equipment or material. He shall be responsible for providing the necessary instructions regarding radiation hazards and safe working practices to all employees using or handling radioactive substances or radiation producing machines.
h. (The Director) may require the user of any new or altered radiation installation to prepare plans and specifications of the proposed installation and submit them to the Department for review and approval prior to starting construction or operation.
i. Each user shall maintain records showing the radiation exposures of all individuals for whom personnel monitoring is required in accordance with these ("RAD") regulations. Such records shall be kept...in accordance with the instructions contained in that form or on clear and legible records containing all the information....
j. Records of individual radiation exposures which must be maintained...shall be preserved until five years after the effective date of this regulation, or until a date five years after termination of the individual's employment or association with the user, whichever is later. Records which must be maintained pursuant to this regulation may be maintained in the form of microfilms.
k. No x-ray apparatus or other radiographic sources shall be left unattended without locking the apparatus itself, or the room or building in some manner which will prevent its use by unauthorized persons.
l. Any person possessing or using a source of ionizing radiation shall furnish to each employee, for whom personnel monitoring is required, a copy of such employee's personal exposure record annually, at any time such employee has received excessive exposure, and upon termination of employment.
m. If a dentist would use radioisotopes he is no longer a registrant but a licensee and must comply with all the requirements of a specific licensee as under (e).

The practitioner has responsibility for following the x-ray equipment manufacturer's maintenance schedule since failure to do so releases the manufacturer from any responsibility for future adherence of the equipment to the standards.

The federal performance standard places the ultimate responsibility for compliance on the individual who installs or assembles certified components. This individual, under the terms of Public Law 90-602, becomes manufacturer. Under ordinary circumstances, dentists will not choose to install their own x-ray equipment. An individual who does undertake this task, however, must file a form FD-2597, "Report of Assembly of a Diagnostic X-ray System," which certifies that the unit has been installed in compliance with the instructions of the manufacturer and which also requires that any evidence of noncompliance or malfunction be reported.

In some circumstances, a practitioner may find that the constraints of the performance standards prevent the performance of specialized diagnostic techniques. Under such circumstances, an individual may request a variance from the standard by applying directly to the Food and Drug Administration or through the cooperation of the manufacturer of the equipment. The subject of federal regulations has been reviewed by Johnson and Barone,[4] and additional information can be obtained from the Food and Drug Administration, Bureau of Radiological Health, Division of Compliance (HFX-400).

REFERENCES

1. Council on Legislation of the American Dental Association. Radiation hygiene and practice in dentistry. *J Am Dent Assoc.* 76:107, 1968.

2. National Bureau of Standards Handbook No. 76. *Medical x-ray protection up to 3 million volts.* Washington, DC: US Government Printing Office, 1961.

3. National Council on Radiation Protection and Measurements Report No. 35. *Dental x-ray protection.* Washington, DC: US Government Printing Office, 1970.

4. Johnson, O.N., and Barone, G.J. What the federal x-ray regulations mean to the dentist. *J Am Dent Assoc.* 95:810–813, 1977.

INDEX

20/83
28/83
28/83
29/83